Navigating the Maze of Research

ENHANCING NURSING AND MIDWIFERY PRACTICE

6th Edition

Navigating the Maze of Research

ENHANCING NURSING AND MIDWIFERY PRACTICE

6th Edition

DEBRA JACKSON AO, RN, PhD, SFHEA, FACN

ELIZABETH HALCOMB RN, BN (HONS), PhD, FACN

HELEN WALTHALL RN, BSC (HONS), PGDIP, PhD

ELSEVIER

Elsevier Australia. ACN 001 002 357
(a division of Reed International Books Australia Pty Ltd)
Tower 1, 475 Victoria Avenue, Chatswood, NSW 2067

ISBN: 978-0-7295-4439-9

Notice

Practitioners and researchers must always rely on their own experience and knowledge in evaluating and using any information, methods, compounds or experiments described herein. Because of rapid advances in the medical sciences, in particular, independent verification of diagnoses and drug dosages should be made. To the fullest extent of the law, no responsibility is assumed by Elsevier, authors, editors or contributors for any injury and/or damage to persons or property as a matter of product liability, negligence or otherwise, or from any use or operation of any methods, products, instructions or ideas contained in the material herein.

National Library of Australia Cataloguing-in-Publication Data

 A catalogue record for this book is available from the National Library of Australia

Senior Content Strategist: Natalie Hunt
Content Project Manager: Kritika Kaushik
Copy edited by Leanne Peters
Proofread by Tim Learner
Index by Straive

Typeset by GW Tech

Printed in China

Last digit is the print number: 9 8 7 6 5 4 3 2 1

CONTENTS

ACKNOWLEDGMENTS

We couldn't have produced this exemplary text without the assistance of some very talented people who we would like to acknowledge. We say a big thank you to all of our contributors for their excellent work on this edition, while not forgetting to acknowledge those contributors whose work appeared in earlier editions. This new edition is the product of five earlier editions and so builds on the work of numerous nurse scientists and scholars.

We would also like to acknowledge Dr Tamara Power, who was involved in the early work of this edition and who unfortunately had to withdraw. We thank her for her contribution. Thanks also to Professors Jennifer Carryer CNZM, Sandy Middleton and Jill Maben OBE for their useful comments highlighting the purpose and scope of the book. We also want to thank the peer reviewers for their thoughtful and helpful critique, Natalie Hunt (Content Strategist), Kritika Kaushik (Content Project Manager) and Leanne Peters (Editor) for their support and encouragement. Finally, we congratulate you, the reader, for wanting to better understand what research can bring to your professional practice. We hope you find this book an informative and engaging stimulus to your life of learning and we wish you all the very best for your future career in nursing and/or midwifery, whether as a consumer of research or indeed as a consumer *and* researcher.

DEBRA JACKSON AO
ELIZABETH J HALCOMB
HELEN WALTHALL

FOREWORD 1

N ever before in my lifetime has the value of nursing research been so evident as over the preceding pandemic years. The crushing demands placed on nurses, midwives and the health system during the COVID-19 outbreak clearly demonstrated the need for nurses and midwives to provide care that is steeped in a strong evidence base. Delivering evidence-based care means giving patients the best chance of recovery. It also means judicious use of scarce healthcare resources. Nursing and midwifery research can impact on individual patient care and also on systems of healthcare delivery. Yet, our evidence base remains thin. Many systematic reviews of nursing and midwifery care end with recommendations for 'further research'. Nurses and midwives comprise over 60% of the healthcare workforce, yet the number of nursing and midwifery researchers remains disturbingly low. There is a clear international groundswell of support calling for the provision of fully funded clinician researcher academic pathways in both nursing and midwifery to address this gap.

The latest edition of this seminal text has been prepared by expert nursing and midwifery researchers and edited by experienced nurse academics. It fulsomely covers critical components of the research pathway. It is an invaluable guide to those nurses and midwives commencing their research careers and for educators teaching them.

For those who may not intend themselves to lead research, this book explains key research concepts to help them become informed research collaborators and end users. Not all nurses and midwives need to become active researchers, but all nurses and midwives should be research informed. This is particularly important for healthcare leaders seeking an understanding of the quality of available evidence to drive practice and systems change.

I urge nurses and midwives to 'Navigate the Maze of Research', understand the components of quality research and support the call for more-defined research career pathways for nurses and midwives. Importantly, for some, this may be the starting point to becoming active researchers, further growing and developing the evidence base for nursing and midwifery care.

Professor Sandy Middleton RN PhD FACN FAAN FAHMS
National Health and Medical Research Council Investigator Leadership Fellow
Director, Nursing Research Institute
St Vincent's Health Network Sydney, St Vincent's Hospital Melbourne and Australian Catholic University
Director, Implementation Science
Director, Nursing and Midwifery Implementation Science Academy
Maridulu Budyari Gumal (Sydney Partnership for Health, Education, Research and Enterprise [SPHERE])
Advanced Health Research and Translation Centre
Honorary Clinical Professor, University of Central Lancashire (UK), Research Institute for Global Health and Wellbeing (LIFE)

FOREWORD 2

C uriosity in nurses and midwives is essential for exemplary practice, for excellent scholarship and for improving care to patients and their families. It is also an essential ingredient of good research. This new 6th edition of *Navigating the Maze of Research* stimulates and supports nurses and midwives to be curious, to ask questions of their practice and to question and understand published research as research consumers.

This new edition updates and adds to previous editions, further explaining and demystifying research paradigms, methodology and methods, and provides challenges and resources to build confidence and support greater understanding of research in nursing and midwifery. Importantly, it also addresses and updates issues around ethical approaches to research, developing evidence-based solutions, research pathways, approaches to Indigenous research, diversity and inclusion in research and cultural competence in the use of research.

Debra Jackson AO, Elizabeth J Halcomb and Helen Walthall are all active researchers, and in this textbook they have assembled a stellar group of researchers from across Australia, New Zealand and the United Kingdom (UK) to produce a set of accessible and clear chapters that explain and unpack the salient issues in research debates today. The key terms, abstracts and learning objectives provide clear introduction to each chapter, and the content and format, along with the case studies, help embed learning for each key topic.

Research literacy is increasingly important for undergraduates, clinicians and postgraduates and this research textbook is a key resource and 'go to' text for both novice and established researchers to generate new knowledge and to understand and interpret existing research evidence.

This illuminating and contemporary text should be read not only by students and clinicians, but will, I believe, also prove very useful to research teachers and established researchers.

Professor Jill Maben OBE
Professor of Health Services Research and Nursing,
School of Health Sciences, University of Surrey,
Guildford, Surrey, England, UK
Visiting Professor of Nursing Research, Florence
Nightingale Faculty of Nursing, Midwifery and
Palliative Care, Kings College London,
London, England, UK
Visiting Professor of Nursing, School of Health
Professions, Murdoch University, Perth,
Western Australia, Australia
Adjunct Professor of Nursing, Faculty of Health,
University of Technology, Sydney,
New South Wales, Australia

PREFACE

■ ■

I have spent a long career both as a researcher and as a teacher of research methodology and methods. I have vivid memories of what seemed initially to be an impenetrable soup of complex terminology, seemingly rigid rules and philosophical conundrums or challenges. It was a slow process as things fell into place, the various approaches to research came to life in my mind and the jigsaw of terminology settled into a satisfying orderliness. Good research texts were a critical support for this journey.

The conduct of research is underpinned by wide-ranging political and epistemological differences. They are what make the process of research so fascinating. But what matters most in research is the selection and application of the right approach to the question to be answered. The sheer breadth and complexity of nursing means there are a great many wide-ranging questions that need to be explored, and resolved where possible, if we are to provide the best care to those for whom we are responsible. This means that almost all research approaches are relevant to nurses.

This book draws on a wide range of nurse experts who have brought together a wonderful breadth of background and experience. Their contributions exemplify and capture the richness and diversity that is nursing.

Just as research requires us to be methodical, the format of this book takes us through the research process in a logical and comprehensive manner. Every aspect of the process is captured chapter by chapter. I believe this book is a gift to students of research from any background. Most importantly it is a treasure in the ongoing quest to grow and support the passion and capacity for research focused on solving the multiple questions and challenges that arise from nursing practice, health policy and service development.

PROFESSOR JENNY CARRYER CNZM
NZRN, PhD, DipSocSc, BA
Professor of Nursing,
Massey University,
New Zealand
Executive Director,
College of Nurses (NZ)

CONTRIBUTORS

PARVEEN ALI RN, RM, MSCN, PhD, SFHEA, FFPH
Professor of Nursing and Professor of Gender Based Violence, Health Sciences School, University of Sheffield and Doncaster and Bassetlaw Teaching Hospitals, Sheffield, England, UK

JANE V APPLETON RGN (RETIRED), RHV (RETIRED), BA(HONS), MSC, PhD, PGCEA, FiHV
Retired Professor of Primary and Community Care, Oxford Brookes University, Oxford, England, UK

KAY ARANDA BSC(HONS), MSC, PhD
Reader, School of Sport and Health Sciences, University of Brighton, Falmer, East Sussex, England, UK

HELEN AVEYARD BSC, MSC, PhD
Principal Lecturer for Student Experience, Programmes in Adult Nursing and Professional Doctorate in Nursing, Oxford Institute of Nursing, Midwifery and Allied Health Research (OxINMAHR), Faculty of Health and Life Sciences, Oxford Brookes University, Oxford, England, UK

ANN BONNER BAPPSC(NURS), MA, PhD
Professor and Head of School, School of Nursing and Midwifery, Griffith University, Brisbane, Queensland, Australia

CAROLINE BRADBURY-JONES BSC, MA, PhD
Professor of Gender Based Violence and Health, School of Nursing, University of Birmingham, Birmingham, England, UK

GEARÓID BRENNAN RN, BA(HONS), BN, PGCERTHE, MN, PhD, FHEA
Lecturer in Mental Health Nursing, Faculty of Health Sciences and Sport, University of Stirling, Stirling, Scotland, UK

MICHELLE BRIGGS RN, MSC, PhD
Florence Nightingale Foundation Chair, Division of Nursing and Social Work, The University of Manchester, England, UK

JOANNE BROOKE RN, MSC, DPROF
Professor of Nursing, Faculty of Health, Education and Life Sciences, Birmingham City University, Birmingham, England, UK

TIFFANY CONROY RN, BN, MNSC, GRADCERTUNIVTEACH&LEARN, PhD, FRCNA
Professor of Nursing, Deputy Dean for Nursing Leadership and Innovation, Academic Lead for Nursing, College of Nursing and Health Sciences, Flinders University, Adelaide, South Australia, Australia

MARILYN CRUICKSHANK RN, PhD, FACN, FACIPC
Professor of Nursing (Research), School of Nursing and Midwifery, University of Technology Sydney, Sydney, New South Wales, Australia

ANDREA DONALDSON BSC, BN, MSC, PhD, CATE
Senior Lecturer, School of Nursing, Massey University, Palmerston North, Manawatu, New Zealand

ALI DRUMMOND RN, BNSC, MINTERNATIONALPH, FHEA
Acting CEO, Congress of Aboriginal and Torres Strait Islander Nurses and Midwives (CATSINAM), Australia

LEAH EAST RN, BN(HONS), GRADCERTAP, PhD
Professor in Nursing, University of Southern Queensland, Faculty of Health, Engineering and Sciences, School of Nursing & Midwifery, Toowoomba, Queensland, Australia

KATE FRAZER BSC, MPH, PhD, RGN
Associate Professor, School of Nursing, Midwifery and Health Systems, University College Dublin, Dublin, Ireland

LESLIE GELLING RN, BSC(HONS), PGCERT, MA, PhD, FHEA, FRSA
Associate Professor in Adult Nursing, Department of Nursing Science, Bournemouth University, Bournemouth, Dorset, England, UK

JULIAN GRANT BN(HONS), GRADCERTPAEDS, GRADCERTCCHN, PhD
Associate Dean (Research) / Professor of Nursing, Faculty of Science and Health, Charles Sturt University, Bathurst, New South Wales, Australia

ELIZABETH HALCOMB RN, BN(HONS), GRADCERTHE, GRADCERTICNURS, PhD, FACN
Professor of Primary Health Care Nursing, School of Nursing, University of Wollongong, Wollongong, New South Wales, Australia

RUTH HARRIS RN, BSC(HONS), MSC, PhD
Professor of Health Care for Older Adults, Florence Nightingale Faculty of Nursing, Midwifery and Palliative Care, King's College London, London, England, UK

VANESSA HEASLIP DN, RN, DIPHE, BSC(HONS), MA, PhD
Professor of Nursing and Healthcare Equity, School of Health and Society, University of Salford, Salford, Manchester, England, UK

MARIE HUTCHINSON RN, RM, BSC, GRADDIPHA, MHSC, PhD
Professor, Faculty of Health, Southern Cross University, Coffs Harbour, New South Wales, Australia

ROB ION RN, PhD
Independent Scholar, UK

DEBRA JACKSON RN, PhD, SFHEA, FACN
Professor, Faculty of Health, University of Technology Sydney, Sydney, New South Wales, Australia

TRACY LEVETT-JONES RN, BN, PhD, MED WORK
Distinguished Professor and Head of School, School of Nursing and Midwifery, University of Technology Sydney, Sydney, New South Wales, Australia

RHONDA MARRIOTT AM, RN, CM, BSC(NSG), MSC(NSG)DIPPSYCHNSG, PhD
PVC Aboriginal and Torres Strait Islander Leadership and Director, Ngangk Yira Research Centre for Aboriginal Health and Social Equity, Murdoch University, Perth, Western Australia, Australia

DEBBIE MASSEY RN, PhD
Senior Research Fellow, Nursing, Griffith University, Gold Coast, Queensland, Australia

EAMON MERRICK BHEALTHSCI(NURS), MHEALTHSERVMAN, GRADCERTEDSTUDIES(HIGHERED), PhD
Senior Lecturer, Faculty of Health and Environmental Sciences, Auckland University of Technology, Auckland, New Zealand

CLAIRE MINTON RN, MN, PhD
Senior Lecturer and Director of the Bachelor of Nursing, School of Nursing, Massey University, New Zealand

CALVIN MOORLEY RN, BA, PGCE, PhD
Professor and Chair of Diversity and Social Justice, Institute of Health and Social Care, Adult Nursing Department, London South Bank University, London, England, UK

GAYATRI NAMBIAR-GREENWOOD RGN, BSc, MA, PGCAP, PhD
Senior Lecturer, Faculty Lead for Inclusive Curriculum, Department of Nursing, Faculty of Health and Education, Manchester Metropolitan University, Manchester, England, UK

STEPHEN NEVILLE RN, PhD, FCNZ(NZ)
Professor of Health, Wellbeing and Ageing, Head of Department, Department of Nursing, Auckland University of Technology, Auckland, New Zealand

RUTH NORTHWAY RN(LD), CertEd(FE), MSc(Econ), PhD, FRCN, PHEA, FLSW
Professor of Learning Disability Nursing, Faculty of Life Sciences and Education, University of South Wales, Wales, UK

NEESHA OOZAGEER GUNOWA RN, MSc, PhD
Senior Lecturer and Pathway Lead in Community Nursing, School of Health Sciences, Faculty of Health and Medical Sciences, University of Surrey, Guildford, England, UK

RUTH OSHIKANLU MBE, RN, RM, RHV, QN, FRCN, FRSA, FRSPH
Honorary Doctor, London South Bank University, London, England, UK

KATH PETERS BN(Hons), GCHE, PhD
Professor and Associate Dean (International and Engagement), School of Nursing and Midwifery, Western Sydney University, Penrith, New South Wales, Australia

LUCIE RAMJAN RN, BN(Hons), PhD
Associate Professor, School of Nursing and Midwifery, Western Sydney University, Penrith, New South Wales, Australia

JULIA SLARK RN, PhD
Associate Professor, Head of School, School of Nursing, University of Auckland, Auckland, New Zealand

JENNY SIM RN, BAppSci(Nurs), GradDipBA, GradDipClinNurs, PhD
Associate Professor, School of Nursing and Midwifery, University of Newcastle, Newcastle, New South Wales, Australia

KIM USHER RN, BA, DipAppSc(Nsg), MNSt, PhD, AM
Professor of Nursing, University of New England, Armidale, New South Wales, Australia

HELEN WALTHALL RN, BSc(Hons), PGDip, PhD
Director of Nursing and Midwifery Research and Innovation, Corporate Nursing, Oxford University Hospitals NHS Foundation Trust, Visiting Professor of Nursing, Oxford Brookes University, Oxford, England, UK

TINEKE WATER RN, DipCompNsg, DipCTNsg, GradDipChild&FamilyHealth, PstGradDip HSc, MDS, PhD
Senior Lecturer in Nursing, Auckland University of Technology, New Zealand; Director of Research, University of Puthisastra, Phnom Penh, Cambodia

DENISE WILSON RN, BA(SocSc), MA(Hons), PhD
Professor in Māori Health, Associate Dean Māori Advancement, Faculty of Health and Environmental Sciences, Auckland University of Technology, Auckland, New Zealand

ROCHELLE WYNNE RN, GradDipCritCare, GradCertAppSci(Stats), MEd, PhD
Clinical Nurse Consultant, Cardiothoracic Surgery, The Royal Melbourne Hospital, Melbourne, Victoria, Australia; Honorary Professor of Nursing, The University of Wollongong, Wollongong, New South Wales, Australia

REVIEWERS

BENJAMIN HAY RN, BN, GRADCERT(CRITCARE), GRADCERT(UNITEACH), MN, PhD
Senior Lecturer, The University of Notre Dame
Australia, Fremantle, Western Australia, Australia

ROSEANNE SADD MM(HEALTH), PGCERTADVNURSPRAC, PGCERTTERTTEACH
Lecturer, Department of Nursing, Toi Ohomai
Institute of Technology, Tauranga,
New Zealand

ASHLYN SAHAY BN(HONS), GRADCERTLEARNTEACH, PhD
Postgraduate Research Coordinator, Director Health
Workforce Academy, Central Queensland University,
Rockhampton, Queensland, Australia

GRAEME D SMITH RN, BA, PhD
Professor of Nursing, School of Health Sciences,
Caritas Institute of Higher Education, Hong Kong

ABOUT THE EDITORS

Debra Jackson, Elizabeth Halcomb and Helen Walthall are registered nurses, all with a passion for research. Debra and Elizabeth met many years ago in Sydney (Australia), when Elizabeth was doing her honours degree in nursing, and have worked together over the years since. Helen and Debra first met as colleagues in Oxford (United Kingdom) and have subsequently collaborated for several years, particularly to support research training activities.

FROM THE EDITORS

Over the years, we have worked in Australia, New Zealand and the United Kingdom teaching research and evidence-based practice to student groups at baccalaureate, master and doctoral levels. We have also worked with practising clinicians with various levels of education, clinical experience and research knowledge to make research less mystifying and more readily applicable to clinical practice. As teachers, we have experimented with several different pedagogies/learning practices to make research come alive for students and clinicians. This learning package is, in part, a result of that experimentation, stemming as it did from the original edition of Rae Langford's book, published first in the United States some decades ago. Sally Borbasi and Debra Jackson collaborated on the first four editions. Leah East joined the team for the fifth edition. In this latest edition, the sixth of our collaboration on this title, Sally had retired and Leah was not available and so we formed a new team of editors. In addition, we have reshaped and advanced the work of previous editions and added some significant new content. Once again, we have sought contributions from a range of highly experienced nursing and midwifery academics and scholars from Australia, New Zealand and the United Kingdom. Many of our contributors (and reviewers) have been using this book with their students for years and therefore have first-hand knowledge of how the material could be expanded and improved. Each of our contributors has carved their own path as a researcher and scholar. Working through the book, readers will note that contributors present their own approaches to elements of the research process. We have encouraged this as we feel it is important that readers can understand multiple perspectives and ways of doing things.

We are pleased to have incorporated new material on developing evidence-based solutions, diversity and inclusion in research, knowledge translation and research career pathways for nurses and midwives. We have again included case studies as a key learning tool to encourage readers to apply the knowledge within the book to real-world clinical practice. Together, we have produced a cutting-edge collection of work to inform, challenge and stimulate. We believe we bring you a book that is even better geared to making you, the student, understand and navigate the maze we call research. We make research accessible!

Many of the challenges included in this edition have been tested with undergraduate nurses and midwives, who have found them fun and engaging. Students have commented that this approach makes research seem more real and relevant and helps them to feel more confident in reading and making sense of research articles. Academics have given us positive feedback, reporting that their students are increasingly discussing and applying research findings to clinical situations and classroom activities.

The goal of this book is to equip you, as a student and beginner research consumer, with the skills to enable you to quickly find, critically read and readily identify possible uses for relevant clinical research. The book aims to introduce you to the research process and provide insight into how and why research is conducted. Importantly, this book highlights that not all nurses or midwives will actually conduct or *do* research but that we all need to be able to *use* the findings from research in our daily practice to ensure safe, effective and high-quality care. To do this, clinicians need to understand the foundations of basic research and be able to evaluate critically and, if appropriate, implement research evidence. Knowledge is constantly 'moving', and this book provides the latest facts and tips about how you can keep on top of it and use it to your best advantage. The approach taken is a logical progression of concepts and interactive and multimodal content, aimed at getting students actively involved in the learning process with the provision of multiple opportunities to practise and integrate the newly acquired skills. We hope you find this approach as useful as we and our students have.

Finally, as we prepared this book the world was held tight in the grip of the COVID-19 pandemic. This pandemic required nurses and midwives to rapidly change their practice to meet the changing health needs of their communities. This has reinforced the vital importance of nurses and midwives as researchers and consumers of research, and the role of research in shaping and informing clinical practice.

Happy navigating!

DEBRA JACKSON AO
ELIZABETH J HALCOMB
HELEN WALTHALL

TO THE READER

W e hope you will find this text useful. This book is an introduction to research for nurses and midwives. It is designed to meet the needs of those who are beginning their foray into health research and who seek to be able to better understand research findings. This book will help you to begin to be a critical reader of research and to be able to decide whether or not particular research findings will be useful to enhance and inform practice. In preparing this edition, we have amassed a group of skilled and experienced researchers in nursing and midwifery.

To promote your understanding of the comprehensive material provided in this book, we will walk you through the chapters as a precursor to your own navigation of the text. Let's start at the very beginning. The first chapters sketch the research backdrop. This section introduces you to research as a strategy for generating knowledge and is devoted to honing your library, internet, reading, abstracting and research appreciation skills. The important distinction between conducting research yourself and informing your practice through other people's research is made. Using research in the provision of care is called 'evidence-based practice' and its implementation is mainly due to a process described as 'knowledge translation' (research utilisation). To conduct or use research, students need to become skilled research consumers. Research consumers can find and understand research articles, evaluate their relevance and apply the results/knowledge to their practice. **Chapter 1** sets the scene by introducing you to the concept of research as an important avenue for gaining disciplinary knowledge on which to base professional practice. To do this requires some understanding of what is called the 'research process'. In this chapter, you will be introduced to the fundamental concepts associated with the research process, particularly

around designing and conducting research studies. This is a really important chapter for laying the foundations of your understanding, so make sure you read it well.

To practise from an evidence (research) base, clinicians need to understand the research literature and how to find it. **Chapter 2** navigates the library and its many assets, providing insights for efficient and effective database searching (knowledge access) while also explaining the core features of a library and how they have changed rapidly in recent years and continue to change. This chapter will provide you with important insights for enabling research proficiency.

Chapter 3 builds on the concepts explored in the previous chapters by showing you the processes involved in conducting a literature review as an integral part of the research endeavour.

Chapter 4 goes on to explore how nurses and midwives can draw on research and use research findings to help improve direct care of individual people.

The middle chapters of this book are designed to give you the vocabulary necessary to read, understand and appraise research by introducing you to the main types of research designs: quantitative, qualitative and mixed methods. As an introductory research textbook, **Chapters 5**, **6**, **7**, **8** and **9** explain fundamental concepts for beginners in the field. We introduce you to more critical reading and to the major approaches to research that you will encounter in the literature. Over time, as you grapple more deeply with research content through your ongoing study, your ability to feel comfortable with this material will inevitably increase.

Having provided some hints and tips for evidence searching and explored some of the major research paradigms described in the literature, the next important steps for appreciating, undertaking and applying research are presented in the final chapters of this book.

Chapter 10 introduces readers to indigenous perspectives in nursing and midwifery research. In Chapter 11, diversity and inclusion are considered in relation to the conduct of research and the generation of knowledge. In so doing, the text builds on some of the basic concepts and principles learned in earlier chapters of the book.

Chapter 12 extends the idea of evidence being considered worthy of implementation by looking at just how that might take place and why a lot of good/'best' evidence is not carried over into practice, but sits in journals underutilised. Once we have established what research is good research, we need to think about how we get that research evidence into practice. How do we translate that knowledge to practice so that patients benefit? What are the barriers and facilitators to that end?

Chapter 13 discusses research career pathways for nurses and midwives. This chapter highlights the range of opportunities for nurses and midwives to build their careers, with a focus on research opportunities and pathways.

Finally, to show you how it all falls into place, Chapter 14 brings together much of what has been covered beforehand to show how it can inform your practice as a nurse or midwife. This brings you to the end of the book.

In our experience, many students tend to approach research as a topic that doesn't seem to have much relevance to them. They will ask: 'Why do I need to know this?' However, they will soon discover their professional associations consider research so vital to nursing and midwifery that they expect all practitioners, regardless of their educational preparation, to be research consumers. As a nurse or midwife, you need to continually keep abreast of the knowledge that forms the basis of your professional practice, and to do that you need to know the information we present in this book. In addition, you will need to update your knowledge and skills constantly as you move through your career as a lifelong learner. This is where this learning package (textbook and website) takes off! It is designed to enhance your skills in finding information quickly and using that information effectively so you can successfully read, understand, evaluate and apply research findings in your everyday clinical practice. It encourages you to examine what you do in the clinical area and to pose questions such as: 'Am I providing the best possible care?', 'Why am I doing this intervention?' and 'Is this the best way to carry out this intervention?'. It seeks to involve you as an active participant in this learning process. Student challenges and critical-thinking opportunities feature throughout the text, along with interactive exercises and quizzes on the Evolve website. The more you participate in the various activities, exercises and discussions about the identified research content, the more confident and competent you will become in using research as a tool to improve your practice and/or argue for change. Most importantly, this book represents an excellent starting point for you to become the kind of lifelong learner that is expected of you as a health professional.

By the final pages, we hope you will have gained a much better understanding of research and why it is such an important avenue for the development of nursing and midwifery. Understand too, that research as a form of knowledge-making is subject to constantly shifting sands.

Whatever you do, don't overlook the many special features of this book as they are specially designed to boost your learning. Used well, you may find you not only learn how to translate research effectively in your midwifery or nursing practice, but that you also increase your ability to read and think critically, to analyse situations and to use and manage available resources better.

Okay, that's enough from us! We invite you now to begin the first step in your journey to navigate the maze that is nursing and midwifery research. Bon voyage!

SPECIAL FEATURES

- Case studies: Several case studies are provided to help you learn about the concepts we describe as part of the research process in the book. Three of these are used as consistent scenarios throughout the text. We hope that Ahmed, Jamie and Martha's activities will help build your understanding of how to apply the material throughout the book.
  - Case study 1: Ahmed (he/him) is an undergraduate nursing student in the second year of his degree. His current subject involves learning about the conduct of research and its implications for practice. For an assignment,

he has to explore best practice in caring for an 87-year-old man, living with chronic heart failure and newly diagnosed chronic obstructive pulmonary disease (COPD), who also has carer responsibilities for his 85-year-old wife who is living with dementia.

- **Case study 2:** Jamie (they/them) is a final-year undergraduate nursing student undertaking a core research subject. Jamie has to undertake a mini-research project to demonstrate their understanding of evidence-based practice applied to a case study. They have been assigned to investigate the care required by a 14-year-old young woman, living with learning disabilities and who is newly diagnosed with type 1 diabetes. She is currently living in foster care and has a history of mental health issues, including self-harming behaviours.
- **Case study 3:** Martha (she/her) is a second-year nursing student caring for a 75-year-old woman from India in a care-home placement experience. The woman was diagnosed with Alzheimer's disease 10 years ago. She is well supported by her family with daily visits from her devoted husband and family members. Martha notes that the woman has lost 12 kilograms in weight in the past few months and is presently very underweight. When Martha talks to the woman's husband and his daughters during their daily visit, she realises that the family are very distressed about this and have asked if they can do anything to help.
- **Community case study:** Saint Peter's Street is situated on the edge of the City of London; it is a lively street with a corner pub opposite the Seacole Estate (a welfare housing development), where the residents socialise. There is a small greengrocer's shop on the Estate and a general practice. There is a large park 5 minutes' walk away, a church and a mosque all within walking distance. The Seacole Estate is made up of six buildings, including a 20-floor tower block, apartments and terrace houses. On the same street are private houses and apartment blocks. There is a shared community space used for social activities, including a community garden project. The community is a mixture of people from different backgrounds. The residents look out for each other through the neighbourhood watch group, collect each other's mail, and assist each other through citizenship.

- **Student quotes:** These quotes are designed to help you identify with other students' feelings about research.
- **Abstracts:** Just as a research article has an abstract—an introductory paragraph that summarises the article—so too does each chapter of the book.
- **Learning objectives:** These describe what you should be able to do after reading each chapter and working through the activities.
- **Chapter outline:** Each chapter contains a list of the major headings to give you an idea of the topics covered.
- **Key terms:** A list of the terms that are important to know is provided for each chapter.
- **Student challenges:** Try these activities to apply what you are reading and learning.
- **Additional resources:** These provide a list of materials to refer to for further information.
- **Glossary:** A list of all the key terms in the book is provided at the back of the book.
- **Evolve website:** This website includes quizzes and learning activities for each chapter, as well as a test bank and PowerPoint slides for faculty members.

DEBRA JACKSON AO
ELIZABETH J HALCOMB
HELEN WALTHALL

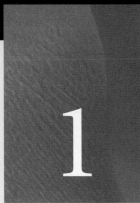

1

INTRODUCTION TO NURSING AND MIDWIFERY RESEARCH

JANE V APPLETON ■ TRACY LEVETT-JONES

CHAPTER OUTLINE

LEARNING OBJECTIVES

After reading this chapter and following critical reflection, readers should be able to:

■ explore preconceived ideas about research

■ define the term 'research'

■ understand what nursing and/or midwifery research means

■ understand what is meant by 'evidence-based practice'

■ describe ways to acquire knowledge

■ describe the historical development of nursing and/or midwifery research

■ discuss why nursing and/or midwifery research is important

■ discuss the contribution research can make to inform and change practice.

KEY TERMS

deductive reasoning

epistemology

evidence-based practice

inductive reasoning

intuition

knowledge translation

mixed methods research

qualitative research

quantitative research

reasoning

research

research questions

ABSTRACT

Research is one way to acquire knowledge in order to make sense of the world. Research offers a systematic method of confirming what is already known in a profession and building new knowledge. Nursing and midwifery research is a way to explore and discover new knowledge that clinicians, managers, policymakers and educators can draw on to develop clinical practice. Nurses and midwives use research findings, professional experience and patients' values and expectations to provide quality care based on the best and most up-to-date available evidence. This is known as evidence-based practice. Research is essential for the complex and rapidly changing healthcare landscape. In this chapter, you will be introduced to the concept of nursing and midwifery research and learn how it has developed over time. Research and evidence-based practice will be discussed and there will be opportunities for you to begin to develop your understanding of the importance of research.

STUDENT QUOTE

I expected to learn about research at university and I am delighted I have been able to link it to both my studies and my clinical practice.

INTRODUCTION

Nursing and midwifery educators often pose a series of the following types of questions to students when they are studying research for the first time.

- What image comes to mind when you hear the word 'research'?
- What are your feelings about studying research?
- How is research important to nursing and/or midwifery?
- Who should conduct research?
- How does research relate to evidence-based practice?

Many students will have preconceived ideas about what research is but might be unsure about its application in day-to-day nursing and midwifery practice. Although students probably agree that research has a place in nursing and midwifery, they might think someone else should be doing it or using it. Students

are often excited and curious about studying research but can be anxious about getting started.

STUDENT CHALLENGE

Preconceived Ideas About Research

Consider each of the following questions and record your answers.

1. What images come to mind when you think of the term 'research'? Paint a word picture or draw an image.
2. How do you feel about studying research? Use 'feeling' words such as happy, sad, scared or anxious. Try to examine why you might be feeling this way.
3. Do you think research is important to nursing and/or midwifery? Why or why not?
4. Who do you think should conduct nursing and/or midwifery research?
5. What characteristics should a researcher possess? List the traits you think a researcher needs.
6. Who should use the findings of nursing and/or midwifery research?
7. How does research relate to evidence-based practice? Can you 'do' evidence-based practice without understanding the basics of research?

Compare your answers with those of two or three of your peers. Discuss similarities and differences. What do your answers tell you? Did you learn anything that might be useful as you begin your study?

This chapter conceptualises research as an integral component of safe and effective healthcare provision. Nurses and midwives learn about research as part of their undergraduate and postgraduate studies and are expected to apply this learning to their clinical practice so the care they provide is effective, current and evidence-based. Students will also find that effective use of research findings is an essential requirement of academic writing.

One of the hallmarks of a profession is that its members (in this case, nurses and midwives) base their practice on a strong foundation of evidence. For instance, a qualified nurse should know the answer to the question 'What are the most effective ways to prevent pressure ulcers in hospitalised older people?', while a midwife should know the answer to the question 'What are the advantages of breastfeeding?'.

To maintain public trust in both nursing and midwifery and to ensure best-practice patient care, it is the responsibility of professionals to ensure that their knowledge is contemporary and complete. The way that knowledge is generated and tested is through a process called research.

Research is an essential tool in the rapidly changing practice of nursing and midwifery.

Nurses and midwives have worked hard to establish a research tradition and to find answers to questions that can inform their clinical practice, workforce issues and nursing and midwifery education. However, unless research evidence is read, appraised and used by clinicians to develop their own individual knowledge and care delivery, research does not achieve its potential impact. Limited translation of research findings into practice is a problem shared by all healthcare professions and, as such, encouraging research utilisation has become a priority. The process of applying evidence from research into practice is called **knowledge translation**. If nurses and midwives translate research findings into their own individual practice, the results will be the incorporation of the evidence for best practice at the point of care (see Chapter 12 for further reading on this topic). Using best practice will ensure that patient care is efficacious, cost-effective and acceptable to both patients and health professionals.

STUDENT CHALLENGE

How Do We Know What We Know?

1. Either alone or with a small group of friends, brainstorm how you as a student nurse or midwife came to know what you know.
2. When you have finished, compare your findings to the list in Box 1.1.
3. Did you come up with other sources of knowledge that are not listed?
4. Can you think of examples of how you use each of these sources of knowledge in your daily life?

To develop your knowledge about a particular area of interest to apply research findings, it is necessary to make judgments about the quality of the research and its relevance to a particular context or purpose. Understanding the research process allows health

---

BOX 1.1
SOURCES OF KNOWLEDGE

Tradition and custom
Authority and role models
Trial and error
Personal experience
Intuition
Reasoning
Research

---

professionals to determine the quality of various studies. Accessing research papers from peer-reviewed journals may reassure some less-informed readers about the quality of these studies, as peer-reviewed journals only publish papers that have been critically reviewed and judged acceptable by experts. However, the review process in journals is not always perfect and, during their undergraduate education, students will be expected to learn the skills to critique research for themselves. This book is designed to help nursing and midwifery students understand how research is conducted and how to critically appraise research findings then apply these findings in their clinical practice.

Before embarking on the study of research, readers are reminded that research is one source of knowledge among several different sources (Box 1.1). Understanding how people came to know things helps nurses and midwives make informed choices about the type of evidence they can safely apply in their practice.

WHAT IS KNOWLEDGE?

Knowledge is the understanding of facts, truths or principles. It is the information used to conduct our personal and professional lives. The study of knowledge (or theorising knowledge) is called **epistemology**. People acquire knowledge in several ways and may use more than one of these methods at a time when working on a solution to a problem or seeking the answer to a question. All methods of acquiring knowledge are viable options and are valid at various times. Each form of knowledge offers a way to understand the world and possesses strengths and weaknesses. The following sections discuss each method of knowledge acquisition in more depth.

HOW DO NURSES AND MIDWIVES KNOW WHAT THEY KNOW?

Tradition and Custom

Knowledge derived from tradition is sometimes considered to be a 'truth' as it is passed on from previous generations; however, this type of knowledge is informed by history, culture and heritage. It involves those things known or done because 'this is the way it has always been'. These truths are often accepted without question. However, many practices that evolve from this kind of knowledge are ritualistic and ill-informed. The reason or rationale for such practice may have been lost or may have disappeared over the years and the practice may be outdated or not best practice.

In nursing and midwifery, some practices have evolved based mainly on tradition. Although perhaps originally instituted for good reasons, the reason for the practice may no longer be appropriate or effective. Thus, nurses and midwives must remain curious and engage in lifelong learning to ensure that their practice remains based on current evidence.

CASE STUDY 1.1

Ahmed is an undergraduate nursing student in the second year of his degree. As part of his current subject, he has to learn about the conduct of research and its implications for practice. For an assignment, he has to explore best practices in caring for an 87-year-old man living with chronic heart failure and newly diagnosed chronic obstructive pulmonary disease (COPD), who also has carer responsibilities for his 85-year-old wife who is living with dementia.

As Ahmed begins to plan for his assignment to identify the best practices for caring for the couple, he recognises that they are facing many challenges to their health and wellbeing. In addition to the couple's physical health needs, including the new diagnosis of COPD, Ahmed also reflects on the importance of assessing the couple's cultural backgrounds and the impact this might have on their care preferences. Tradition can influence not only nurses and midwives, but also the expectations of the people they care for. The couple is of Italian descent and migrated to Australia 60 years ago. One of the major challenges Ahmed has identified is that the man's wife, who has dementia, now speaks to him only in Italian. Therefore, her husband needs to translate for her, and much of what she says seems to indicate that she is very confused. This is a distressing situation for everyone and made more challenging by the fact that the family's cultural preferences are to care for their parents at home. Ahmed needs to think about how he might integrate the most up-to-date evidence for dementia care in this context to get the best outcomes for everyone.

Authority and Role Models

'Experts' are authorities who are relied on to provide information to guide decision-making and the performance of certain skills. The first authority figures most children encounter are their parents. At school, children begin to rely on teachers, textbooks and other resources to expand their knowledge base. Adults also rely on the opinions of authorities who have expertise in areas they do not. This is a natural evolution, as it would be impossible for all people to be knowledgeable about all things.

When first embarking on a new professional path, people often look to authorities in the field to teach them what they know, or imitate the example set by authority figures who serve as role models. In nursing and midwifery, these authority figures are often senior nurses or midwives. Students and novice clinicians can learn attitudes, knowledge and skills through the role modelling of senior people including discipline academics or expert clinicians (Baldwin et al 2017). While this can perpetuate learning, it can sometimes result in sharing and perpetuating poor practice.

When using knowledge gleaned from authority figures, or when replicating their behaviours, care must be taken to choose these role models wisely by asking questions such as: What makes this person an expert? What is their educational background and experience? How did they acquire this knowledge? Do I accept the word of my lecturers and tutors or practising clinicians without question? How well-read and current are my nursing and midwifery lecturers? Are they involved in scholarly activity and research? Are their clinical skills current? What about the health professionals I see in the clinical area? Do they keep up with the latest discoveries in their clinical area? Do they show evidence of critical thinking in their clinical decision-making, or do they justify actions with 'That's the way we do it here'?

Textbooks and other information sources, including the internet and social media, can provide what is often viewed as an authoritative source of evidence for nursing or midwifery students. Although a lot of credibility is assigned to the written word, it is not always well supported by evidence. This type of information must be examined and critiqued by asking questions such as: Is the information the best source available? Where is the evidence for this information and is it a credible source?

It is not possible for textbooks to always have the most up-to-date information because the information may be replaced by new research as the book ages. This must be a consideration for people reading research. Similarly, while the internet offers access to copious amounts of information, there is limited control over the information available and no guarantee it is accurate or of high quality. To ensure practice decisions are based on the best evidence, nurses and midwives need to be certain their sources are reliable and accurate. However, the high rate at which material is added to the internet makes it difficult for clinicians to sift through the information to determine what is relevant, and to assess its reliability (Aveyard 2019). Information must always be viewed with a critical eye. One might ask the following: Is the information supported by a sound rationale? Is it presented clearly and logically? Is it current? Is the evidence for this information derived from a rigorous study or respected organisation such as the World Health Organization or Heart Foundation.

Trial and Error

The process of trial and error involves trying out a successive number of ideas to solve a problem until one works. The successful idea is adopted until it ceases to work, whereupon it is rejected and the process is started again. This method is often used when someone has a limited frame of reference from which to draw, when seemingly equal options are easily accessible or when standard approaches have been exhausted. Trial and error tends to be a haphazard approach, and often results cannot be reproduced. For example, try to reproduce a meal originally thrown together with a little of this and a little of that—it can be a futile task.

In using trial and error, one might also end up using one option when another would actually work better. This occurs because the selected option solves the problem adequately, leaving the better option unexplored. For example, a teenager has produced a longed-for result on his computer and proudly shows the results of his handiwork to a more computer-literate friend. The friend shows the teenager how to get the same result in one or two keystrokes.

Using a system of trial and error might also entail a certain amount of risk although in some situations, trial and error or prototyping can bring about surprising results. When an obstacle is approached from a 'let's try this and see what happens' perspective, the process is not bound by the constraints of logic and can provide solutions that might not have been discovered with a more logical approach. However, in healthcare, trial and error can often be both irresponsible and dangerous.

Personal Experience

Knowledge derived from the cumulative experiences of being in the world is familiar and powerful. It comes from seeing, hearing, touching, tasting, feeling and doing something ourselves. It is first-hand knowledge: known because one has been there before and experienced the same thing before. Every person is intimately acquainted with using personal experience as a reliable method of knowing, and most people trust personal experience and value it highly in the decision-making process. The more experience is gained in a situation, the greater the comfort and skill in future situations. As the number and variety of these experiences increase, so too is knowledge transferred, adapted and extended from previous situations to fit new situations. As the depth and breadth of a person's experience grows, their operating knowledge base becomes increasingly complex. Personal experience is individual and is often hard to translate or explain to others, particularly to those people who have no similar experiences to draw on. Students from a range of backgrounds study nursing and midwifery, and their past experiences can influence the way that they work, the way that they view health, illness and wellbeing and the care that they provide.

Patricia Benner, the author of a very famous nursing theory (Benner 1984, Benner, Tanner & Chesla 2009) and many seminal nursing books, describes five levels that a nurse goes through to develop clinical expertise: novice, advanced beginner, competent, proficient and expert. Movement from one level to the next occurs with experience. Experience is only gained when previous knowledge is refined or challenged by clinical evidence. The novice nurse or midwife begins with knowledge gained from their own lived experience and from authoritative sources, and uses that knowledge and reason to solve problems. Experience and new knowledge are then added to their baseline knowledge. Expertise then develops over time as the nurse or midwife tests and refines this body of knowledge in real-world situations; thus, says Benner, experience is a necessary prerequisite for developing expertise. However, Benner also cautions about becoming an experienced non-expert—that is, a nurse who has many years of experience but who does not regularly review what they know and how they practise with regards to contemporary knowledge and evidence.

Intuition

Intuition is a 'hunch' or 'gut feeling' about a situation that is not readily explained or easily backed up by logic or facts. It is an insight or understanding of the whole, seen apart from its component parts. Intuition is closely tied to personal experience. Extensive experience in a particular situation allows knowledge to be so ingrained that it becomes second nature. Acting on this deeply embedded knowledge often occurs automatically and quickly, appearing to be a flash of insight or an immediate recognition of the whole. For expert nurses and midwives, it is often difficult even to recall or recount what produces this insight.

Intuition has long been discounted as an evidential source of knowledge because it is not easily examined or readily categorised. It also appears to occur independently of the consideration of available facts and the use of reasoning processes. So, in a society that holds logic at a premium, intuition is labelled as unreliable or as a 'lucky guess'.

Benner (1984) proposed that intuition is a perceptual awareness. She asserted that rather than being a 'lucky guess', intuition reflects deep knowledge derived from long hours of clinical observation and experience. Intuition is about being attuned to very subtle shifts that may be important only in the case of a specific patient. This type of clinical knowledge continues to be recognised as an important element of decision-making in nursing and midwifery practice (Chilcote 2017, Miller 2018).

Reasoning

Reasoning is a way of using the mind to work out puzzles and present ideas and plans. To reason is to think through an issue or a problem in an objective, systematic and logical way. It involves taking stock of what appears to be happening, making associations between things and determining the likely consequence of a range of responses (Levett-Jones 2018). For example, a nurse or midwife might see a urine sample and notice it is much clearer than it was the day before. As they know the patient is taking antibiotics, they can determine that the treatment for urinary tract infection is beginning to work. The clinician is thus making associations between different pieces of information and reaching a plausible conclusion.

Research

Research is a systematic process used to confirm and refine existing knowledge and to build new knowledge both inductively and deductively. **Inductive reasoning**, where reasoning moves from the particular to the general, underlies qualitative research. **Deductive reasoning**, where two or more variables form the basis for assuming the existence of a relationship that can be tested, underpins quantitative research. Inductive research is useful when little is known about a particular area. Through the process of exploration, investigators using inductive methods of research construct concepts or theories that can explain what is going on in a particular context. Deductive research begins with a proposed theory about the effect of an intervention, which an investigator then tests and verifies before recommending it as an evidence-based practice.

Quantitative research is used to describe, explore, explain, measure or predict observable or measurable conditions with as much objectivity as possible. **Qualitative research** allows investigators to identify, examine and explain the experiences of an individual or group from numerous subjective viewpoints. Quantitative and qualitative research approaches are presented in more detail later in the chapter and in Chapters 7 and 8 respectively.

WHAT IS NURSING AND MIDWIFERY RESEARCH?

Nursing and midwifery research addresses problems or questions that are encountered in practice, in education or are concerned with the nursing and midwifery workforce. The results from nursing and midwifery research inform and guide future practice, whether the users of research findings are in management, education or clinical settings. Nurses and midwives use the research process as a tool to search for, develop, refine and expand the body of knowledge that shapes and enhances professional practice. The research process challenges practice based solely on tradition and provides evidence to either accept or reject taken-for-granted norms.

In contemporary healthcare environments, nursing and midwifery research often overlaps with research from other professions including medicine, allied health professionals and health services because of increasing numbers of multidisciplinary interventions and therapies. The increasing importance of teamwork in healthcare means many questions that arise in practice are often interdisciplinary and involve a team of researchers from a range of disciplines, including nursing and midwifery. Additionally, collaborating with team members from disparate professions (e.g. human geographers, social scientists, business academics or engineers) can help to find solutions to complex problems by looking at them through different professional and disciplinary lenses.

Nurses and midwives collaborate and make important contributions through multidisciplinary teamwork. For example, a large, randomised control trial, led by an academic midwife, involved a multidisciplinary team that examined the impact of position during the late stages of labour for nulliparous women who chose to have a low-dose epidural for pain relief (Bick et al 2017). This study provided evidence that when given epidural anaesthesia, nulliparous women with epidural analgesia benefited from a lying-down (lateral) position during the second stage of labour and there were no short- or long-term disadvantages of this positioning (Bick et al 2017).

Research is a process of systematic discovery undertaken to establish things such as the incidence of problems, effectiveness or appropriateness of interventions, and feasibility of implementing interventions. Table 1.1 connects research examples with the aim of finding out how often things occur (incidence), whether things work (effectiveness), whether they are acceptable (appropriateness) and whether it is possible to implement them (feasibility).

WHY IS RESEARCH IMPORTANT?

The development of knowledge that is evidence-based allows nurses and midwives to make better-informed decisions and choices concerning their practice. Research findings may validate existing practices created from

TABLE 1.1		
Connecting the Examples		
Research Examples	**Findings**	**Questions**
Breastfeeding	Health issues, medications	What are some of the circumstances in which breastfeeding may be difficult?
Wound healing	Effectiveness of dressing	Is there an association between moist wound dressings and improved healing of wounds?
New practices	Feasibility	How will a team accept, implement and evaluate change?
Person-centred care	Appropriateness	Do older people value hospital visiting hours in an acute stroke unit?

tradition, intuition and personal experience. Importantly, research may examine such tried-and-true practices and make them more efficient, less expensive or less complicated. It also may explore ways of tackling newly evolving problems in an increasingly complex world. Ultimately, nursing and midwifery research ought to contribute to better healthcare outcomes for consumers.

Nursing and midwifery research findings provide reliable evidence to inform professional practice, education or workforce issues. Professions are commonly judged by the body of knowledge they generate, and a clearly defined evidence base built on a strong research foundation lends credibility to nursing and midwifery as distinct professions. Practising nursing or midwifery in today's litigious society demands increasing accountability for one's actions. Healthcare consumers expect nurses and midwives to have sound rationales for their decisions and actions. Thus, nurses and midwives require a current knowledge base drawn from research to provide evidence for best practice. This connection is the rationale for evidence-based practice (Fig 1.1) and is written into the Nursing and Midwifery Board of Australia (NMBA 2016) and the Nursing Council of New Zealand (NZNC 2007) registered nurse standards and competencies for practice and the United Kingdom's (UK's) Nursing and Midwifery Council's code for professional standards of practice and behaviour (NMC 2018).

Nurses and midwives are expected to provide care that is both safe and cost-effective, and they must be able to justify their decisions based on the best available evidence. For example, although many healthcare organisations have tried to reduce costs by substituting nurses with untrained staff, research has shown that appropriate numbers of nurses with a degree-level qualification results in fewer patient complications, shorter hospital stays and fewer re-admissions (Griffiths et al 2019).

Healthcare research is a big business with huge financial investments made each year. Imperatives that drive healthcare research can be either philanthropic or commercial. For some, the pursuit of knowledge is to improve health, minimise risk and alleviate suffering. For others, research is undertaken to develop new drugs and innovative technologies that can be sold on the free market. During the COVID-19 pandemic the RECOVERY study, an international trial of COVID-19 therapies for hospitalised patients with suspected or confirmed COVID-19, tested known drug therapies in an attempt to find a drug intervention that would improve mortality and morbidity rates. (See https://www.recoverytrial.net.)

KEY HISTORICAL INFLUENCES

Although known by many people as the 'Lady with the Lamp', Florence Nightingale was a political activist and a highly effective researcher. She advocated for those

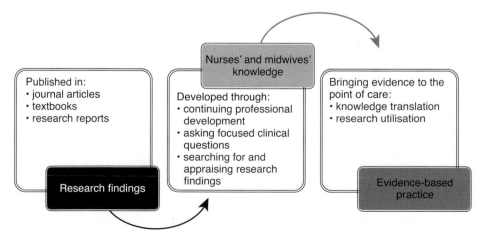

Fig. 1.1 ■ Linking the domains of research, knowledge and evidence-based practice.

who were disadvantaged and researched extensively about the environmental and social causes of poor health. Nightingale's views on the need for an educated nursing workforce formed the foundation of contemporary education programs. Examples of Nightingale's research are documented in her classic book 'Notes on Nursing' (Nightingale 1859). However, relatively little formal research was carried out by the nurses and midwives who followed Nightingale, until the late 1940s.

The progress of nursing research has been closely tied to the development of nursing and midwifery education. When nursing and midwifery began to move towards advanced education and affiliation with university settings in the mid-1980s, a research culture began to develop. Ironically, it was research by investigators from other professions that exposed deficiencies in the preparation of nurses and urged better educational opportunities and a move to university-based education. Sociologists found the study of nurses and nursing as a work culture particularly fascinating and, as a female-dominated occupation, nursing held a special appeal for sociological investigation. Nursing work, habits, roles and attitudes were dissected and reported for decades in the sociological literature (Russell 1990).

During the 1960s and 1970s, in the United States (US), the number of nurses with advanced degrees and research skills continued to increase, and the push for doctoral preparation in nursing began. Formal support mechanisms for research and research funding in nursing increased. Nursing practice became more standardised, complex and specialised. Nursing education at a master level became more common and emphasised specialisation in rapidly emerging specialty areas. Research was carried out to establish standards for specialty practice. Nurse researchers began to turn to nursing care and clinical practice to provide questions for research, and the focus shifted from the study of nurses to the practice of nursing. Nursing theories evolved that attempted to describe and explain the practice of nursing (Alligood 2013). These theories then began to be tested by nurse researchers.

In Australia, New Zealand and the UK, such developments took longer. The move to tertiary education only began in earnest in the mid-1980s. In the US, there was already a critical mass of nurses with doctoral degrees and research skills by this time, and many

nurses went to the US to study for higher degrees because these were not available in their home countries. In Australia, the Dawkins reforms of the late 1980s saw the merger of colleges of advanced education and universities. This resulted in the basic entry for nursing in Australia becoming an undergraduate degree, with nursing research identified as a crucial component of this process of the professionalisation of nursing.

In the UK, the introduction of Project 2000 saw the transfer of all nursing education from hospital-based schools of nursing to universities and higher education institutions. This prompted an increasing focus on research and a move to degree-level preparation for all nurses in 2009. Across all three countries, the inception of postgraduate degrees led to further growth in nursing research, although in the early stages, much of this research was about nursing education and nurses themselves.

In Australia, New Zealand and the UK, undergraduate students currently study research as part of their nursing and/or midwifery degrees. Internationally, there are increasing numbers of doctoral programs in nursing and midwifery. Centres for nursing and midwifery research are beginning to proliferate in many hospital and university settings, and clinical professors of nursing and midwifery have been established through university and health service partnerships. The quality and quantity of nursing and midwifery research continues to grow and an increasing number of research journals have been launched to help disseminate research findings. Clinical practice specialty groups progressively fund, promote and publish research in their respective specialty areas. Furthermore, there is an increasing focus on supporting the development of a skilled clinical academic research workforce in nursing and midwifery (see Chapter 13).

Much health-related research is now driven by national health priority areas and the funding is strategically aligned. While research remains predominantly initiated and conducted by nurses and midwives affiliated with the university sector (academics and students), **research questions** are being increasingly generated by clinicians and clinical academics. Indeed, many clinicians are joining with academics to form research teams. Moreover, research teams are increasingly being expected to be multidisciplinary and cross-institutional.

Traditionally, Australian and New Zealand researchers have relied on the Australian Research Council, the National Health and Medical Research Council (NHMRC) and the Health Research Council of New Zealand, Te Kaunihera Rangahau Hauora o Aotearoa, to support research. The New Zealand Nurses Organisation (NZNO), the New Zealand College of Midwives and the Nursing Education and Research Foundation offer advice about research activities, and some offer grants and scholarships. The NZNO has an excellent index of New Zealand nursing research that can be accessed free of charge. In the UK, the Royal College of Nursing (RCN) and the Royal College of Midwifery (RCM) maintain a list of research funding opportunities for nurses and midwives and the National Institute for Health and Care Research (NIHR) is funding a range of research training opportunities for nurses and midwives. Internationally, organisations such as Sigma Nursing provide opportunities for international networking of researchers.

QUESTIONS NURSING AND MIDWIFERY RESEARCHERS ASK

Earlier in the chapter, we stated that research is a systematic way of generating knowledge in response to questions posed about nurses and midwives and their practice. It is reasonable to suggest that nursing and midwifery research questions arise from an identified clinical problem, education or workforce issue, curiosity or a practical need. Developing an appropriate research question and refining it for research requires a person to have a good grasp of practice and research. Nursing and midwifery research questions can arise from many different sources (Box 1.2).

BOX 1.2
SOURCES OF RESEARCH QUESTIONS

- Clinicians' experiences
- Literature
- Patients' experiences
- Pregnant women and their partners
- Relatives and carers
- Theories
- Social media
- Context of practice

Often the researcher's personal experience as a nurse and/or midwife helps to identify research questions that should be investigated. At other times, research questions are formulated when a gap in the literature is identified and recommendations have been made for further research to be undertaken. The context of nursing and midwifery practice, and existing or emerging theories about various aspects of practice, can also prompt questions for research.

To demonstrate how the research question leads the researcher to the next step in the research process, it is necessary to use the major classifications of research. They are qualitative research, quantitative research and mixed methods research. These are discussed later in this book (see Chapters 7, 8 and 9).

Here are some examples of how different research approaches may be used.

- How do women and their partners in a rural Indigenous community experience support during treatment for gynaecological cancer? The best way to find this out is to ask the women and their partners, so the research may involve interviews and use a qualitative approach.
- How effective is a partner support program for reducing stress for women receiving treatment for gynaecological cancer and their partner? The way to address a 'how effective is this' question is to make a comparison. Therefore, this study may be set up as an experiment with a control group and a group participating in the partnership support program. This would be a quantitative study.
- How can a partner support program, designed for rural women with gynaecological cancer, be customised by Indigenous communities to respect the distinctive nature of their ways of life? The best way to answer this question is to take it to the community and generate data from their discussions and understandings of the problem and its solutions. The data collected might be a mixture of qualitative and quantitative data and so this would be **mixed methods research**.

EVIDENCE-BASED PRACTICE

Evidence-based practice (EBP) can be defined as a 'problem-solving approach to the delivery of healthcare that integrates the best evidence from research with a clinician's expertise, including internal evidence from patient data, and a patient's/family's preferences and values' (Melnyk & Fineout-Overholt 2019, p. 5). Internationally, many current competency standards for registered nurses and midwives include a requirement to implement EBP based on critical review of research findings. This shows an expectation that a nurse or midwife will be able to access research findings (often called 'evidence'), demonstrate an ability to evaluate the research that produced the findings and then make a decision about using these findings at the point of care. The thought processes involved in reading, appraising and making a decision about using research findings in practice are part of knowledge translation. Deciding to go ahead and use research findings in practice is called research utilisation.

CASE STUDY 1.2

Jamie has negotiated a supervisor for their core research project and is beginning to feel much more confident and excited about the project. Jamie will investigate the care of a 14-year-old young woman with learning disabilities, living in foster care, and who is newly diagnosed with type 1 diabetes. The young woman also has a history of mental health issues including self-harming behaviours. As Jamie is nearing the end of their undergraduate degree, they are very aware of the need for EBP, as opposed to basing practice on tradition and custom. Jamie knows it is important to begin any study with a thorough search of the literature. After talking to supervisors, Jamie makes an appointment with the university librarian to seek advice on how to design a search strategy for the electronic databases that will identify research articles and clinical practice guidelines to identify the current evidence for practice and any potential gaps that a new study might be able to answer.

Some of the barriers to EBP are time pressures, limited access to electronic databases and the internet during work hours and limited skills and resources to access and appraise all of the evidence required to answer a focused clinical question. Cochrane set up a systematic process for research teams to find, appraise and summarise research evidence ready for use by clinicians (Sackett 1996). This process became known as the systematic review and is explained more fully in Chapter 3. Reports of systematic reviews can be found in a range of EBP sites listed at the end of this chapter. For everyday use, the systematic review report may be too long to digest, so summaries of evidence are also prepared and come in a range of guises such as best-practice information sheets and practice guidelines. These materials are a valuable resource for nursing and midwifery students, as well as busy clinicians who do not have the time or spare resources to access and critique research for themselves. However, even such summaries need to be reviewed critically before being used to guide practice.

STUDENT CHALLENGE

Sourcing Potential Evidence for Practice Searching the Joanna Briggs Institute EBP Database— Evidence-based practice tutorials

1. Go to the following website: https://www.youtube.com/watch?v=aCcd96UoF7I
2. Go to your university library database and search for JBI EBP (Ovid).
3. Scroll through the titles and choose one of interest.
4. Look at the information source for the title and identify whether it is based on a systematic review of the literature. (Chapters 2 and 3 discuss searching the literature in greater detail.)

Nurses and midwives need to keep up to date with the research outputs in their specialties by subscribing to journals, either personally or through the hospital or university library, or by signing up to journals' new content alerts. When reading papers, it is important to critique the quality of the research. If a nurse or midwife judges the research to be of high quality, they might then consider relevance and workplace policies, practices and processes before deciding whether and how to adopt the findings into practice. Information about how to critique research is included in Chapter 5. Following their pre-registration education, nurses and midwives will be able to make some judgments about the quality of research reports, including journal articles. Try the next challenge: it gives you some tips on how to identify and critique a research report.

STUDENT CHALLENGE

Identifying Evidence You can Use in Practice

1. Find a research report in the form of a journal article. Check the journal to see whether the papers included in it are peer-reviewed before publication, as this is an indicator of quality.
2. What year was the paper published? How might the currency of the paper affect the usefulness of the findings?
3. As you skim-read the paper, ask yourself the following questions.
   a. Are the sections of the paper clearly marked (introduction/background, literature review, research design/methodology, results, discussion, conclusions)?
   b. Can you find the research question and/or aim early in the paper?
   c. Are you persuaded by the author's claims about the significance of the work?
   d. Is there a section on the study limitations? (Hint: this could be a separate section or may be in the discussion section.) Does this information tell the reader where it is limited and what this study adds to current knowledge?
   e. Are there recommendations for further research?

The point of this exercise is to make you aware that, even at this early stage of your studies, you can identify the parts of a research paper and make preliminary judgments about the quality of the findings. With additional research training, you will become more confident in critiquing the design and conduct of a study.

CONCLUSION

Research is an important source of knowledge to be used by nurses and midwives and by nursing and midwifery students. Research is a complex process in which one cannot expect to be an expert straight away. However, there are many elements of research that can be grasped immediately. Completing the challenges in this chapter has enabled the reader to learn how to start to appraise a research report. EBP organisations, such as JBI (formerly known as the Joanna Briggs Institute) and Cochrane, have repositories that are a great resource for students. Lastly, nursing and midwifery students must always remember that evidence-based practice has a significant impact on the quality of patient care.

Acknowledgments

This chapter builds on an earlier chapter by Kim Usher, Jane Mills and Jane V Appleton.

ADDITIONAL RESOURCES

Useful Evidence-based Practice Sites

Excellence in Research for Australia: https://www.arc.gov.au/excellence-research-australia
GRADE: http://www.gradeworkinggroup.org
JBI: https://jbi.global
Cochrane: https://www.cochrane.org

Recommended tool for Critical Review of Academic Papers

Critical Appraisal Skills Programme (CASP): https://casp-uk.net/casp-tools-checklists

RECOMMENDED READING

Aveyard H, Sharp P: A beginner's guide to evidence-based practice in health and social care, ed 3, Maidenhead, 2017, Open University Press.
Ellis P: Evidence-based practice in nursing, 2019, SAGE.
Dang D, Dearholt SL, Bissett K, et al: Johns Hopkins evidence-based practice for nurses and healthcare professionals: model and guidelines, Indianapolis, 2021, Sigma Theta Tau.

REFERENCES

Alligood M: Nursing theory, utilization and application, ed 5, 2013, Elsevier.
Aveyard H: Doing a literature review in health and social care: a practical guide, ed 4, London, 2019, Open University Press.
Baldwin A, Mills J, Birks M, et al: Reconciling professional identity: a grounded theory of nurse academics' role modelling for undergraduate students, Nurse Education Today 59:1–5, 2017.
Benner PE: From novice to expert: excellence and power in clinical nursing practice, Menlo Park, 1984, Addison-Wesley.
Benner PE, Tanner CA, Chesla CA: Expertise in nursing practice: caring, clinical judgment, and ethics, New York, 2009, Springer Publishing Company.
Bick D, Briley A, Brocklehurst P, et al: A multicentre, randomised controlled trial of position during the late stages of labour in nulliparous women with an epidural: clinical effectiveness and an economic evaluation (BUMPES), Health Technology Assessment 21(65):1–206, 2017. doi:10.3310/hta21650.
Chilcote DR: Intuition: a concept analysis, Nursing Forum 52(1): 62–67, 2017.
Griffiths P, Maruotti A, Recio Saucedo A, et al: Nurse staffing, nursing assistants and hospital mortality: retrospective longitudinal cohort study, BMJ Quality & Safety 28:609–617, 2019.

Levett-Jones T. (ed): Clinical reasoning: learning to think like a nurse, ed 2, Sydney, 2018, Pearson.

Melnyk BM, Fineout-Overholt E: Evidence-based practice in nursing & healthcare. A guide to best practice, ed 4, Philadelphia, 2019, Wolters Kluwer.

Miller EM, Hill PD: Intuition in clinical decision-making: differences among practicing nurses, Journal of Holistic Nursing Dec;36(4):318–329, 2018.

Nightingale F: Notes on nursing: what it is and what it is not, London, 1869, Harrison and Sons.

Nursing and Midwifery Board of Australia: Registered nurse standards for practice, 2016. http://www.nursingmidwiferyboard. gov.au/Codes-Guidelines-Statements/Professional-standards/registered-nurse-standards-for-practice.aspx.

Nursing and Midwifery Council: The Code: Professional standards of practice and behaviour for nurses, midwives and nursing associates, London, 2018, NMC.

Nursing Council of New Zealand: Competencies for registered nurses; 2007. http://www.nursingcouncil.org.nz/Nurses.

Russell L: From nightingale to now: nurse education in Australia, Sydney, 1990, Harcourt Brace Jovanovich.

Sackett D: Evidence-based medicine: what it is and what it isn't, The BMJ 312:71–72, 1996.

2

FINDING AND USING RESEARCH

KATH PETERS ■ GEARÓID BRENNAN ■ LUCIE RAMJAN

CHAPTER OUTLINE

LEARNING OBJECTIVES

After reading this chapter and following critical reflection, readers should be able to:

■ use the different services and resources offered by the library

■ understand how the library filing and classification systems can support locating resources

■ access, compare and contrast electronic databases to obtain nursing, midwifery and health information

■ conduct a basic information search using library resources

■ identify which electronic databases and other electronic resources, such as eBooks and online journals, will best address an information need.

KEY TERMS

call number

catalogue

citation database

electronic database

grey literature

index

information literacy

interlibrary loan/ document delivery

journal

microform

peer reviewed

PICO

PICO(T)

reference collection

reserve collection

search engine

search strategy

seminal works

social media

ABSTRACT

Libraries collect, store and organise information and make it readily accessible for use. Libraries can also direct users to other profession-specific repositories of information. Hard-copy materials within the library are organised using a classification system and located by searching the catalogues. Electronic data is accessed using databases or, in some cases, via a library catalogue. Successful searches for information about a particular topic demand certain skills. These include the ability to define the topic of interest, select appropriate electronic search tools and conduct a basic search of databases and the catalogue system to identify and access the information required.

STUDENT QUOTE

The vast array of electronic databases the library offers is excellent. The ease of use and the support the library staff offer assists me in finding information with minimal problems!

HOW CAN THIS CHAPTER HELP YOU?

Take the following quiz to find out if this chapter will help you.

1. Do you know what professional libraries are available to you and if there are resources available to you remotely?
2. Do you know what kinds of materials your local professional library has and what kinds of services they offer?
3. Do you find it easy to locate what you are looking for when you use a library?
4. Do you know what an electronic database is? Can you identify the most appropriate databases for nursing, midwifery and allied health?
5. Do you know how to search an electronic database?
6. Do you know the advantages of using electronic databases compared to internet search engines such as Google Scholar?
7. Do you know how to effectively use social media to source and disseminate information?

If you answered 'yes' to most of these questions, you may want to skim this chapter. If you answered 'no' or if you have ever said to a lecturer or colleague, 'There wasn't any information available on the topic', then it would be useful for you to read this chapter and complete the student challenges.

INTRODUCTION

In the 21st century, almost limitless access to information is available via the internet. With access to vast amounts of information, people need appropriate skills to determine which information is useful and appropriate for use in their studies. Central to these skills is **information literacy**. This includes the capacity to know when information is needed, and the ability to find, appraise, organise and use the information effectively (Sample 2020). Possessing these skills can also enhance lifelong learning beyond completion of courses and is regarded as central to education and professional practice (Goodsett 2020).

TYPES OF LIBRARIES

Contemporary libraries can be described as either physical or virtual libraries. The physical library is the actual library building with the collections of different resources for borrowing and library staff to assist you in person. The virtual library is an electronic library, accessed by a computer or mobile device, consisting of online resources such as eBooks, online **journals**, newspaper articles and various other electronic documents. These online resources can be accessed by members remotely via a library homepage. These types of resources do have an advantage over print resources in that they cannot be misplaced on the shelves and more people can use them from distant locations. To access some electronic resources, you may be prompted for a username and password as some articles or journals may only be available to subscribers or library members. Always check with your library if you have any problems accessing and using electronic resources. Many libraries offer specialist librarians in nursing, midwifery or health, an online chat service or even online question services to assist you with your information needs. Overall, the traditional view of a library as a place where information is physically housed has been relegated to history and libraries are now places that facilitate information access regardless of where you are.

Academic libraries are connected to academic institutions and collect information of interest to staff and students. The types of material collected are strongly associated with the degrees offered at that individual institution. In other words, the resources held support the curricula taught. The library also usually has a physical presence on campuses where students are attending classes. Specialty libraries are formed by organisations with specialised information needs. They collect information on specific topics dictated by the needs of the organisation. These may include business and corporate libraries or professional libraries, such as hospital libraries. The information collected is based on the needs of the specific population being served. If you are employed in a hospital or other healthcare facility, you may have access to an onsite library, which is usually a cross between an academic and a specialty library. Many professional organisations, such as the Australian College of Nursing, New Zealand Nurses Organisation and the Royal College of Nursing in the United Kingdom (UK), offer either their own library or subscriptions to electronic resources as part of their membership. Information about member benefits can usually be found on a library or organisation's website.

WHAT'S IN THE LIBRARY?

Libraries use very precise systems to organise all the information they collect. These organising systems are called classification schemes. Libraries use two major classification schemes: the Dewey Decimal Classification (DDC) and the Library of Congress Classification (LCC). Both systems use number–letter combinations to label their collections. These labels are known as **call numbers**. Some libraries put call numbers on all their materials, while others label books only. Each hard-copy book has a call number, and ranges of call numbers are clearly marked on library shelves to make books about a specific subject easy to locate. As a rule of thumb, in Australia, New Zealand and the UK, most public and academic libraries use the DDC. Specialty libraries may use a scheme adapted to handle large volumes of material in relatively few subject areas. Medical libraries may use the National Library of Medicine Classification system, adapted from the LCC. The key point is that all the physical material in the library is carefully organised to make it easy to find.

Library users need to know what physical and human resources exist within the library as well as what external resources may be accessed from the library. Every library is arranged differently but there are usually some common features. The main section of the library typically contains a loans (circulation) desk, an information/reference/research inquiries desk and an area set aside for computer workstations where you can search in catalogues, indexes, abstracts, **citation databases** and full-text databases. Other key areas include a reference collection, a current and bound periodicals section and the main collection shelves. Most libraries also have a media or audiovisual centre, reserve collection section and special collections. Most modern libraries have a variety of learning spaces to accommodate the study needs of individual students. Students can access computers with internet, and printing and photocopying facilities. Space is available for interactive learning with others as well as for private reading time.

The loans (circulation) desk is where you borrow books and other materials to use outside the library. The information/reference/research inquiries desk is the place to go when you don't know where to look for needed materials or when you have questions about various library services and resources. Many libraries combine the functions of the information/reference research inquiries desks. The names used to describe these services may vary between libraries. Most libraries have help guides available either in print or online from the library homepage, including virtual tours of the library. Library staff will demonstrate how to access various databases and may offer consultations for further assistance. There may be classes where you can learn about the services the library offers. Smartphone and mobile device applications provide other options to give library users access to information and resources.

The **reference collection** contains materials such as encyclopedias, dictionaries, statistical reports, directories, handbooks and other materials that are handy for quick reference. These materials are referred to as 'library use only' because they are for use within the library and may not be borrowed and taken outside the library.

While most journals are now available online, some continue to be available in hard copy. Journal issues frequently start with the first issue of the current year and contain all the issues for the year to date. The bound journals contain single issues of a particular journal, published in previous years, bound together in book form, called a volume. The number of years contained in a volume depends on the size of the journal and number of issues published annually. Typically, 1 year of a journal constitutes a volume, and the specific volumes or issues of journals the library owns are referred to as its holdings. This section is usually arranged by call number (e.g. DDC), but in some libraries it is arranged alphabetically by journal title. It is common practice for libraries to have current and bound journals housed together on the same shelf. Most journals are also now available online via the library catalogue. It is useful to find out what journal resources are available in full text at the libraries accessible to you.

In addition to books and journals, many libraries have an audiovisual section containing DVDs and computer software. Some libraries may also have a **microform** section consisting of microfilm and microfiche that allows the reader to view different documents stored on film (e.g. newspapers). This may be especially useful for those involved in historical research.

The **reserve collection** section contains materials that have been put aside by the library or faculty staff for special use. The function of the reserve section is the sharing of limited resources needed by numerous users (e.g. prescribed textbooks). Typically, these materials can only be checked out of the library for a few hours, overnight or for 1 or 2 days. Some material can only be viewed in the library. These materials are often heavily used, so a reserve system allows a greater number of people to access them.

Special collections, or archives, contain rare materials that are not easily replaced. These might include collections of items such as: government and professional documents; old, rare or one-of-a-kind books; or materials of historical importance. Access to these materials is usually restricted and they often are not able to be borrowed.

Sometimes, if the library you are a member of does not have a specific resource, book or journal, you may be able to access a document delivery or interlibrary loan service. This may involve the library either providing a copy of a journal article or a hard copy loan from another affiliated library service.

You may have visited your university or health centre library; however, if you have only a vague idea about where things are located or how to use the library in general, please take time to do the following student challenge. It can save you a lot of time and energy when you need to use the library and want to quickly locate the resources or services you need.

STUDENT CHALLENGE

Exploring Library Layouts

Your online library should provide online guides to accessing essential services and resources. Most also have an online librarian who can assist you with your enquiries.

To explore your online library, open your library website. Allow an hour for this experience.

- Locate the online guides to finding resources.
- Identify what online services and tutorials your library provides.
- Determine what resources are available to you.
- Discover how you borrow and renew books.
- Locate the electronic databases your library allows you to access.
- Identify some of the key journals in your area of interest that are available in full-text format.

To explore your physical library, visit your university campus or health centre library. Allow at least an hour for this experience. Become comfortable with the space and with the library before attempting to undertake the following tasks.

1. Make a mental note of the physical layout (the library may already have a map for users). Then:
   a. locate and visit the loans desk, information/reference/research inquiries desk, reserve desk and study areas
   b. find a library workstation; find the search tool section (e.g. indexes, abstracts, databases and catalogues) available via the internet

Continued

STUDENT CHALLENGE—cont'd

Exploring Library Layouts

   c. find several journal titles and their holdings that are available via the library catalogue for your area of interest

   d. visit the special collections and archives

   e. locate the section containing theses and dissertations

   f. locate the audiovisual resources collection (microfilm, microfiche, CDs, DVDs)

   g. find the photocopiers and determine how you pay for copies.

2. Find out about library operations.

   a. What are the library's opening hours?

   b. Find out if there is a specialist nursing/midwifery librarian. Locate their contact details and find out what sort of help they provide.

   c. Are tours or classes available in the library to learn about searching the literature and, if so, when and how do you enrol?

   d. Identify what interlibrary loan or document delivery services you can access.

   e. What are the policies for borrowing and returning materials? Is there a self-checkout system, text reserve system, drop-off box or loan extension system?

   f. Is this library connected or affiliated with other libraries you can use?

   g. Can you access library search tools from computers in other locations on campus or from your home computer?

3. Where are the nursing or midwifery resources located? Locate the following: nursing and/or midwifery books, nursing and/or midwifery journals, professional documents (such as those from the Australian Nursing and Midwifery Accreditation Council [ANMAC], Nursing Council of New Zealand [NCNZ], Nursing and Midwifery Council [NMC], Royal College of Nursing [RCN], Australian College of Nursing [ACN] or New Zealand Nurses Organisation [NZNO]) and government publications (such as those from the Australian Institute of Health and Welfare [AIHW] and the National Health Service [NHS]).

SEARCHING FOR INFORMATION IN CATALOGUES

Libraries have specific filing systems called **catalogues** to assist you in locating specific materials so you may retrieve the information you seek. It is worthwhile spending time exploring your library's catalogue, as it will list all items held in the library online. The titles of newspapers, scholarly journals and other library materials, such as government or professional documents, will be listed. However, information about the specific content contained in those periodicals or documents is not usually found in the catalogue.

Books are listed with bibliographical information, location, collection, call numbers and borrowed status. Books may be located by searching for a specific title, author, keyword(s), call number, International Standard Book Number (ISBN), government document classification number or subject matter.

Using Electronic Catalogues

Most catalogues are now available electronically. They may be accessed directly from library workstations or from any internet connection, either on or off campus.

You may be asked to provide a username and password to authenticate yourself as someone authorised to use the system. Connection to the catalogue enables you to search for books and other library materials. You simply need to follow the onscreen directions, which tell you how to search for a book by title, author, keyword and so on. Many libraries external to your own university also offer free access to their catalogues where you can search and discover which resources are held.

These online systems offer the added advantage of providing the latest information on all new materials coming into the library, and usually carry additional useful information such as whether a book is available on the shelves or if it has been borrowed. In cases where books have been borrowed, the due date for return will often be indicated in the catalogue. Catalogues may have a holds/reservations system that you are able to use when an item you require is out on loan. This will allow you to place a reservation on the resource for when it is returned. Some catalogues may also allow virtual shelf-browsing that shows which resources are shelved nearby; for example, naming the five books held on either side of a selected text.

Using your library's electronic catalogue, complete the following challenge.

Indexes, Abstracts and Electronic Databases

Historically, the term '**index**' was used for a list of citations to journals and other publications such as newspapers and government or professional documents. It is important to note that terminology has changed over the years. While the electronic versions of indexes still perform the same function as their paper-based predecessors, they are now more commonly referred to as **electronic databases**. Multiple databases exist that provide publications for a wide variety of discipline-specific and specialty areas. You can use keywords and specific search terms to locate publications on a topic of your choice. Choosing the right keywords is important to ensure that your search retrieves all the resources around your topic and to reduce the number of irrelevant resources identified. A librarian can help you outline a search strategy that will suit your database and topic area.

Once you have located a publication, you can read the abstract. An abstract is a short summary and is useful in helping you decide whether the publication contains the information you are seeking. These summaries are virtually always available as part of the

citation information provided to users as part of their search results after they search a database. The library will probably not hold full-text versions of all the materials identified in search results, but it should have access to them through **interlibrary loan/document delivery**. Some databases may provide links to other databases, which may enable you to access the full text of an article.

Some common and useful databases are listed in Boxes 2.1 and 2.2. Please note that, although the word 'index' remains in titles, these electronic resources are also known as databases.

A major advantage of electronic databases is that they are available online from any location and offer access to a wide range of information. EBSCOhost is an online research platform that offers access to multiple full-text databases relevant to a variety of disciplines including nursing and midwifery (EBSCO Information Services 2021a). These databases include Cumulative Index to Nursing and Allied Health Literature (CINAHL) and MEDLINE, the two main research databases that provide online access to materials related to research and practice in the disciplines of nursing, midwifery, medicine and allied healthcare.

CINAHL includes indexing for over 3000 journals and provides full-text articles for more than 1500 journals in the areas of nursing, midwifery, consumer health, medicine, complementary medicine and multiple other allied health disciplines (EBSCO Information Services 2021b). Journal articles, eBooks, book chapters, practice guidelines, dissertations/theses, conference proceedings, educational software and audiovisual content can all be accessed via CINAHL. While CINAHL focuses on nursing, midwifery, allied health and psychosocial issues, MEDLINE focuses more on biomedicine and health. MEDLINE contains more than 21 million references from journals in the life sciences including, but not limited to, medicine, nursing, dentistry, veterinary medicine and behavioural sciences (National Library of Medicine 2021). There is some overlap between CINAHL, MEDLINE and other databases that specialise in similar health topics, so many researchers will search multiple databases to identify all relevant literature. These database searches are generally described in literature reviews under a heading such as 'search strategy' or similar.

Other useful electronic platforms include ProQuest Central, which provides access to more than 12,000 scholarly journals (ProQuest LLC 2021b). ProQuest Central offers specific collections titled Health and Medicine and Applied Social Science Index and Abstracts (ASSIA) which provide scholarly resources focused on health, medicine, nursing, psychology and social science (ProQuest LLC 2021a). Various other electronic databases and **search engines** are available covering a variety of disciplines; for example, Google Scholar, which enables broad searches of multidisciplinary scholarly literature (Google 2021), and Intermid, a database that allows browsing of two reputable midwifery journals (MA Healthcare Ltd 2021). Further databases you may find useful to search during your studies include Scopus, PsychInfo and Evidence-Based Medicine Reviews (EBMR). EBMR is a specialised database for locating full-text evidence-based publications by searching seven evidence-based medicine review databases, including Cochrane Database of Systematic Reviews and the Database of Abstracts of Reviews of Effects (DARE) (Cochrane Library 2021). Additionally, the JBI Evidence-based Practice database is a convenient online database that provides best-practice guidance for healthcare professionals for a diverse range of clinical issues (JBI 2021).

Most electronic databases have introductory lessons to guide you in your search and a help function to troubleshoot any difficulties you may encounter. However, if you require additional support, you may wish to contact the library staff who can assist you in learning how to identify the database(s) that best suit your needs and how to best search it.

Using Apps to Search

There are now dedicated academic literature search applications (apps) available for most mobile internet access devices. Increasingly, these apps are being used by healthcare professionals to access literature (Johnson & Howard 2019). There are many apps available designed for both Apple and Android devices which allow you to search multiple search engines, libraries and databases simultaneously, which can save you time. The search apps allow you to view and download full-text versions of articles returned by your searches. There are also apps that facilitate access to specific journals; for example, the *Journal of Advanced Nursing*, *Journal of Nursing Scholarship* and *MCN: The American Journal of Maternal/Child Nursing*. Full-text access may, however, require you to log in with a subscription or via your library.

Using Social Media

It's difficult to discuss apps and not say something about the role of **social media**. Social media can be used in nearly all stages of the research journey. With appropriate ethical approvals and consent procedures, it can be used to advertise studies and aid participant recruitment. The interactions users have on platforms can even become research data (Thomas 2020). However, in this chapter we are going to focus on the role of social media for discovering, sharing and disseminating research findings.

You will be aware that social media has many pitfalls, such as people (including unverified users) posting whatever they want, even if it is not scientifically valid. Social media can be a source of disinformation and misinformation. However, it is not always acknowledged that social media can be harnessed to share scholarly works (McNamara & Usher 2019, Luc et al 2021). It can also be an incredibly engaging and accessible way to find key studies to inform your research and practice.

One of the advantages of social media is that it can be an equal playing field between academics, clinicians, students, consumers of healthcare and the general public. All parties can interact together on the same platform, helping to shape debate and discourse. Indeed, it can bring scientific findings directly to members of the public in a couple of clicks.

Platforms such as Twitter only allow a limited number of characters to be used. This means people must be able to summarise their findings succinctly. However, people can provide links to scholarly work, meaning that research can be downloaded and shared instantly across the globe. Linking with researchers on social media can allow people to ask questions about their work and develop links with others working in the same area.

Traditionally, publishers would track how many times each article was cited by other researchers and academics. However, a new form of metric, known as Altmetric, has become common. Altmetric also tracks how many times a paper has been shared or discussed across various social media platforms such as Facebook, Twitter and blog sites (Altmetric 2020). This has become a very popular way of capturing the impact a study has by looking at how many times it has been tweeted and shared through social media. It is for this reason that several journals have social media managers and social media strategies for prompting the dissemination of articles the journal publishes (McNamara & Usher 2019).

The following are some top tips for using social media to find articles.

- It may be helpful to set up a separate professional account that you just use for work.
- Think about who the key scholars and clinicians are in your area of interest and start following them.
- Follow the top five journals for your area of interest.
- Find out the names of the editor-in-chief and editors for these journals and follow them too.
- Large research groups or studies will often have their own social media accounts. They may post when there have been new developments, meaning you may be one of the first to learn of key findings.
- Key clinicians and academics might not just discuss their paper but may also link to a blog or online event about their work. This can help in communicating key findings to the public in an accessible manner.

- You can also follow hashtags (#). This can also be a good way to keep up to date with key issues, because anyone who uses a hashtag in their post can make it accessible to those who follow the hashtag.
- Journals or other relevant professional groups may host discussions. These are normally advertised in advance, and anyone can join in by using the relevant hashtag. This is a great way to engage with key scholars in the field.
- Conferences and events will often have their own hashtag, which is a great way of following the discussion even if you are not attending the event.

STUDENT CHALLENGE

Examining Electronic Databases

Consider the following using a computer workstation in the library or your own personal computer.

1. How do you switch between searching the catalogue and electronic database searches?
2. Look at all the electronic databases available online from your library. Which ones look like they would be most relevant to nursing, midwifery or healthcare?
3. Explore at least two databases you consider relevant to your area of interest. Can you locate a description of each database? Can you find a list of the journals that are indexed?

TIPS FOR SUCCESSFUL SEARCHING

As previously discussed, a search can be conducted using electronic databases, internet search engines and catalogues to find information about specific subjects. Searching for a particular book or article by title or by author is straightforward. Searching for unknown materials on a subject or topic you have interest in is slightly more complicated. Trying to do a search and receiving a message that says, 'there are 21,346 matches' or 'there are no matches meeting your search parameters' can be very frustrating. This section is designed to provide tips for effective searching so that you are more successful and productive and can develop a **search strategy**. During your search, you need to be mindful of publication bias (where knowledge published may be misleading for a variety of reasons,

including flawed methodologies; see Dowdy, Tincani & Schneider 2020) and salami slicing (where multiple publications from the one study dominate the area; see Gray et al 2021), both of which can either skew or provide an inaccurate representation of results.

Clearly Define Your Search

Start the process with a clear idea of your search topic or subject area. Tip: it can be helpful to write down what you would like to explore in sentence form [written description] or summarise your topic in the form of a question. What are the key concepts and subconcepts for that subject or topic? Which concepts are most important? Concepts should usually be verbs and nouns. Tip: it can be useful to underline or highlight the main concepts in your written description and in the question you have developed. Next, think of other keywords that mean the same as your key concepts or subconcepts (synonyms) and think of the alternative spelling of these words; for example, paediatrics or pediatrics, labor or labour. Truncate words or use wildcards to expand a search. Truncation involves formulating other words by using the base of a word (e.g. nurs* = nurse, nurses, nursing, nursery). Wildcards are symbols that replace characters in a word (e.g. wom?n = woman or women) (MIT Libraries 2021). Tip: it is worthwhile creating a table with the keywords and associated phrases and listing truncated words and/or wildcards that you may decide to use in your search. Some databases have specific MeSH headings (**Me**dical **S**ubject **H**eadings), which are easily recognised and matched by the database.

Consider the information you currently have. Reading your own textbooks, reference books or articles for background information before you access databases and catalogues can help focus and direct your search. Look at the references listed in these books and articles. You may find pertinent sources on your topic that you can look up electronically or in the library. You should also refer to subject guides produced by your lecturers, as these are often a good starting point to find the information you need. If you are using an evidence-based frame of reference, you may prefer to adopt either the PICO(T) (discussed below) or SPIDER (discussed in Chapter 3) approach to searching for specific knowledge.

	Population or Problem	Intervention	Comparison Intervention	Outcome
TABLE 2.1 Using the PICO Framework: What is the Best Care Management for a Young Woman With a Learning Disability and Type 1 Diabetes?				
Concept	Young woman with learning disability and type 1 diabetes	Management of type 1 diabetes	N/A	Improved diabetes care
Keyword	Learning disability Type 1 diabetes	Diabetes management Medication adherence Blood glucose monitoring	Non-pharmaceutical Diet Exercise	Self-management interventions

Identify Key Search Terms

One approach commonly used in nursing and midwifery research to identify key search terms is the PICO model. **PICO** stands for **P**opulation/**P**roblem, **I**ntervention, **C**omparison, **O**utcome. In some cases, 'T' for **T**imeframe is also included—**PICO(T)**.

Using the PICO framework, consider the question in Table 2.1.

Choose Appropriate Resources

Books tend to provide good reference information on a particular subject or topic, which is especially useful if the subject area is new to you. It is important that the books you use are current, unless they are **seminal works**. Journals provide more current and specific information than books as they report changing trends and practices. Research journals are particularly valuable for providing the results and outcomes of the latest research (MIT Libraries 2021). If you require definitions, statistics, trends, professional or government documents or policies (**grey literature**) then these are usually found in electronic reference materials available on the internet. For example:

- Australian Bureau of Statistics: https://www.abs.gov.au
- Australian Government Department of Health: https://www.health.gov.au
- National Health Service: https://www.nhs.uk
- New Zealand Ministry of Health Manatū Hauora: https://www.health.govt.nz.

Alternatively, such reports may be found in the special documents section of the library.

Choose Appropriate Databases

Choosing an appropriate database is imperative for success in searching. Each database has a primary area of focus, plus advantages and limits. A description of the purpose of a particular database may be listed in the catalogue or there may be further information next to or underneath the name of the database on the library homepage. A list of the included journals is usually provided with the database. Think about three issues when selecting a database. First, what subjects are covered in the database? Tip: as indicated, the database description will help you decide which database to use and provides information on subjects. Second, what years does the database cover? Tip: some databases only index recent articles while others index older publication years. For earlier seminal publications, you may need to source the print index. Third, what sources does the database include (e.g. peer-reviewed literature and/or grey literature)? Tip: the database description should provide this information and indicate whether the database searches articles only or other sources such as book chapters, theses or newspapers (Benedictine University Library 2021).

Place Limits on Your Search

Use limits to narrow your search so it is as precise as possible. If you have several key terms, use them. Limits you can apply include language, type of resource, publication date and full-text only (Benedictine University Library 2021). You can always remove some of the limits if the results are not what you want or if the search yields too many hits, as occurs in the following case study.

CASE STUDY 2.1

Ahmed's assignment requires him to explore best practice in caring for an 87-year-old man living with chronic heart failure and newly diagnosed COPD. If Ahmed enters the term 'chronic obstructive pulmonary disease' to search in PubMed, the result yields 88,062 different citations. If the search term 'chronic heart failure' is entered, the result yields 56,464 results, and if the term 'best practice' is searched, Ahmed will get 193,216 results. If the three individual search terms 'chronic obstructive pulmonary disease', 'chronic heart failure' and 'best practice' are combined, the search results are reduced to 115 citations. If Ahmed further limits the search to full-text articles written in English, he will get 95 citations. A further limitation to include the most contemporary literature (last 5 years) yields a manageable 39 citations. (See Fig. 2.1.)

All electronic databases have rules for use that can save time and effort when searching. The more you know about these rules and how to use them, the more successful you will be with refining your searches. For instance, most databases use Boolean operators (Clarivate Analytics 2020). These operators or joining words allow you to combine terms with the words 'AND', 'OR', 'NOT' or 'NEAR' to retrieve a specific result. The term 'AND' narrows a search by ensuring that all search terms are present. The term 'OR' broadens a search by ensuring that any of the search terms are present. However, this term needs to be used with caution as it retrieves multiple categories, some of which may not be relevant to your search. The term 'NOT' limits a search by removing a particular search term that you do not want (Benedictine University Library 2021). Finally, the term 'NEAR' ensures the search terms are found within close proximity (usually within 10 words) of each other (see Table 2.2). Other operators or joining words may be used to place limits on things such as age, gender, type of journal, years of publication and so on. Note that it is not always necessary to use uppercase letters.

When searching within a database, you may find a limit option that will only return references in your search results that are **peer reviewed**. Peer-reviewed articles are articles that have been subjected to a process of critical evaluation by one or more experts on the subject material.

A few databases use a technique that gives you a list of articles ranked in order of relevancy; that is, from most to least likely to be relevant, based on a set of supplied search terms (e.g. 'COPD', 'best practice'). Articles containing all the terms would be high on the results list and those containing one term would be at the bottom of the results list.

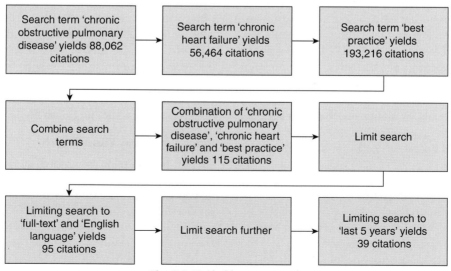

Fig. 2.1 ■ Limiting your search

TABLE 2.2

Examples of Boolean Operators (Joining Words) for Conducting a Search

Boolean Operator (Joining Word)	Example	What Happens
OR	COPD OR males	Retrieves all citations containing 'COPD' or 'males' in an article
AND	COPD AND males	Retrieves all citations containing both 'COPD' and 'males' in an article
NEAR	COPD NEAR males	Retrieves all citations containing both 'COPD' and 'males' within close proximity (usually within 10 words) of each other in an article
NOT	COPD NOT males	Eliminates any citations containing 'COPD' that also contain 'males'

The best way to increase proficiency with using search operators is through regular practice and consultation with an expert to guide your attempts. Many students do not make full use of the electronic database system's capabilities, so make sure you review the available materials on conducting a search to guide your practice. Library assistance is always available if you are experiencing difficulties.

An equally important skill is locating electronic repositories of professional data and knowing what types of data may be found in these repositories. It is important to realise how public-access internet search tools can assist you in literature searching. One highly recommended search tool is SUMSearch 2, a free medical meta-search engine (Chandran et al 2020), which simultaneously submits your search terms to some highly reputable medical information within, for example, DARE, National Guideline Clearinghouse and PubMed. These sites are government-sponsored and therefore likely to have limited bias due to conflicts of interest.

View Your Search Results

Once you have defined and run your search, you will want to view the results. The first page of results will list each citation with the option to view an abstract or full text if available. Simply looking at article titles or journal names helps you eliminate more articles from your search. If a citation seems promising, you may want to look at the abstract. You should save, email, export or print the full-text version if available, to retain the original pagination, tables and figures. As you build your personal library on this search, it can be stored electronically using software programs such as EndNote, RefWorks or Mendeley. This referencing software can help you manage the literature and citations.

CASE STUDY 2.2

After completing the search and reviewing the titles and abstracts of the papers, Ahmed identified 39 articles worth further examination. The next step Ahmed will need to take is to access the full text of each of the 39 articles.

The next step is to access the full text, which can be retrieved automatically using referencing software. However, if this is not available, you will need to check the database and library catalogue to identify if online access to the full-text paper is available. If there is no online version, sometimes the library will have a print copy or full-text access via another means. If the article is only offered in print, it will require a visit to the library. The library may also have special library services such as document delivery to assist you in accessing a full-text copy from an affiliated library.

CASE STUDY 2.3

Jamie is a final-year student undertaking a core research subject. Jamie must undertake a research project to demonstrate understanding of evidence-based practice applied to a case study. They have been assigned to investigate the care required for a 14-year-old young woman with learning disabilities, who has been newly diagnosed with type 1 diabetes. She is in foster care and has a history of mental health issues, including self-harming behaviours.

Returning to Table 2.1, if we search ProQuest Central using only the word-string 'learning disability and diabetes', limiting to English, full-text, evidence-based healthcare, peer-reviewed publications in the last 12 months, the search yields 84 citations. By adding 'type 1' to the term 'diabetes' to limit articles specifically relating to type 1 diabetes, the citations are reduced to 74 articles.

Tip: if you do find important and relevant articles on your topic, check the reference lists at the end of each article. The reference list will guide you to other good topic-specific resources. Additionally, some search engines identify articles related to the one you are reading. If any of the references, be they in the reference or related article lists, look useful, check and see if you can access the full text. Check the source (the journal in which the article is published) in your catalogue to see if your library has full-text access either electronically or in print. These references could be very useful when writing up your paper. Your library may be able to assist if you are having difficulties finding the references.

Now that you have had step-by-step information, try the following student challenge and do another search using the computer and whichever electronic resources you deem most appropriate. Use the information from the Tips for successful searching section and the knowledge gained from the previous student challenges to assist you.

STUDENT CHALLENGE

Use Your Knowledge to Practise a Basic Search

Search for updated information on a basic nursing or midwifery skill (such as handwashing, blood pressure readings or taking a fetal heart rate).
1. Define what you are looking for.
2. What resources will you use? Why did you choose them?
3. Describe how you conducted your search. What parameters did you use? How did you limit the search? Did you limit your results to peer-reviewed articles?
4. How many different searches did you do? What guided your decision-making processes during the search process? What aspects of your search approach worked and what aspects did not work?
5. Save the results of your search. Locate the articles you think are most pertinent to your selected topic. Do they contain the information you need?

CONCLUSION

In this chapter, we have introduced you to the library and its related functions, including: how to search using catalogues and databases; choosing appropriate search strategies and databases; how to place limits on your search; and searching via apps. By working through this information, hopefully you are now equipped with the fundamental skills to locate resources and use filing and classification systems to undertake your own search for relevant study materials.

ADDITIONAL RESOURCES

Help Button

Electronic databases have an online help button. It is designed to help you make the best use of that database. Click on it whenever you require assistance and need guidance while conducting an electronic search.

Librarians

There are specialist librarians for nursing and midwifery—seek their expert help. They field all kinds of questions and are willing to assist. Librarians also run classes on conducting searches and specialist librarians offer consultations by appointment. There are also online librarians available on most electronic library websites via a chat facility to seek advice. Alternatively, you can phone or email for support.

Library Help Guides

Many libraries offer a range of guides to make library use easier. Increasingly, libraries provide online workshops or videos to show you how to use various services. These are an important resource if you take the time to use them.

REFERENCES

Altmetric: How outputs are tracked and measured, 17 September 2020. https://help.altmetric.com/support/solutions/articles/6000234171-how-outputs-are-tracked-and-measured.

Benedictine University Library: General library research tutorial: module 4: searching a database, 2021. https://researchguides.ben.edu/general-research/searching.

Chandran VP, Khan S, Kulyadi GP, et al: Evidence-based medicine databases: an overview, Journal of Applied Pharmaceutical Science 10(7):147–154, 2020.

Clarivate Analytics: Web of Science core collection help. 2020. https://images.webofknowledge.com/images/help/WOS/hs_search_operators.html.

Cochrane Library: Centre for Reviews and Dissemination (CRD) databases. https://www.cochranelibrary.com/about/CRD-database-info.

Dowdy A, Tincani M, Schneider WJ: Evaluation of publication bias in response interruption and redirection: a meta-analysis, Journal of Applied Behavior Analysis 53(4):2151–2171, 2020.

EBSCO Information Services: EBSCO Research Platform, 2021a. https://www.ebsco.com/products/ebscohost-research-platform.

EBSCO Information Services: Full-text database CINAHL Complete, 2021b. https://www.ebsco.com/products/research-databases/cinahl-complete.

Goodsett M: Best practices for teaching and assessing critical thinking in information literacy online learning objects. The Journal of Academic Librarianship 46(5):102163, 2020.

Google: About Google Scholar, 2021. https://scholar.google.com/intl/en/scholar/about.html.

Gray R, Mackay B, Waters A, Brown E: Reporting the results of a clinical trial across multiple papers, does it matter? European Journal of Cardiovascular Nursing 20(6):618–619, 2021.

JBI: Products and services, 2021. https://jbi.global/products#database.

Johnson EM, Howard C: A library mobile device deployment to enhance the medical student experience in a rural longitudinal integrated clerkship. Journal of the Medical Library Association 107(1), 30–42, 2019.

Luc JGY, Archer MA, Arora RC, et al: Does tweeting improve citations? One-year results from the TSSMN prospective randomized trial, The Annals of Thoracic Surgery 111(1):296–300, 2021. https://doi.org/10.1016/J.ATHORACSUR.2020.04.065.

MA Healthcare Ltd: About Intermid, 2021. https://www.magonlinelibrary.com/page/collections/intermid/about.

McNamara P, Usher K: Share or perish: social media and the International Journal of Mental Health Nursing, International Journal of Mental Health Nursing 28(4):960–970, 2019. https://doi.org/10.1111/INM.12600.

MIT Libraries: Database search tips: Boolean operators, 2021. https://libguides.mit.edu/c.php?g=175963&p=1158594.

National Library of Medicine: MEDLINE: Overview, 2021. https://www.nlm.nih.gov/medline/medline_overview.html.

ProQuest LLC: Health & Medicine, 2021a. https://about.proquest.com/en/subjects/health-medicine/.

ProQuest LLC: ProQuest Central, 2021b. https://about.proquest.com/en/products-services/ProQuest_Central/.

Sample A: Historical development of definitions of information literacy: A literature review of selected resources, The Journal of Academic Librarianship 46(2):102116, 2020.

Thomas N: Little quick fix: get your data from social media, London, 2020, SAGE.

CONDUCTING AND WRITING A LITERATURE REVIEW

KIM USHER ■ HELEN AVEYARD ■ CAROLINE BRADBURY-JONES ■ TIFFANY CONROY

CHAPTER OUTLINE

LEARNING OBJECTIVES

After reading this chapter and following critical reflection, readers should be able to:

■ understand the purpose of a literature review

■ understand the different types of reviews

■ discuss new and emerging developments in literature review methods

■ develop a clear question to guide a literature review

■ identify the main components of a literature review

■ critically evaluate the values and assumptions within contemporary literature reviews.

KEY TERMS

critical appraisal

data collection

data extraction

electronic database

focused mapping review and synthesis (FMRS)

integrative review

literature review

literature search

realist review

research question

sample

scoping review

search terms

systematic review

systematic review with meta-analysis

umbrella reviews

ABSTRACT

Now that the previous chapter has introduced you to using library resources, we are going to put some of these skills into practice. In this chapter, we are going to take you step-by-step through the process of undertaking a literature review. We start with some background information about literature reviews, describe some of the different types of literature reviews and emerging developments in this field and explain when they may be used. Mostly though, we focus on the 'how to', taking you stepwise through developing a focused research question and how it can be used to search the literature. We describe how to develop search terms, screen the literature against inclusion/exclusion criteria, critically appraise the literature and extract data. Important considerations about how to record your literature search and how to prioritise the literature are also discussed. Even if you are not ready to undertake a literature review right now, having a good understanding of the steps involved will stand you in good stead for future research projects.

STUDENT QUOTE

I know the general topic. I want to review the literature to understand what is already known on this topic so that I can identify any gaps in the evidence.

INTRODUCTION

Once you are familiar with using the library, you have a wealth of academic resources at your fingertips that you will soon be using within your written work. Academic study usually involves delving further into research papers (peer-reviewed research reports published in reputable academic journals) rather than relying solely on textbooks, which might have previously been your main source of knowledge. However, once you start accessing and using a wider range of resources, you will realise the extent of resources available. This can make it hard to know where to start. Undertaking a literature review is an integral part of the research process. It can also be considered research in its own right, because it needs to be done in a systematic manner. In fact, doing a literature review follows the research process and the fundamental IMRaD formula: Introduction, Methods, Results and Discussion.

A literature review presents a summary of the available evidence at a certain point in time on a particular topic. As a result, it provides the researcher with an overview of the similarities and inconsistencies in the literature and identifies areas where further research is needed. In order to do so, a review should contain the best available evidence which addresses the review question. This is usually primary research rather than secondary data. Primary data is data collected by the researcher firsthand and directly from the source, while secondary data is data collected by someone else, such as data collected for other research purposes (e.g. literature review, census data). What is known as grey literature may also be included in some types of literature reviews. Grey literature is produced by organisations outside of the traditional academic or commercial publishing approaches and consists of reports, government documents and evaluations.

The type of research included in a review depends on the question guiding the review. In this chapter, we provide an overview of how to read, understand or undertake a review of the literature. We also explore some of the issues that you need to be aware of when thinking about or doing your own literature review.

WHAT IS A LITERATURE REVIEW?

A **literature review** is a piece of work that summarises the available and relevant work undertaken in an area. It usually has a very specific focus on a question or topic. There are several recognised steps in the process of doing a literature review that reflect the research process. These include identifying a question to guide the review, searching for literature, recognising what you find and its relevance to your review, assessing the strength of the evidence, analysing the literature and writing up your results.

This might seem quite a challenge if you are starting out as a student, but you are unlikely to be required to undertake a very detailed literature review in your first semester. However, you may be required to use the principles of doing a literature review in your academic work and it is important that you understand the processes involved.

WHY DO A LITERATURE REVIEW?

A literature review generally has two purposes. It can be undertaken prior to commencing research, to identify a gap in knowledge. You will often see this type of review prior to the reporting of the findings when you read a research paper. Alternatively, a literature review can be a piece of research in its own right. This is where you use the literature to answer a specific question. In both cases, the purpose is to provide a critical analysis and synthesis of all available evidence (Aveyard 2019). As a nurse or midwife, literature reviews are valuable to clinical practice. Literature reviews are undertaken to identify the best possible care, supported by the current best available evidence. Implementing evidence into practice requires being able to identify and critically appraise relevant literature and then synthesise or summarise this evidence.

LITERATURE REVIEW METHODS

Like all research methods, the methods for undertaking a literature review have developed in recent years. Traditionally, when writing a literature review, researchers would have gathered pertinent information about a topic and presented it in an essay-like format. This may have included details about how they searched and critiqued the papers, but formal reporting of this step was often omitted. This largely unstructured process allowed for 'cherry picking' or selectively choosing papers that might have supported the pre-held views of the researcher and may not have been representative of the comprehensive body of research.

In the past two decades, the approach to literature reviews has become more systematic, largely due to the influence of the evidence-based medicine movement and organisations such as Cochrane, JBI and the Campbell Collaboration, which have developed systematic methods for various types of literature reviews (Higgins et al 2019). These systematic approaches help to eliminate bias in selecting literature for inclusion and introduce rigour in the methods used, which means that we can have more confidence in the results.

The 'first' systematic literature reviews were pioneered by the Cochrane Collaboration (now Cochrane), which worked to develop methods for the systematic identification and synthesis of research findings, enabling clinicians to make sense of data from various trials, especially when they report conflicting results (see www.cochranelibrary.com). These **systematic reviews** focused on questions of effectiveness and typically included a meta-analysis, which is the numerical combination of the results from the different studies. The success of Cochrane has led to more attention being given to the literature review process and has resulted in greater rigour and transparency in the conduct of reviews. There is currently an expectation that authors of published reviews be explicit about their search strategy and process for the selection, appraisal and analysis of literature. The EQUATOR guidelines have enhanced the quality of reporting in literature reviews (Reporting Guidelines, https://www.equator-network.org/) and are likely to be a useful resource for readers of this chapter.

TYPES OF LITERATURE REVIEWS

There are a number of different types of literature reviews (Table 3.1). If you scan some of the leading nursing and midwifery journals, you will find excellent examples of these. Review types include, but are not limited to, systematic review, integrative review, scoping review, realist review, umbrella review and focused mapping review and synthesis (FMRS). (See Aveyard and Bradbury-Jones [2019] for details of the different types of literature reviews.) The titles of the different reviews are not always consistent, and the word 'systematic' is often added even when the review is not a systematic review with meta-analysis as defined by Cochrane. This can lead to confusion. Different types of reviews have different purposes. For example, the goal of a **systematic review with meta-analysis** is usually to review the available research about the effectiveness of interventions. These reviews tend to exclusively use empirical studies such as randomised controlled trials (RCTs), non-randomised controlled trials and case-control studies. They use a focused question and a comprehensive search strategy. **Integrative reviews** generally have a focused question though a broader remit than the effectiveness of interventions and often include a wider range of study types. A **scoping review** is used to indicate the size and nature of the available literature on a particular topic, and often has a broad research question. The goal of a **realist review** is to

TABLE 3.1
Common Types of Literature Reviews

Review Type	Overview	Appraisal Required	Reviewers Involved/Analysis
Systematic review with meta synthesis	Combines the results of quantitative studies—usually RCTs—to determine the effect of results	Yes	Two or more reviewers; usually numerical analysis of measures assuming heterogeneity of results
Scoping review	Preliminary assessment of the potential size and scope of the available literature	No	One or more; characterises quantity and quality of literature and other key features
Umbrella reviews	Brings together reviews that answer different questions about a shared topic	Yes	One or more; what is known and recommendations for practice
Mixed studies review	Reviews a combination of methods within the review	Yes—needs to use appraisal relevant to types of studies	Two or more; analysis addresses both types of evidence and then produces a synthesis
Qualitative systematic review with synthesis	Integration of findings from qualitative studies	Yes	Thematic analysis including two or more reviewers
Realist review	Why something works, in what circumstances it works and with or for whom it works	Not usually	One or more reviewers; involves preliminary understanding of an issue, applies evidence to refine theory

build explanation or to clarify evidence of complex interventions applied in diverse contexts or settings. This type of review seeks to unpack why complex interventions work (or fail) in different contexts or settings. With an ever-increasing number of reviews available, **umbrella reviews** (or systematic reviews of reviews) compare and contrast already-published reviews. The **FMRS** focuses on specific sources of information within a specified timeframe. Regardless of the type of review, all reviews need to be conducted in a systematic way to ensure the results are reliable, quantifiable and reproducible.

Using the following case studies as examples, we can see two situations when nursing/midwifery students may be required to undertake a literature review.

CASE STUDY 3.1

Literature reviews can be undertaken in different ways. Ahmed is a second-year undergraduate student who is seeking to learn about research for an assessment. To do this he will need to look at the evidence around people's experiences of these conditions and will be identifying the most up-to-date research on these topics. This needs to be done in a systematic way to ensure he does not selectively choose the evidence, but instead gets a comprehensive view of the available literature.

Similarly, Jamie is a final-year undergraduate undertaking a core research subject. Jamie has to undertake a mini-research project to demonstrate understanding of evidence-based practice applied to a case study. They have been assigned to investigate the care required for a 14-year-old young woman with learning disabilities, who is newly diagnosed with type 1 diabetes. She is in foster care and has a history of mental health issues, including self-harming behaviours. Jamie needs to explore the evidence behind caring for people with learning disabilities. In their subsequent research proposal, Jamie will need to write this up as a literature review to justify the ongoing project.

What types of review should Jamie and Ahmed consider?

WHERE DO I START?

The first task is to identify your literature review question and how detailed your approach needs to be. This will depend on your year of study and the purpose of the review. Start reading generally around your topic and identify if any reviews have already been undertaken. This will help you to become familiar with key knowledge and ideas in your topic area. If you have not been given a focused question on which to base your review, reading around the topic will help you to focus your review question. Prior to conducting a literature search, search review databases—such as JBI, PROSPERO and Cochrane—for prospectively registered systematic literature reviews, to ensure the proposed review has not already been undertaken and to identify whether a review has already been conducted in a similar area. It is good practice to develop a literature review protocol as this helps to reduce bias and limit overlap with other reviews. PROSPERO, Cochrane and JBI have frameworks for developing protocols that are registered on their platforms (see Additional resources at the end of the chapter for relevant links). Registering protocols at the commencement of the review process is also good practice. If the protocol is not registered, you can add it to a personal or university site for others to read. Some journals also offer opportunities to publish review protocols.

DEVELOPING A FOCUSED RESEARCH QUESTION

A clear literature review question is vital, otherwise your review will be too broad and you will find yourself needing to discuss a wide range of literature without a specific focus. You need to be very clear about the scope and purpose of your review, otherwise you will not be able to identify which research is relevant to your review. Hence, although we often talk about a 'comprehensive review', this generally means a comprehensive search on a very focused review question rather than the review being a comprehensive overview of a broader topic. A good review question is clear, focused, can be answered by collecting and analysing data and assumes the possibility of different outcomes. If you ask a question that cannot be answered by gathering and analysing research papers, you will not have a researchable question. Fortunately, there are tools that can assist in designing a good **research question**.

Jamie (Case study 3.1) wants to learn more about type 1 diabetes. They may want to be able to identify strategies to reduce the incidence complications associated with type 1 diabetes, but first they need to know what risk factors contribute to the number and severity of complications. This is quite a broad topic and Jamie will need to refine it further by focusing on either extrinsic factors (e.g. financial considerations, family and support systems, access to healthcare) or intrinsic factors (e.g. patient age, gender, self-care abilities). For example, 'What is the best way to prevent complications associated with diabetes?' is too broad and requires a decision about what 'best' means and how it can be measured, it requires questions about the causes of infections (intrinsic and extrinsic) and so on.

Using a Tool to Develop the Research Question and Search Terms

Once the basic review question is identified, there are a number of tools that can ensure the question is specifically focused. A well-formulated question provides focus for your literature search and guides the selection of literature sources. Methods to design review questions for intervention studies were developed by Richardson and colleagues (1995) who used the acronym 'PICO' to assist researchers in developing a focused question. The PICO formula is often used by students who are designing their own research or review question. PICO stands for: **P**opulation (or **P**atient), **I**ntervention, **C**omparison and **O**utcome. Remember to consider the elements of PICO when creating your question.

Example:

Does short-acting insulin *(I) compared with* long acting insulin *(C) among* adolescents with type 1 diabetes *(P) reduce* the incidence of complications *(O)*?

The PICO and PEO frameworks (**P**opulation, **E**xposure, **O**utcome) are widely used in nursing, midwifery and health research and in professional practice. To address a literature review question, PICO can be expanded to determine the types of study designs that will be included in the review; this is known as PICO(T) (see Table 3.2).

TABLE 3.2		
Developing a Research Question: A Worked Example Using the PICO(T) Formula		

Initial Broad Focus: 'What is the Best Management of Mothers with Hyperemesis Gravidarum?'

Focused Research Question: 'Does Fluid Resuscitation with Added Potassium Reduce the Length of Hospital Stay for People with Hyperemesis Gravidarum?'

Population	People with hyperemesis gravidarum
Intervention/**I**ssue	Fluid resuscitation with added potassium
Comparison/**C**ontext	Fluid resuscitation without added potassium
Outcome	Reduced length of hospital stay
Types of studies	1. Randomised controlled trial (and quasi-randomised controlled trial)
	2. Controlled before and after studies

An alternative tool for qualitative/mixed methods research is the SPIDER framework (**S**ample, **P**henomenon of **I**nterest, **D**esign, **E**valuation, **R**esearch type) to develop a qualitative research question (Cooke, Smith & Booth 2012). An example of a qualitative research question using the SPIDER framework is: 'What are the *experiences* (**E**) of *a diagnosis of type 1 diabetes* (**PI**) for *people living with learning disability* (**S**)?' The design (**D**) (focus groups or interview) and research type (**R**) (qualitative or mixed methods) elements are used in the literature search as **search terms**.

SEARCHING FOR LITERATURE

One of the main tasks of conducting a review is searching for relevant literature. Generally speaking, the **literature search** should be comprehensive, which means identifying all the relevant literature, rather than a small subset of available literature. This is because it is important that the review is balanced and inclusive.

The main approach to searching is usually through relevant academic **electronic databases**. Commonly used databases include MEDLINE, CINAHL and PsychInfo, but there are many more available at your academic library. All databases operate slightly differently and a librarian can help adjust the search strategy to the specific database. Librarians are expert in literature searching, and can offer invaluable advice about the most appropriate databases to search and the identification of keywords and search terms. You can set up

alerts so that if your search identifies any new papers, these will be sent to you automatically. (See Chapter 2 for further information about using library resources and searching databases.)

Once the relevant databases are identified, the search strategy is considered. All databases are searched using key **search terms**. Search terms are developed based on the review question. Broadly speaking, the literature can be searched using free-text terms, which can be combined with the Boolean operators 'AND', 'OR' and 'NOT'. Free-text terms can be used with controlled headings such as MeSH (**Me**dical **S**ubject **H**eadings), which have been pre-identified by the database. Alternatively, only controlled headings might be used. There are advantages and disadvantages of each approach to be considered, depending on the review type. For example, when searching for a very popular topic, searching in the full text (whole paper) is likely to produce an excessive number of results, whereas if the search term is relatively unusual, the whole text may need to be searched to find any reference at all. Getting advice from a librarian is very useful to help develop the best search terms for your specific purpose.

The development of search terms is crucial to the type and number of papers that will be retrieved. It is important to consider the use of Boolean commands. Inappropriate use of 'AND' will limit the search extensively, as the search engine attempts to retrieve references that cover all included topics/terms. When

---

BOX 3.1
AN EXAMPLE OF A SEARCH STRATEGY

Question: What is the impact of long shifts on quality of nursing care?
'long shift' OR 'long-shift' OR '12 hour shift' OR 'twelve hour shift'
AND
'quality of care' OR 'quality of patient care' OR 'standard of care' OR 'safety'

---

searching for similar terms or synonyms, it is preferable to use 'OR'. Unless there is an unreasonably long list of hits from the search with 'OR', there is no need to limit further. 'NOT' enables you to remove a term from a search. A common error many students make is to assume every term in the research question must be specifically searched for and combined with the Boolean operator 'AND'. This is not necessarily the case. If your search terms are refined to retrieve fewer results, it is important to consider what may be potentially lost from the results. It is often better to have a larger list to work through manually than to limit the search inappropriately using Boolean operators. An inappropriate use of 'OR' will also widen the search extensively (see Box 3.1). For example, there are many synonyms that might be used with 'quality of care', and it is the job of the reviewer to decide when these synonyms stray too far from the original context or meaning of the keyword.

The Boolean operator 'NOT' can be useful to exclude articles that do not fit the topic. If the research question is about children, terms such as 'child AND/OR adolescent' may be used and include 'NOT adults' to increase the number of papers that are relevant. It is important you determine your inclusion and exclusion criteria to guide your search (see the next section).

Using a truncation symbol such as an asterisk (*) in a search broadens the search by locating terms that start with the same letters, which is called the stem. If you use the stem nurs*, the search will find *nurses* and *nursing* as well as *nurse*. Truncation symbols vary across different databases, so check with your librarian or the database help menu.

When using a phrase in a search, ensure quotation marks surround the phrase; this instructs the database that all the results must contain the exact phrase. For example, the phrase 'kidney failure' will provide more relevant search results than kidney failure without quotation marks, which would find anything with the words 'kidney' or 'failure', meaning a lot of irrelevant material would be generated.

Students often question how many papers should be retrieved from a search and how many papers it is reasonable to look through. This depends on the purpose of the review, the nature of the topic area and the research question. However, it does not take as long as you might imagine to look through a list of results from a database search.

Inclusion/Exclusion Criteria

Determining the inclusion and exclusion criteria for the review will help determine the specific literature that is relevant to the review question. Some criteria are pragmatic, such as date of publication. Other criteria may focus on the type of literature that might help answer the review question; for example, qualitative interview studies will give insight into patient experience, so the inclusion criteria may require that papers be reports of qualitative studies, if this insight is required. Some of the most common inclusion criteria are: published in English language, peer reviewed, age of participants (adult or child studies), study design, setting (hospital, emergency department, community care), exposure or intervention, and reported outcomes.

Identifying Relevant Literature

Once the inclusion and exclusion criteria are identified, it is important to ensure only papers that meet inclusion criteria are included. Eligibility for inclusion can often be ascertained through a review of titles and abstracts. This is sometimes referred to as a 'title search' and the vast majority of titles retrieved from the electronic databases will not be selected at this point, as it becomes apparent they do not address the review question. Inclusion/exclusion criteria can be used to develop a tool to assess if papers are eligible to be included in the review. This is an important step to ensure that all the papers meet the criteria for inclusion. Fig. 3.1 shows an example of studies that were assessed against inclusion/exclusion criteria. Creating a table like this also provides a record of reasons for excluding papers. The next stage is to review the

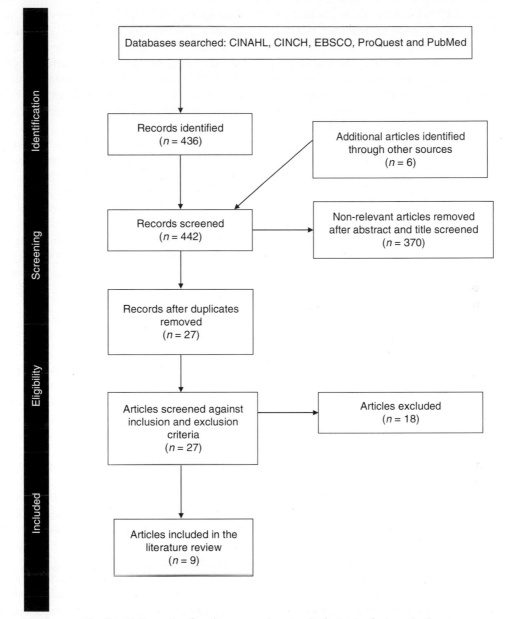

Fig. 3.1 ■ Example of studies assessed against inclusion/exclusion criteria

remaining papers in more detail. The abstracts of these titles can be read and compared against the inclusion and exclusion criteria. Duplicate publications are identified and removed at this stage.

The reviewer then needs to obtain the full text of papers that appear to meet the inclusion criteria. Even at this stage, not all the selected papers will be relevant for inclusion in the review; however, it is not always possible to tell without reading the full paper. Many authors choose to use a reference management system, such as EndNote, Mendeley, Rayyan or RefWorks, to organise the papers/references. Many university libraries offer training courses on how to use these kinds of software. With EndNote, it is easy to store a copy of each paper in an EndNote library and to identify any duplicate papers. Other software systems are available to assist with the management of the entire review process. Covidence, developed by Cochrane, is a screening and **data collection**/extraction tool that can be used to screen titles and abstracts of potential papers by allowing you to highlight keywords, import citations and upload papers, screen full-text papers and record reasons for exclusion, create data extraction forms, populate risk of bias tables and extract outcomes data. These data can then be exported in Microsoft Excel format. Covidence is primarily for Cochrane authors but a free trial can be accessed at www.covidence.org, or your institution may have a licence for use.

At this point, the list of papers or studies (in an EndNote or Covidence library) for inclusion in the review are identified. It is often productive to read the reference lists of the included papers to check for additional papers that might be relevant but were not identified through the database searches. Some authors also do 'hand searches', or look through the contents pages, of key journals or the reference lists of included papers to identify additional sources.

Documenting the Search

It is important to record all the details about the search, such as the date the search was completed, keywords and synonyms used and how these were combined, which databases were searched and how many articles were retrieved. Many databases will allow you to save the search strategy and results. The titles excluded and the reasons for the exclusions, the number of duplicates, the number of full-text versions of the potential papers reviewed and the number of papers finally included must also be recorded. Many researchers use the PRISMA (Preferred Reporting Items for Systematic Reviews and Meta-Analysis) flow chart to document their search strategy and results (Page et al 2021). See Figs 3.2 and 3.3 for examples of a completed PRISMA flowchart and documenting a search strategy and search results.

DATA SUMMARY TABLES

Data summary tables are a useful tool, enabling each paper to be summarised and its relevance to the review question be stated. This process can be referred to as

'**data extraction**', and can be presented in a form sometimes referred to as a 'table of evidence' (Aveyard 2019). This table needs to show basic information about the study (e.g. aim, **sample**, method), as well as the study outcomes. For quantitative studies, it is important to record both outcomes that are significant ands outcomes in which there were no differences. This makes it easy when reporting results to specify how many studies showed a significant difference in the selected outcome and how many showed no difference. (See He et al [2022] for an example of reporting quantitative outcomes.) Fortunately, tools like Covidence and Rayyan can assist with the screening and data extraction process. When writing the review report, the completed data summary for each paper is useful to refer to rather than having to keep re-reading each entire paper (see Table 3.3).

QUALITY APPRAISAL

Quality appraisal involves identifying the strengths and weaknesses of each paper to assess how useful it is to the review. This is because more weight will be given to the results from good-quality research papers and less weight to the poorer-quality papers. If a paper is of very poor quality, it may be excluded altogether.

Quality appraisal involves a judgment process with appraisal tools used to reduce variance in these judgments. There are many available tools. Critical Appraisal Skills Programme (CASP) tools (CASP 2018) are well known and available online (see the next student challenge), with tools for different types of research approaches. The JBI website also has a range of **critical appraisal** tools that can be downloaded (https://jbi.global/critical-appraisal-tools). These generic tools can be used to appraise all types of study designs (Effective Public Health Practice Project [EPHPP] 2009a, Hawker et al 2002, Hong et al 2018). A dictionary or guidelines is usually available with these tools to guide the researcher in the appraisal process (EPHPP 2009b). In some review types, such as systematic reviews, quality appraisal is often undertaken independently by more than one person before findings are compared to add to the rigour of the assessment process.

	A	B	C	D	E	F	G	H	I	J	K	L	M	N	O
1		CINAHL		EBSCO Academic search complete		PUBMED		PROQUEST—HEALTH & MEDICINE		CINCH—Health informit		Google Scholar		Scopus	
2	SUBJECT HEADINGS/KEYWORDS (ENGLISH, 2002–2012)/SEARCH STRING	No. of hits	No. relevant	No. of hits	No. relevant	No. of hits	No. relevant	No. of hits	No. relevant	No. of hits	No. relevant			No. of hits	No. relevant
3	nurs* AND discharge AND 'telephone follow up'	149	103	157	118	0	0	105	19	0	0	273		144	58
4	nurs* AND telephone AND 'follow up' NOT survey	589	82	98	45	0	0	65	16	0	0			49	13
5															
6	'nurse-led' AND 'telephone follow up' AND discharge AND hospital	10	8	12	9	36	15	6	3	0	0			29	9
7	'nurse initiated' AND 'telephone follow up' AND discharge AND hospital	6	5	6	4	0		2	0	0	0			18	4
8	nur* AND discharge AND 'telephone follow up' NOT pharmacy	101	61	156	118	0	0	85	22	0	0				
9															
10															
11															
12															
13	TOTAL	855	259	429	294	36	15	263	60	0	0	273		240	84
14	Limiters: peer reviewed, English language														
15	Total number hits	2096													
16	Total number of relevant		712												
17															
18															
19															
20	*reduced to terms in abstract to limit search														

Fig. 3.2 ■ Example of a flowchart

	A	B	C	D	E	F	G	H
	Reference of article	Are post-discharge telephone calls made by a nurse?	Are post-discharge phone calls used as an intervention within 7 days of discharge?	Are post-discharge telephone calls made for at least one of the reasons listed in the inclusion criteria?	Are post-discharge telephone calls discussed separately?	Are post-discharge telephone calls evaluated separately?	Included/excluded	Reason for exclusion
2	Paquette, Le May, Fiola, Villeneuve, Lapointe, Bourgault, 2013	Yes	Yes	Yes	Yes	Yes		Patients are children; calls were made to parents
3	Polek, Hardie, 2012	N/A	No	N/A	N/A	N/A	Excluded	Calls were not made within the 7 days
4	Stolic, Mitchell, Wollin, 2010	N/A	N/A	N/A	N/A	N/A	Excluded	Paper is a literature review
5	Szöts, Konradsen, Solgaard, Østergaard, 2014	N/A	N/A	N/A	N/A	N/A	Excluded	Protocol paper
6	Yang, Chen, 2012	N/A	N/A	N/A	N/A	N/A	Excluded	Patients are children, calls were made to parents
7	Tang, Fujimoto, Karliner, 2014	Yes	Yes	Yes	Yes	Yes	Included	N/A
8	Szöts, Konradsen, Solgaard, Bogø, Østergaard, 2015	Yes	Yes	Yes	Yes	Yes	Included	N/A
9	Zhang, Wong, You, Zheng, 2011	Yes	Yes	Yes	Yes	Yes	Included	N/A
10	Zhang, Wong, You, Zheng, Li, Zhang, Huang, Ye, Liang, Liu 2013	Yes	Yes	Yes	Yes	Yes	Included	N/A

Fig. 3.3 ■ Example of recorded search terms and search results

TABLE 3.3

Data Extraction Table

Title	Author/Year	Design	Methods	Sample	Study Site	Results	Quality Rating	Level of Evidence	Risk of Bias
Follow-up telephone calls to patients discharged after undergoing orthopaedic surgery: double-blind, randomised controlled trial of efficacy	Clari et al (2015)	Double-blind RCT	2 groups: usual care plus telephone call vs usual care	Sample: N = 219 Elective low- or medium-intensity orthopaedic surgery patients	Orthopaedic teaching hospital, northwest Italy	**No difference:** Premature contact with healthcare system **Significant difference:** Frequency of problems reported Received more useful information Patient satisfaction	Strong	Level 1 evidence	One site sample may not be representative Readmissions not measured

For experimental quantitative studies, quality is assessed by the risk of bias. Thus, a high-quality study is one that: uses a randomised sample; mentions the power analysis to determine sample size; blinds participants and assessors to the intervention and usual care allocation; uses valid and reliable data collection tools; and controls potential confounders. Processes of randomisation should be clearly described in the paper. Some of the areas that different quantitative quality appraisal tools assess are:

- selection bias
- study design
- confounders
- blinding
- data collection methods
- withdrawals and dropouts.

See also Fig. 3.4.

For qualitative studies, assessing bias is less straightforward. There is debate on this issue, but the quality is generally associated with having clear aims and a suitable design, being conducted ethically, using appropriate and rigorous methods, with sufficient details about methodological rigour, and clarity and coherence in reporting.

It is important to remember that it is not possible to appraise a study unless you are familiar with the research design used in the study. So the first step in quality appraisal is to understand the research design used in the paper being appraised. These issues will be explored in Chapters 7, 8 and 9. There is more about reading and appraising research in Chapter 5.

Clinical Significance Versus Statistical Significance

In the meta-analysis component of systematic reviews, the statistical significance of interventions

Author	Design and data collection	Selection bias	Study design	Confounders	Blinding	Data collection methods	Withdrawals and dropouts	Final score
Lavesend et al (2016)	RCT	Strong	Strong	Strong	Weak	Weak	Moderate	Weak
Gaines-Dillard (2015)	Case/control Study	Moderate	Moderate	Weak	Moderate	Moderate	Weak	Weak
Hannan (2012)	RCT	Moderate	Strong	Strong	Moderate	Weak	Strong	Moderate
Li et al (2014)	Case/control Study	Moderate	Moderate	Weak	Moderate	Weak	Strong	Weak
Tang et al (2014)	Quality improvement intervention	Moderate	Weak	Weak	Moderate	Weak	Moderate	Weak
Zhang et al (2013)	RCT	Strong	Strong	Strong	Moderate	Strong	Strong	Strong
Clari et al (2015)	Double-blind RCT	Strong	Strong	Strong	Strong	Strong	Strong	Strong
Miller & Schaper (2015)	Case-control Intervention study	Moderate	Moderate	Weak	Moderate	Weak	Strong	Weak

Fig. 3.4 ■ Example of quality appraisal

is reported and interpreted. Statistical significance indicates a relationship between two events that is not a result of chance. Clinical significance indicates the level of importance of the relationship from the clinical perspective. It is important in nursing and midwifery research to consider the clinical significance of results. That is, whether the findings make a difference to the person's health or well-being. In essence, a study could have statistical significance but not be clinically significant. However, determining clinical significance is not straightforward as ultimately it requires some degree of value judgment.

Which Evidence is Best?

For all reviews, it is necessary to assess the quality of evidence included and for reviewers to give more weight in the analysis to the stronger papers. Traditional systematic review and meta-analysis uses a hierarchical system of classifying evidence known as the levels of evidence (Burns, Rohrich & Chung 2011). This system ranks studies according to the probability of bias. Systematic reviews of RCTs are considered the highest level of evidence because they represent the strongest possible evidence. RCTs are ascribed the highest level of evidence for an individual study because they are designed to have a low risk of bias and systematic errors. Cross-sectional studies, expert opinion and case reports involving one subject are given a lower level due to the possibility of researcher/author bias and lack of control of confounding factors.

Levels of evidence are also an important component in quantitative or mixed studies literature reviews as more weight is given to the results of level 1 to 3 studies than level 4 to 5 studies, and this assists to prioritise information, especially when there are mixed results (positive and negative) from different studies. It is important to note that the concept of levels of evidence applies only to systematic reviews with meta-analysis and **not** to other types of review.

DATA ANALYSIS

Once relevant papers that address the literature review question are identified, data has been extracted into a table and the critical appraisal has been undertaken, the papers with the best quality of evidence will be apparent. The next step is analysing the literature and writing up the review findings (see Box 3.2). The PRISMA Checklist provides important guidance on the elements to include when writing the literature review (Page et al 2021) (see the next student challenge).

There are different approaches to analysis within literature reviews. For quantitative studies, it is sometimes possible to do a statistical analysis, often referred to as a meta-analysis, that combines the findings of multiple papers. However, this can only be undertaken when the included studies are sufficiently similar to combine. For qualitative or mixed methods studies, or quantitative studies that are too heterogeneous to combine, a thematic or content analysis is usually undertaken. For mixed studies reviews that include both qualitative and quantitative studies, a combination of the two approaches is required.

STUDENT CHALLENGE

Identify Guidelines for Reporting Literature Reviews

Go to the EQUATOR (Enhancing the QUAlity and Transparency Of health Research) Network site (https://www.equator-network.org). Identify the PRISMA reporting guidelines for literature reviews.

BOX 3.2
SUMMARY OF AN INTEGRATIVE REVIEW OF NURSES' CONTRIBUTION TO SHORT-TERM HUMANITARIAN CARE IN LOW- TO MIDDLE-INCOME COUNTRIES: AN INTEGRATIVE REVIEW OF THE LITERATURE

AIM AND OBJECTIVES

To appraise the literature related to voluntary humanitarian work provided by international nurses in low- to middle-income countries.

DESIGN

Integrative review.

SEARCH STRATEGY

Electronic databases between 1995 and 2015 using Pro-Quest Health and Medicine
   Academic Search Complete (EBSCO), PubMed, MEDLINE, Embase,
   ScienceDirect and Scopus.

SEARCH TERMS

'nursing', 'humanitarian', 'international' and 'volunteer'.

INCLUSION/EXCLUSION CRITERIA

- Primary research related to charitable healthcare provision in low- and middle-income countries (LMIC), including medical capacity building.
- Peer-reviewed papers of primary research related to short-term humanitarian care (short-term medical mission—STMM).
- Published 1995–2015 in English language.
- Assistance was short term (<2 years duration).
- Participants were qualified health professional international volunteers that specifically included nurses as part of the STMM team.

- Excluded studies that addressed a response to an acute disaster (including military efforts for terrorism or war) or focused on team learning with undergraduate and/or postgraduate teams.

RESULTS

Twenty-five papers were critically appraised; six were excluded, as they did not meet the accepted criteria for detailing the research process, research method or ethics requirements. Therefore, 19 papers were retained following critical appraisal (eight qualitative, four quantitative, three mixed methods and four systematic reviews).

ANALYSIS

Findings revealed limited data describing the care nurses provide and the professional roles and tasks they fulfil within the context of international humanitarian short-term medical trips. Issues raised included a description of demographic data regarding participants and sending agencies, motivation for volunteer participation, perceptions of effectiveness of particular programs and sustainability issues related to cultural, ethical or moral obligations of foreign health professionals working in low- to middle-income countries.

Source: Dawson S, Elliott D, Jackson D: Nurses' contribution to short-term humanitarian care in low- to middle-income countries: an integrative review of the literature, Journal of Clinical Nursing 26(23–24):3950–3961, 2017.

Meta-Analysis

Meta-analysis is used when the results of trials, usually RCTs, are similar enough to be combined in statistical analysis. This approach is used in systematic reviews for Cochrane, when the review question is about effectiveness. By using a summary statistic, the results from different randomised trials can be brought together, demonstrating the results across all of the included studies in a cumulative statistic. This summary statistic will indicate how confident we can be in the result by showing confidence intervals. Cochrane has produced a handbook that can be downloaded and shows all the steps in conducting a review (Higgins et al 2019). This approach requires significant experience and skill and so is not normally undertaken by those new to doing a literature review.

Thematic Analysis

Thematic analysis is often used when qualitative studies are being reviewed or when it is dictated by the quality and extent of available literature. There are many approaches to thematic analysis (Braun & Clark 2019), although students new to the literature review process are encouraged to undertake a simple thematic analysis (Aveyard 2019). With this approach, each paper is examined for the main themes within the results. Once this has been undertaken, the researcher looks across all papers to identify themes or common findings. Common themes or findings are then summarised, synthesised and critiqued (Aveyard 2019).

Analysis when Both Quantitative and Qualitative Research is Included

When there are both qualitative and quantitative papers in a review, the qualitative and quantitative studies are usually analysed separately, and then the results are combined or synthesised (Pluye & Hong 2014). The results from the qualitative studies can be presented as themes and incorporated with the quantitative analysis to create a synthesis of all included studies.

Emerging Developments in Literature Reviews

We have already discussed how popular literature reviews have become in nursing and midwifery over the past few decades. As the field has evolved, so have the methodologies associated with it, including the development of the FMRS as a new approach to reviewing. You are encouraged to access the original article if you are interested in finding out more (Bradbury-Jones et al 2019). Like all other forms of literature review, the FMRS is systematic and has a focused question, but unlike the all-encompassing, wide searches of other reviews, the FMRS is concerned with mapping the existing research in an area and therefore looks only within a predefined set of literature. It is ideal for answering questions such as 'What is happening in this area of nursing and/or midwifery?' rather than 'What is the evidence to support this type of intervention?' For FMRS, a patterning chart is developed to present the prominent themes from the review and to show how these are distributed across the included literature (Bradbury-Jones et al 2021).

A way of conducting literature reviews that addresses questions of interest to Indigenous peoples and other marginalised groups has been proposed (Usher et al 2021, Smallwood et al 2022). Decolonisation refers to a way of dismantling colonial impact in countries once oppressed. It also refers to making explicit the ongoing colonial impacts within education, government policies and public perspectives. The decolonised approach has been developed to help overcome the current pathogenic approach to Indigenous health and research; this follows previous developments where Indigenous/Indigenist methods of research have been developed to conduct research with and for Indigenous people. Indigenous approaches to research challenge the dominant position and require researchers to use approaches that prioritise the needs, beliefs and experiences of the research participants. To do so means valuing local knowledge, ways of being and developing awareness of power relationships; it also means working with the local people. While quite a lot has been written about the need to decolonise research overall, less has been written about the need to decolonise literature reviews.

Decolonised literature reviews are, however, beginning to occur in the literature (Usher et al 2021). These reviews recognise the impact of colonialism on Indigenous people and attempt to conduct a review to overcome the westernised approach to the development of evidence by drawing on Indigenous ways of knowledge and practice and respecting that the research must be driven by an Indigenous agenda.

Adoption of decolonised approaches to literature reviews will assist nurses to ensure future literature reviews are conducted in such a way that the research more authentically reflects the perspectives and lived reality of Indigenous peoples and communities. The decolonised approach has synergies with the current agenda that seeks to challenge curriculum and educational theories that propagate educational perspectives of injustice, exclusion, supremacy, socioeconomic inequality and inequity.

CONCLUSION

Literature reviews can be a discrete piece of research in their own right, but they can also be used to provide a synopsis and evaluation of the available evidence at a particular point in time to identify what is known and where there are gaps in the current understanding of a topic. In this chapter, we have presented different methods for undertaking a literature review. There are several features common to all reviews. All follow a systematic approach that includes developing a research question, search strategy, critical appraisal, data extraction and synthesis method. There are many nuances in the different approaches—those undertaking a literature review who are following a specific method need to be aware of the differences and are advised to go to the original sources where the methods are described in detail. All the methodological decisions made should be documented and researchers should justify the approach taken for the review. Whether or not a researcher adopts a specific method, the process undertaken should be transparent and rigorous so that replication is possible.

ADDITIONAL RESOURCES

Further Reading

Aveyard H, Payne S, Preston N: A post-graduate's guide to doing a literature review in health and social care, ed 2, Maidenhead, 2021, Open University Press.

Aveyard H: Doing a literature review in health and social care: a practical guide, ed 4, Berkshire, 2019, McGraw-Hill Education.

Smallwood R, Usher K, Woods C, et al: De-problematising Aboriginal young peoples'

health and wellbeing through their voice: an Indigenous scoping review, Journal of Clinical Nursing 29 Mar:1–16, 2022. https://doi.org/10.1111/jocn.16308.

Effective Public Healthcare Panacea Project: Quality assessment tool for quantitative studies dictionary, 2009b. https://www.ephpp.ca/quality-assessment-tool-for-quantitative-studies/.

PRISMA: PRISMA Flow Diagram, 2020. http://prisma-statement.org/PRISMAStatement/FlowDiagram.aspx.

Systematic Review Protocols and Templates

JBI: https://jbi.global/about-jbi

Cochrane Handbook for Systematic Reviews of Interventions: https://training.cochrane.org/handbook

Schiavo JH: PROSPERO: An international register of systematic review protocols, Medical Reference Services Quarterly 38(2):171–180, 2019. https://doi.org/10.1080/02763869.2019.1588072

REFERENCES

Aveyard H, Bradbury-Jones C: An analysis of current practices in undertaking literature reviews in nursing: findings from a focused mapping review and synthesis, BMC Medical Research Methodology 19(1):105, 2019. https://doi.org/10.1186/s12874-019-0751-2

Aveyard H: Doing a literature review in health and social care: a practical guide, ed 4, Berkshire, 2019, McGraw-Hill Education.

Bradbury-Jones C, Aveyard H, Herber OR, et al: Scoping reviews: the PAGER framework for improving the quality of reporting, International Journal of Social Research Methodology 1–14, 2021.

Bradbury-Jones C, Breckinridge J, Clark MT, et al: Advancing the science of literature reviewing in social research: the focused mapping review and synthesis. International Journal of Social Research Methodology 22(1):451–462, 2019.

Braun V, Clark V: Reflecting on reflexive thematic analysis, Qualitative Research in Sport, Exercise and Health 11(4):589–597, 2019.

Burns PB, Rohrich RJ, Chung KC: The levels of evidence and their role in evidence-based medicine, Plastic and Reconstructive Surgery 128(1):305–310, 2011.

Cooke A, Smith D, Booth A: Beyond PICO: the SPIDER tool for qualitative evidence synthesis, Qualitative Health Research 22(10):1435–1443, 2012.

Critical Appraisal Skills Programme: CASP Checklists, 2018. https://casp-uk.net/casp-tools-checklists.

Effective Public Health Practice Project: Quality assessment tool for quantitative studies, 2009a. https://www.ephpp.ca/quality-assessment-tool-for-quantitative-studies/.

Effective Public Health Practice Project: Quality assessment tool for quantitative studies dictionary, 2009b. https://www.ephpp.ca/quality-assessment-tool-for-quantitative-studies/ https://merst.ca/wp-content/uploads/2018/02/qualilty-assessment-dictionary_2017.pdf.

Hawker S, Payne S, Kerr C, et al: Appraising the evidence: reviewing disparate data systematically, Qualitative Health Research 12(9):1284–1299, 2002.

He Q, Zhao X, Wang Y, et al: Effectiveness of smartphone application–based self-management interventions in patients with type 2 diabetes: a systematic review and meta-analysis of randomized controlled trials, Journal of Advanced Nursing 78(2):348–362, 2022.

Higgins JPT, Thomas J, Chandler J, et al (eds): Cochrane handbook for systematic reviews of interventions, ed 2, Chichester (UK), 2019, John Wiley & Sons.

Hong Q, Pluye P, Fábregues S, et al: Mixed methods appraisal tool (MMAT), version 2018 user guide, 2018. http://mixedmethodsappraisaltoolpublic.pbworks.com.

Page MJ, McKenzie JE, Bossuyt PM, et al: The PRISMA 2020 statement: an updated guideline for reporting systematic reviews, BMJ 372:n71, 2021. https://doi.org/10.1136/bmj.n71.

Pluye P, Hong QN: Combining the power of stories and the power of numbers: mixed methods research and mixed studies reviews, Annual Review of Public Health 18(35):29–45, 2014.

Richardson WS, Wilson MC, Nishikawa J, Hayward RS: The well-built clinical question: a key to evidence-based decisions, ACP Journal Club 123(3):A12–13, 1995.

Smallwood R, Usher K, Woods C, et al: De-problematising Aboriginal young peoples' health and wellbeing through their voice: an Indigenous scoping review, Journal of Clinical Nursing: 1–16, 2022. https://doi.org/10.1111/jocn.16308.

Usher K, Jackson D, Walker R, et al: Indigenous resilience in Australia: a scoping review using a reflective decolonizing collective dialogue, Frontiers in Public Health 9: 2021. https://www.frontiersin.org/articles/10.3389/fpubh.2021.630601/full.

4

DEVELOPING EVIDENCE-BASED SOLUTIONS

ANN BONNER ■ JULIA SLARK ■ GAYATRI NAMBIAR-GREENWOOD

CHAPTER OUTLINE

LEARNING OBJECTIVES

After reading this chapter and following critical reflection, readers should be able to:

- identify a potential clinical problem that needs solving
- understand how evidence-based solutions are needed for everyday nursing and midwifery practice
- understand different levels of evidence that inform nursing and midwifery practice
- develop skills in identifying which journals are recognised for publishing nursing and midwifery papers.

KEY TERMS

evidence-based practice

evidence

literature search

peer reviewed

ABSTRACT

This chapter will assist you with finding solutions to a question or problem which you have encountered (or will encounter) when undertaking a clinical placement or working in clinical practice. It will help you to develop a structured method of searching databases to find research that could be used as evidence to inform your practice. In addition, this chapter will develop your skills in recognising whether journals are publishing quality evidence or whether the quality of papers is too poor to be used to guide practice.

STUDENT QUOTE

I am about to go on a clinical placement and I want to provide the most up-to-date care to people. However, I'm worried whether I will be putting good-quality evidence into practice.

HOW CAN THIS CHAPTER HELP YOU?

On clinical placement, many students see other nurses or midwives doing something differently to how they were taught, or they find themselves doing routine tasks and not understanding why they are being done. Consider the following questions to identify how this chapter will be of benefit to you.

1. Do you know how to find a solution to a clinical question or problem?
2. Are you sure that the nursing or midwifery procedures that you have seen in clinical practice are contemporary and based on the best available evidence?
3. Can you confidently use a research report to inform your understanding of the evidence?

Even if you answered 'yes' to all of these, this chapter may give you new insights into evidence-based solutions.

INTRODUCTION

Evidence-based nursing and midwifery practice is about:

- making decisions to inform clinical practice based on the best available scientific **evidence**
- recognising the preferences of patients and their significant others
- the personal judgment of health professionals
- the context in which healthcare is delivered (Pearson et al 2005).

Accreditation bodies for nurses and midwives internationally indicate that the practice of registered nurses and registered midwives must be underpinned by the best available evidence.

There are many reasons for using evidence generated by research in practice, such as improved delivery of the most effective and efficient healthcare, professional accountability to practise in the most of up-to-date way and the increasing expectations of patients and their significant others to receive quality and safe healthcare. In this chapter, you will learn more about evidence-based practice, explore strategies to find evidence and learn what to do with the evidence once you have found it. This chapter will also help you recognise that there are journals which may not publish quality evidence to inform your practice.

I THINK I HAVE A PROBLEM WHILE ON PLACEMENT

CASE STUDY 4.1

Second-year student nurse Martha is caring for a 75-year-old woman originally from India who was diagnosed with Alzheimer's disease 10 years ago. She lives in a care home but has daily visits from her devoted husband and family. Martha notes that the woman has lost 12 kilograms in the past few months and is very underweight. When she talks to the woman's husband and daughters, Martha realises that the family are very distressed about this and have asked if they can do anything to help.

Martha discusses the issue with the registered nurse, who refers the woman to the care homes' dietitian. After the consultation, the dietitian decides to set a goal for the woman to not only maintain her weight, but to gain a minimum of 800 grams per week. The dietitian also explains that it is important that she does not lose any more weight. The dietitian works with the kitchen staff to ensure that they provide a nutrient-rich diet, involving three meals a day. They also suggest that she receive an extra small meal and supplement drinks between meals and at supper, so that she does not go too long without food (as dinner is served at 6 pm, and the residents don't have anything to eat until breakfast).

On the next shift, Martha decides to try and assist the woman at mealtimes. However, after a couple of mouthfuls the woman pushes the food away and won't accept being fed. Martha also notices, over the next couple of days, that she is too tired to eat the supper, but enjoys the biscuits provided for morning and afternoon tea.

WHAT ARE SOME EVIDENCE-BASED SOLUTIONS?

Most nurses and midwives would acknowledge that we should use 'research evidence' to support our practice, but what does that really mean and how can we use it to support the decisions we make? Research evidence is knowledge that is based on research findings and can support us to make well-informed decisions about the care we provide to our patients and their families.

The term **'evidence-based practice'** (EBP) was first introduced by Archie Cochrane in the 1970s (Sackett et al 1996). Cochrane identified a system for doctors to keep up to date with the latest evidence for practice as more and more research was being undertaken. However, it has been suggested that EBP evolved from Florence Nightingale in the 1800s with her *Notes on Nursing* and the idea to provide better outcomes for patients who experienced unsanitary conditions during the Crimean War (Mackey & Bassendowski 2017). An EBP approach for the modern nurse or midwife requires us to ensure that the rationale for our care is clear and that the evidence we use is up-to-date and based on the most reliable sources (Aveyard & Sharp 2017).

To assist nurses and midwives to think about and use EBP, Melnyk and Fineout-Overholt (2017) have suggested the seven steps shown in Box 4.1. Think about how you could use this process to help you make decisions about the care you provide, to ensure that it is based on the best available evidence.

Another approach to EBP has been developed by JBI. The revised JBI approach considers evidence-based healthcare as decision-making that considers the feasibility, appropriateness, meaningfulness and

> **BOX 4.1**
> **SEVEN STEPS TO EBP**
>
> Step 0: A spirit of inquiry to notice internal data that indicate an opportunity for positive change.
> Step 1: Ask a clinical question using the PICO(T) (population/problem/phenomenon, intervention/issue, comparison/context, outcome, [timeframe]) question format.
> Step 2: Conduct a systematic literature search to find out what is already known about a clinical issue.
> Step 3: Conduct a critical appraisal (rapid critical appraisal, evaluation, synthesis and recommendation).
> Step 4: Implement best practices by blending external evidence with clinician expertise and patient preferences and values.
> Step 5: Evaluate evidence implementation to see if study outcomes happened in practice and if the implementation went well.
> Step 6: Share project results, good or bad, with others.
>
> Source: Adapted from Steps of the evidence-based practice (EBP) process leading to high-quality healthcare and best patient outcomes. © Melnyk & Fineout-Overholt, 2017. Used with permission in Fineout-Overholt E: A guide to critical appraisal of evidence, Nursing Critical Care 14(3), 24–30, 2019.

effectiveness of healthcare practices (Jordan et al 2019). For evidence-based decision-making to occur, we should find the best available evidence, consider the context in which care is delivered, involve the individual patient and utilise our professional judgment and expertise as the health professional providing the care.

HOW TO USE EVIDENCE TO INFORM PRACTICE

Learning in the clinical environment is a dynamic, two-way process. We acquire the science of nursing and midwifery knowledge from coursework and skills workshops at university. We then apply, observe and watch the application of the art of nursing and/or midwifery in clinical placements. These experiences bring with it a range of personal, professional and academic questions that often need answering.

CASE STUDY 4.2

Martha decides to look up the available literature about food, diet and the nutritional needs of people who live with dementia. She searches several sources to uncover how she can help improve the care she gave the woman and finds the following information.

1. Using the search terms 'dementia' and 'nutrition' in an electronic database, Martha found a study by Heelan and colleagues (2020) which reported that many people with dementia prefer frequent opportunities to eat small amounts. The paper also suggested that finger food that the person can hold in their hand, such as cheese and crackers or sliced fruit, would ensure the availability of regular healthy foods that could be easily chewed and swallowed.

2. Martha discussed these research findings with her mentor and the team during handover. The nurse in charge and the team thought that these strategies would be a good way to improve the diets of many residents, as there was often quite a lot of leftover food at mealtimes. One of the team also felt that the fruit would help with the residents' bowel movements and improve their ability to fight infections.

3. When Martha used the search terms 'dementia' and 'improving diet', she found a study by Oldknow and colleagues (2019) which stated that people living with dementia often experience a change in their taste buds and so some of them prefer strongly flavoured foods. This made Martha think of the woman and the kind of cultural diet that she may have eaten at home. The food provided at the care home was very different from the smell, flavours and textures she was used to in her Indian cookery at home. Martha also discovered an Australian study by McGrath and colleagues (2021), which suggested the provision of culturally appropriate food was one of many actions that could be taken to provide a more appropriate and ethical way of caring for people from diverse backgrounds living in care homes.

4. Martha spoke to her mentor and the team during handover about these ideas. They agree that staff would talk to the woman's husband and his daughters during their visit about potentially bringing in small meals and snacks that she would have enjoyed previously. The woman's husband was delighted with this suggestion, and over the next few days he started bringing in some food to share with his wife.

5. Martha also came across research by Watkins and colleagues (2017) and information from the Alzheimer's Society website that malnutrition in care homes was a well-documented subject and that a variety of interventions, creativity and sensitivity to cultural practices is required to address and improve residents' health and wellbeing.

Table 4.1 shows some case studies where seeking evidence would have enhanced culturally appropriate care and reduced harm to patients.

HOW DO WE EFFECTIVELY IMPLEMENT EBP INTO OUR EVERYDAY DECISION-MAKING?

To implement EBP effectively, we should consider all aspects of the current evidence available to us through our **literature search**, as well as nursing or midwifery knowledge and patient and family preferences and values. Fig. 4.1 demonstrates the links between the research evidence, the knowledge of the health professional and the patient and family's preferences and values which are vital to evidence-based nursing and midwifery practice.

HOW TO ASK THE RIGHT QUESTIONS TO DEVELOP THE BEST EVIDENCE-BASED SOLUTIONS

The first step in using research in practice is identifying areas of practice that could or should be improved. Observations of clinical practice, deep and considered reflection of personal and clinical experiences and an inquiring mind are good foundations for a well-developed research question (Considine et al 2017).

How can you identify a good research question?

1. *Observation.* Look for practice gaps in processes or outcomes of care. Has the gap been identified through new research or guidelines, clinical audit outcomes or patient feedback?

2. *Reflection.* Why is there a failure in that practice? What has gone wrong? Why doesn't what you are doing work any more? Has the patient demographic, techniques, procedures or equipment changed?

3. *Enquiry.* Ask the people around you, other nurses/midwives and health professionals. Search the literature and read local policies, databases and clinical guidelines.

4. *Scrutiny.* You must not change practice based on poorly performed research or weak evidence. Check the quality of the studies you are reading to ensure that they represent high-quality research (more on this in Chapter 5).

TABLE 4.1
Case Studies

Subject of Concern	Context	Evidence that Would have Informed
Diagnosis of Orthodox Jewish people 'rocking' as psychologically disturbed in psychiatric care	Swaying during prayer is considered to help concentration and is culturally normal	Loewenthal and Marcus (2020) Jewish community websites, such as JewishCare NSW (https://jewishcare.com.au)
An Australian First Nations woman feeling like a burden was 'all tied up together' with her identity as a First Nation Australian and the (erroneous and racist) stereotype that First Nation Australians go to hospitals to 'get drugs'	Racially prejudiced stereotype of First Nations peoples (globally) has a significant impact on the quality and safety of clinical and broader healthcare practice	Malatzky and colleagues (2020)
The ineffective and lack of belief of pain experience/pain-management of young Black men with severe pain in sickle-cell crisis, due to racial bias including concerns of drug addiction that are unfounded but informed by racist stereotypes	In sickle-cell anaemia patients, neuropathic pain is caused either by the occlusion of blood vessels that supply nerves, resulting in nerve cell damage, or by persistent chronic pain that results in inflammation	Wakefield and colleagues (2017)

Fig. 4.1 ■ Linking the domains of research, knowledge and evidence-based practice.

You could use a framework to help you put a question together. PICO(T) (explained in Chapter 2; see also Table 4.2) is a well-known and widely used framework for developing robust and answerable research questions. It is also useful for framing quality assurance or evaluation projects. PICO consists of four components, which inform the development of a PICO question (Sackett et al 1997).

■ **P**atient type or population: for example, a specific patient or group of patients (gender, age, diagnosis) or a particular setting.

■ **I**ntervention of interest: for example, a specific intervention or treatment which they are

TABLE 4.2
Frameworks to Search for Evidence

Framework	Definition	Explanation
PICO (Sackett et al 1997)	PICO is used for quantitative studies, which make a comparison between groups to study the effects on outcome(s).	■ **P**atient type or population; for example, a specific patient or group of patients (sex, age, diagnosis) or a particular setting ■ **I**ntervention of interest; for example, a specific intervention or treatment that they are undergoing or understanding the patient perspective of their situation ■ **C**omparison; for example, a comparison between two treatments or a control group versus an intervention group ■ **O**utcome; for example, this would include the outcomes that are expected from the enquiry
PICO(T)	PICO(T) is similar to PICO and adds time.	■ **P**atient type or population ■ **I**ntervention of interest ■ **C**omparison ■ **O**utcome ■ **T**imeframe: over what time period*
ECLIPSE (Wildridge & Bell 2002)	ECLIPSE is used to help define search terms for health and social care management-related information.	■ **E**xpectation: What is the information for? (sets the context for the search; might not contribute to search terms) ■ **C**lient group ■ **L**ocation ■ **I**mpact: What is the expected change? What defines success? How is it measured? ■ **P**rofessionals ■ **SE**rvice: What (which) is the service involved? For example, outpatient services, nurse-led clinics, intermediate care
SPIDER (Cooke, Smith & Booth 2012)	SPIDER is designed for searching qualitative and mixed methods studies for topics that do not fit well with the PICO framework categories.	■ **S**ample ■ **P**henomenon of **I**nterest ■ **D**esign ■ **E**valuation ■ **R**esearch type
SPICE (Booth 2004, 2006)	SPICE can also be used for searching for studies which evaluate health services in relation to specific stakeholders.	■ **S**etting: 'where?' (Booth 2006) or 'context of the service' (Booth 2004) ■ **P**erspective: 'for whom?' (Booth 2006) or stakeholders (user, manager, carer, information professional; Booth 2004) ■ **I**ntervention: 'what?' (Booth 2006) ■ **C**omparison: 'compared with?' (Booth 2006) ■ **E**valuation: 'result?' (Booth 2006)

*The 'T' in PICO(T) can also stand for 'Type of study', but 'Timeframe' is more common.

undergoing or understanding the patient's perspective of their situation.
■ Comparison: for example, a comparison between two treatments or a control group versus an intervention group.

■ Outcome: for example, this would include the outcomes that are expected from the enquiry.
As an example of PICO in action, Martha could use the framework to identify the key terms for her search of the literature for the woman she has been

assisting. Using PICO, the search could be narrowed like this:

- Patient: older adults with dementia
- Intervention: strategies to improve nutrition
- Comparison: normal care
- Outcome: improved appetite, dietary intake and weight.

Generating a comprehensive question that targets your clinical query increases your chance of accessing the most accurate and appropriate information. However, not all studies test an intervention/comparison so sometimes there won't necessarily be anything to ask—and that's fine. Some people put a 'T' on the end to make it PICO(T), and that is specific to Timeframe which can be useful to think about; for example, are you searching for studies performed during a specific period of time or only in the last 5 years? Other frameworks are available for different types of problems, such as ECLIPSE, SPIDER and SPICE (see Table 4.2). All frameworks help you to narrow down your question before you start searching the electronic databases for literature. These can also assist with fine-tuning the search terms to use.

LEVELS OF EVIDENCE

When we talk about research evidence, people often refer to the 'levels of evidence' or 'hierarchy of evidence' to classify the quality and trustworthiness of research findings which give us the evidence base for our practice. Historically, there was a strong emphasis on randomised controlled trials and interventional studies as the primary source of high-quality evidence. This was mainly due to a focus on the effectiveness of therapeutic interventions rather than what we understand now as the broader healthcare questions, including patient experience, qualitative research and non-randomised controlled studies, which are all equally important to answer questions posed by nurses and midwives. There are pyramids and tables that depict the research hierarchy of evidence, and these can be useful as it provides a visual and systematic representation. Table 4.3 depicts a pyramid representing the various levels of evidence. The highest level of evidence is the systematic review of randomised controlled trials, and the lowest level of evidence is background information/expert opinion. As qualitative studies are considered descriptive designs, these

TABLE 4.3	
Hierarchy of Evidence	
Excellent	Systematic review
	Multicentre studies
Good	RCT
	Observational studies
	Interpretive studies
Fair	Descriptive studies
	Action research
	Focus groups
Poor	Expert opinion
	Case studies
	Studies of poor methodological quality

Source: Adapted from Evans D: Hierarchy of evidence: a framework for ranking evidence evaluating healthcare interventions, Journal of Clinical Nursing 12(1):77–84, 2003. doi:10.1046/j.1365-2702.2003.00662.x.

are found at lower levels four and five on the pyramid. Quantitative studies produce varying levels of evidence depending on the type of design.

Another method of classifying the quality of research evidence has been developed further with the introduction of the Grading of Recommendations Assessment, Development and Evaluation (GRADE) system (Guyatt et al 2011). The GRADE system assesses the quality of research evidence based on the study design with the strength of recommendations provided by the researchers by considering each of the following:

1. study limitations
2. consistency of results
3. directness of evidence
4. precision and reporting of bias.

The GRADE system promotes evaluation of the quality of the evidence for each outcome and provides an assessment of balance between desirable and undesirable outcomes, which leads to a judgment about the strength of the recommendation.

WHAT DO YOU DO WITH THE EVIDENCE ONCE YOU HAVE FOUND IT?

Nursing and midwifery practice is informed by and draws from a wide range of evidence-based sources from a variety of disciplines including nursing, midwifery, medicine, psychology, sociology, education and others. Evidence itself is found in several sources such as national and international evidence-based guidelines, evidence-based summaries, consensus statements, journal articles and reports.

The way in which journal articles are written can seem quite daunting and is certainly not something that is immediately easy to understand—research articles can leave many of us feeling bewildered. This is because journals have limited space, meaning that authors must compress a lot of information into strict word limits, and to do this, authors have developed and honed their writing skills. They also tend to use scientific jargon—language that you are beginning to become familiar with. So rather than feel overwhelmed or only reading the abstract or skipping the results because it is too difficult, follow these tips on reading journal articles.

1. *Scan* the article for relevance and structure for your purposes.
   a. Notice the headings and subheadings so that you learn the structure of articles and what each section typically contains.
   b. Preview the graphs and tables.
   c. Notice what the article is about and decide whether will it be useful.
2. *Skim read* the paper for the first time.
   a. Focus on the abstract and conclusion to help you gain an overall picture of what the article is about.
   b. Note the date the paper was published, as current research is more relevant.
   c. Is the article published in a reputable journal? (See below for more information.)
   d. Highlight words or phrases that you need to look up to understand their meaning. Look these up so that when you read the article more closely, you are increasing your understanding.
3. *Re-read* the article again, this time doing the following.
   a. Be an active reader—make notes by asking yourself questions such as:
      i. What question (problem) is the study trying to solve?
      ii. Did the authors find an answer to their question?
   b. Sometimes you may find it useful to read the article out of order—reading the recommendations and conclusions first might enhance engagement with the remainder of the paper.
4. *Summarise* by taking notes while reading, as this will improve your reading comprehension and help you to remember key points.
   a. If you have a printed version, highlight key points and make notes directly on the article.
   b. If you have saved an electronic version, learn how to use the highlight and comments functions on your software.

HOW DO I KNOW IF ALL RELEVANT JOURNAL ARTICLES HAVE BEEN FOUND?

As most electronic databases are expanding very quickly, there is no way to really know whether or not everything you are searching for has been found. Some journals publish quarterly or monthly while others might be weekly or even daily. This means databases are constantly being expanded. The point of systematically searching for relevant journal articles is to maximise finding the most relevant and recent evidence.

WHAT ARE THE CLUES TO RECOGNISING IF JOURNAL ARTICLES ARE PUBLISHED BY RELIABLE PUBLISHERS?

In nursing and midwifery (and most other health disciplines), the quality of publishers and publications varies. One of the major threats to finding good evidence to inform practice is the type of journal that publishes the results of research. A common challenge is that readers of research articles may be unaware of the quality of journals and the peer-review process that papers undergo before publication. Some unscrupulous journals contact potential authors (often via unsolicited emails) to encourage manuscripts to be submitted. We call these predatory journals and publishers because they publish work regardless of its veracity or quality, usually following payments from authors to have work published. It is highly likely that in your search you will find articles published in these types of journals (Ashton 2019), especially if you search only in non-academic search engines. Quality journals are indexed in databases such as CINAHL or PubMed (Oermann et al 2018). Ashton (2019) recommends that nursing and midwifery students learn about predatory journals and how to recognise articles published in these journals. It is for this reason that you are reminded in assessments to search for good-quality sources (references) to substantiate claims made in assignments.

An international consensus of journal editors' definition of predatory journals is that these journals prioritise 'self-interest at the expense of scholarship and are characterised by false or misleading information, deviation from best editorial and publishing practices, a lack of transparency, and/or the use of aggressive and indiscriminate solicitation practices' (Grudniewicz et al 2019, p. 211). These publishers accept articles for publication without undertaking quality checks, such as peer-review processes, prior to publication (Oermann et al 2018).

Having a manuscript **peer reviewed** is a process whereby people with expertise in the topic area or research methods are invited to provide a critical review of a manuscript before it is published. The review involves an opinion provided to the journal editor(s) on the quality of the manuscript and whether the manuscript ought to be accepted as it is, improved through revisions or rejected for publication. The peer reviewers may also provide feedback to the author(s) to justify their opinion. This process is repeated until the manuscript is either accepted for publication or rejected. Those journals with a robust and transparent peer-review process are less likely to be predatory journals.

In nursing and midwifery, there are more than 140 predatory journals (Beall 2021). Relying on information from predatory journals that has not been subjected to robust peer review is a potential threat to nursing and midwifery practice (Bourgault 2019) because poor-quality papers could be mistakenly assumed to be good-quality evidence and then put into practice. In the last few years, editors of nursing and midwifery journals have raised awareness of predatory journals and developed guidelines on how to avoid publishing in predatory journals (Darbyshire et al 2016, 2020).

WHAT DO I DO IF I CAN'T FIND ANY RELEVANT ARTICLES?

Usually, when you search electronic databases, it is the search strategy you are using which may lead you to find very few relevant articles. Even experienced researchers who are searching databases have this problem. If this situation occurs, go back, look at your search strategy and try to be less restrictive; for example, use synonyms of similar words or phrases. It is very common for all of us to have a few attempts at developing the search strategy. If you are still struggling to find relevant articles, consulting a librarian to assist with getting the right search terms will help to get you on the right path (see Chapter 3 for more on developing a search strategy).

WHERE TO START WITH IMPLEMENTING EVIDENCE INTO PRACTICE

In everyday practice, nurses and midwives identify problems that need a solution. Often other nurses or midwives who work together have also identified similar problems. As we have seen in this chapter's case study, Martha noticed a problem with a woman's nutritional status. Martha has found some suitable evidence to inform the nursing care provided to the woman but is now wondering how to put the evidence into practice.

Putting evidence into practice frequently requires teams of nurses or midwives to change what they currently do. This requires motivation, time and support from others. In some situations, such as in the case of Martha, this can be relatively straightforward through a discussion at handover, and changes to patient care plans can be made. Other changes to practice may need:

- translation of evidence (i.e. can we use it in practice?)
- a change management process developed (i.e. changes to policies and procedures followed by education/training of staff)
- further study using implementation research techniques (i.e. does the evidence work in practice?).

These are some of the reasons why getting evidence into practice is delayed. Did you know that it can take on average 17 years for research to be translated into practice? (Grimshaw et al 2012, Wensing & Grol 2019). See Chapters 12 and 14 for more information on bringing evidence into practice.

STUDENT CHALLENGE

Reflecting on Practice

While out on placement, find a procedure or task related to the nursing or midwifery care you are providing to patients (or anticipate providing). Examine the procedure or task to determine if it was based on recent good-quality research evidence. Consider who would be interested in knowing what you have discovered and how you might communicate what you have found.

CONCLUSION

In this chapter, we have introduced you to EBP in Chapter 1 and discussed it again in this chapter. The processes of how you find evidence, and what you do when you have found the evidence, are important. We have shown you the importance of questioning of evidence as you think of applying it to your practice. By working through this information, it is hoped that you are now able to ask questions about issues you have identified when on placement, work through how you find evidence and judge which evidence could be used or applied to improve the care of patients.

ADDITIONAL RESOURCES

Fineout-Overholt E: A guide to critical appraisal of evidence, Nursing Critical Care 14(3):24–30, 2019.

Fry M, Attawet J: Nursing and midwifery use, perceptions and barriers to evidence-based practice: a cross-sectional survey, International Journal of Evidence-Based Healthcare 16(1): 47–54, 2018.

Leming-Lee T, Watters R: Translation of evidence-based practice: quality improvement and patient safety, Nursing Clinics of North America 54(1):1–20, 2019.

Spooner AJ, Aitken LM, Chaboyer W: Implementation of an evidence-based practice nursing handover tool in intensive care using the

knowledge-to-action framework, Worldviews on Evidence-Based Nursing 15(2):88–96, 2018.

Cochrane Library: https://www.cochranelibrary.com

JBI, University of Adelaide: https://jbi.global/

JBI: https://jbi.global/sites/default/files/2019-05/JBI-Levels-of-evidence_2014_0.pdf

University of New England—Reading and taking notes on scholarly journal articles: http://www.une.edu/sites/default/files/Reading-and-Annotating.pdf

---

REFERENCES

Ashton KS: Teaching nursing students and nurses about predatory publishing, Journal of Nursing Education 58(11):627–631, 2019.

Aveyard H, Sharp P: A beginner's guide to evidence-based practice in health and social care, UK, 2017, Open University Press.

Beall J: Beall's list of potential predatory journals and publishers, 2021 [Blog Post]. https://beallslist.net/.

Booth A: Clear and present questions: formulating questions for evidence-based practice, Library Hi Tech 24(3):355–368, 2006. https://doi.org/10.1108/07378830610692127.

Booth A: Formulating answerable questions. In Booth A, Brice A (eds), Evidence-based practice for information professionals: a handbook, London, 2004, Facet Publishing, pp. 61–70.

Bourgault AM: Predatory journals: a potential threat to nursing practice and science, Critical Care Nurse 39(4):9–11, 2019.

Considine J, Shaban R, Fry M, Curtis K: Evidence-based emergency nursing: designing a research question and searching the literature, International Emergency Nursing 32:78–82, 2017.

Cooke A, Smith D, Booth A: Beyond PICO: The SPIDER tool for qualitative evidence synthesis, Qualitative Health Research 22(10):1435–1443, 2012. https://doi.org/10.1177/1049732312452938.

Darbyshire P, Hayter M, Frazer K, et al: Hitting rock bottom: the descent from predatory journals and conferences to the predatory PhD, Journal of Clinical Nursing 29(23–24):4425–4428, 2020.

Darbyshire P, McKenna L, Lee SF, East CE: Taking a stand against predatory publishers, Journal of Advanced Nursing 73(7): 1535–1537, 2016.

Grimshaw JM, Eccles MP, Lavis JN, et al: Knowledge translation of research findings, Implementation Science 7:50, 2012.

Grudniewicz A, Moher D, Cobey KD, et al: Predatory journals: no definition, no defence, Nature 576:210–212, 2019.

Guyatt GH, Oxman AD, Sultan S, et al: GRADE guidelines: 9. Rating up the quality of evidence, Journal of Clinical Epidemiology 64:1311–1316, 2011.

Heelan M, Prieto J, Roberts H, et al: The use of finger foods in care settings: an integrative review, Journal of Human Nutrition and Dietetics 33(2):187–197, 2020.

Jordan Z, Lockwood C, Munn Z, Aromataris E: The updated Joanna Briggs Institute model of evidence-based healthcare, JBI, 2019. https://abstracts.cochrane.org/2017-global-evidence-summit/updated-jbi-model-evidence-based-healthcare.

Loewenthal KM, Marcus B: 15 Jewish stereotypes in psychiatric diagnosis and treatment. In Moffic HS, Peteet JR, Hankir A, Seeman, MV (eds): Anti-semitism and psychiatry: recognition, prevention, and interventions, Switzerland, 2020, Springer Nature, pp. 185–192.

Mackey A, Bassendowski S: The history of evidence-based practice in nursing education and practice, Journal of Professional Nursing 33(1):51–55, 2017.

Malatzky C, Haines H, Glenister K: Racism in a place of healthcare: the qualitative case of a rural Australian hospital, Journal of Community Medicine & Health Education 10(3):681, 2020. https://www.omicsonline.org/peer-reviewed/racism-in-a-place-of-healthcare-the-qualitative-case-of-a-rural-australian-hospital-112269.html.

McGrath M, Bagul D, Du Toit SH: Barriers and facilitators of meaningful engagement among older migrants living with dementia in residential aged care facilities: a mixed studies systematic review, Scandinavian Journal of Occupational Therapy 1–12, 2021. https://doi.org/10.1080/11038128.2021.1898675.

Oermann MH, Nicoll LH, Chinn PL, et al: Quality of articles published in predatory nursing journals, Nursing Outlook 66:4–10, 2018.

Oldknow H, Williamson K, Williams E, Palmer L: Dietary intake of people with dementia on acute hospital wards, Nursing Older People 31(6):16–21, 2019.

Pearson A, Wiechula R, Court A, Lockwood C: The JBI model of evidence-based healthcare, International Journal of Evidence-Based Healthcare 3(8):207–215, 2005.

Sackett D, Richardson W, Rosenberg W, Haynes R: Evidence-based medicine: how to practice and teach EBM, New York, 1997, Churchill Livingstone.

Sackett D, Rosenberg WM, Muir GJA, et al: Evidence-based medicine: what it is and what it isn't, British Medical Journal 312:71–72, 1996.

Wakefield EO, Popp JM, Dale LP, et al: Perceived racial bias and health-related stigma among youth with sickle cell disease, Journal of Developmental and Behavioral Pediatrics 38(2):129–134, 2017.

Watkins R, Goodwin VA, Abbott RA, et al: Exploring residents' experiences of mealtimes in care homes: a qualitative interview study, BMC Geriatrics 17(1):1–9, 2017.

Wensing M, Grol R: Knowledge translation in health: how implementation science could contribute more, BMC Medicine 17(88), 2019. https://doi.org/10.1186/s12916-019-1322-9.

Wildridge V, Bell L: How CLIP became ECLIPSE: A mnemonic to assist in searching for health policy/management information, Health Information & Libraries Journal 19(2):113–115, 2002. https://doi.org/10.1046/j.1471-1842.2002.00378.x.

5

READING AND APPRAISING RESEARCH

MARIE HUTCHINSON ■ KATE FRAZER

CHAPTER OUTLINE

LEARNING OBJECTIVES

After reading this chapter and following critical reflection, readers should be able to:

- differentiate between various study designs and their capacity to answer different questions
- explain the importance of appraising research and identifying relevance to practice
- understand the difference between statistical significance and clinical significance
- perform a rapid appraisal to establish whether a study is suited to answer a clinical question
- detail the questions asked in performing a critical appraisal
- follow the steps to critically appraise a qualitative study
- follow the steps to critically appraise a quantitative study.

KEY TERMS

appraisal tool	methodology
bias	primary research
blinding	reflection
clinical significance	reliability
critical appraisal	statistical significance
critical thinking	trustworthiness
data saturation	validity
evidence	

ABSTRACT

Reading and critically appraising research can be a challenging task, particularly for beginners. If you are a newcomer to reading research, it can be difficult to make sense of study designs and methods of data collection and analysis. At first glance, you may also find scholarly papers difficult to read, too complex or full of confusing terminology. The good news is that learning to master the steps in critically reading research is not as difficult as you may think. In this chapter, we address the challenges of becoming an informed and critical consumer of research and provide a step-by-step guide to critically appraising a paper. With a little knowledge and persistence, you will find that understanding how to read and critically appraise evidence is not as complicated as it first appears.

STUDENT QUOTE

It's one thing to find articles, but I need to be able to work out how to choose the right ones and understand how to critique them to know whether I can use them to inform my practice.

INTRODUCTION

Nurses and midwives are the largest group of healthcare professionals and can significantly impact standards of care and clinical outcomes. Within the clinical context, the processes of critical thinking and reflection are employed in decision-making and care planning. A critical component of this process is linking critical thinking to the integration of **evidence**, clinical expertise and patient preferences (Saunders et al 2019). Even though many gains have been made in applying evidence in practice, barriers to uptake and translation of evidence into practice remain. These barriers can lead to a gap of up to 17 years in implementing evidence into practice (Bauer et al 2015, Morris et al 2011, Rogers, De Brún & McAuliffe 2020). One of the factors that contributes to these barriers is the capacity of clinicians to have time to locate, critically appraise and interpret research (Duncome 2018).

Reading and appraising research can be exciting, particularly if you approach reading a paper with some confidence. The appraisal framework provided in this chapter has been developed to give you the confidence to know what questions to ask and help make sense of what you read. A fundamental first step in reviewing evidence and ideas is to do so through a critical lens. The second task is to understand the underlying question that drives you to seek out answers. Learning to focus your question will guide where you look for answers and the types of solutions you are seeking. The third task is to develop the skills to critically appraise what you read, which is vital because not all evidence is useful or even valid (Rosenfeld 2017).

ASKING QUESTIONS AND LOOKING FOR ANSWERS

Nurses and midwives are in a unique situation to translate evidence and new ideas into practice. A key element in this process is to become a critical consumer of evidence. This requires you to be aware of your information needs and the clinical situation, convert this into answerable questions and seek out and appraise the evidence you find. To get you thinking about the types of questions asked in practice, Table 5.1 provides examples of types of foci for clinical questions and how these translate into research questions. Once you learn how to frame questions, the next challenge is to critically and systematically appraise the validity and applicability of what you read.

STUDENT CHALLENGE
Asking Questions

Take a moment to consider the example questions in Table 5.1.
1. Have you asked similar questions during your course of study or in the clinical setting?
2. Can you think of a clinical question that you have raised recently? Do you have an evidence-based answer?
3. How ready do you think you are to engage with new ideas and review evidence to answer your question(s)?

CRITICAL THINKING AND REFLECTION

To think critically is a fundamental skill that clinicians engage in to determine and implement safe and

TABLE 5.1
Types of Questions and Examples of Research Questions

Clinical Scenario	Research Question
For a given patient, what is the better form of treatment?	Is antiemetic therapy in conjunction with antihistamines more effective than antiemetic therapy alone in reducing the effects of hyperemesis gravidarum?
What are the potential risks of missed treatment?	Are nursing home patients with a diagnosis of dementia at increased risk for inadequate pain management?
What is the nature of patient and public involvement and engagement in the research process?	How do Māori and Pacific Islander families experience their engagement in a participatory and experience-based co-design process with multicultural clinicians to design a program to tackle childhood obesity?

quality healthcare (Parker 2017). In practice and in our individual lives, we make decisions daily. Some of these decisions involve more thought and some are easier to make than others. As such, when you make a difficult decision, you have probably engaged in critical thinking, although you may not have been aware of this. **Critical thinking** involves the process of questioning, interpreting, analysing, determining relevance and making judgments on, for example, information, knowledge, professional practice and research (Parker 2017). In addition to actively engaging in critical thinking, students and clinicians engage in **reflection** or reflective practice. Like critical thinking, reflection is a conscious process involving thinking about events, situations and actions, to learn from experience and identify where actions can be taken to lead to better clinical practice (Delves-Yates 2021).

To ensure safe and quality healthcare, nurses and midwives need to engage with literature and research evidence. To determine the relevance, quality and strength of research evidence, we examine the literature through a critical lens. It is easy to read research and think it is credible, unbiased and significant, particularly when it is well written and convincing. However, this is not always the case and there are dangers in accepting what you read at face value rather than being more critical. As Greenhalgh and colleagues (2020) point out, many studies have significant limitations, such as small sample size and poor methodological reporting, many of which are not always apparent without careful examination. It is important to note that although it is essential to review literature and

research through a critical lens, doing so does not equate to criticism, devaluation and negative connotations. Rather, this involves judgment and constructive appraisal of the value of the evidence for application to address your clinical problem. Now that you have learned something about research and research processes, it is time to learn how to critically appraise research to determine its value.

STUDENT CHALLENGE
Reflecting in Action

Reflect on a clinical skill you have recently practised while on clinical placement or in your clinical practice.
1. Did you know why you carried out the skill and what rationale underpinned the action?
2. When you are in clinical practice, how do you verify that the action taking place is the best way to do it?
3. Have you sought out research evidence to use and share when you identify that practice needs to be challenged?

TAKING A STRUCTURED APPROACH: PERFORMING A CRITICAL APPRAISAL

A **critical appraisal** is a structured and systematic process for assessing and interpreting evidence by considering validity, results and relevance to your own context and clinical practice (CASP n.d.). Internationally, a large number of structured **appraisal tools** are available. Both JBI and the Critical Appraisal Skills Programme (CASP) have several appraisal tools that can be used for evaluating quantitative and qualitative studies. The Mixed Methods Appraisal Tool (MMAT) is another example of an instrument that can be used. The MMAT is unique in the assessment of five core quality criteria across different study designs: 1. qualitative; 2. randomised controlled; 3. non-randomised; 4. quantitative descriptive; and 5. mixed methods (Hong et al 2018). For this chapter, we have developed a simple checklist that contains core elements of these appraisal tools to guide you through the foundations of the critical appraisal process. Before conducting an appraisal, an initial preliminary assessment is helpful to establish whether the paper is relevant to your needs.

THE PRELIMINARY ASSESSMENT

Several preliminary questions will help focus your thinking and quickly identify whether a paper is useful or suited to answering your question (see Box 5.1). The answers to these preliminary questions should be evident from reading the abstract, which summarises the aim, study design, important results and conclusions. After the preliminary appraisal, if you consider the study is poorly designed or does not answer your question, you may not proceed to a full appraisal.

BOX 5.1
NINE QUESTIONS TO ASK WHEN PERFORMING A PRELIMINARY APPRAISAL

1. Why was the study undertaken?
2. What is the underlying question: is it relevant to my question or interests?
3. What type of evidence is provided?
4. Is there a clear statement of aims?
5. What was the overall design of the study?
6. Is the study design appropriate for the research question and study objectives?
7. Is the study population relevant to my question or clinical situation?
8. What were the outcomes of the study?
9. Are the results and conclusions relevant?

What is the Underlying Question and is it Relevant to my Question or Interests?

The first questions focus on why the study was undertaken and whether the topic is relevant to your interests. The abstract of a research paper should clearly state the aim of the study or, alternatively, identify the question the study was attempting to answer or why the study was undertaken. This may be written along the following lines: 'This study aimed to establish the acceptability and feasibility of a trial of a sexual health promotion intervention for people with serious mental illness in the United Kingdom'.

What Type of Evidence is Provided?

The type of research evidence provided can be ranked according to the source. Primary sources of evidence document and report on the study, and are usually reported by the people who conducted the research, whereas secondary evidence summarises or re-analyses published findings. The data may be presented in secondary or another processed form such as a narrative, integrative review or systematic review. If you are interested in answering a clinical question about treatment or interventions, you need to locate well-designed primary studies and/or a secondary systematic review (LoBiondo-Wood & Haber 2018). The usefulness of this evidence will be improved if measures of clinical significance are reported; if not, the study may be of less clinical value (Robinson & Haviland 2021). If you want to understand how knowledge is evolving on contemporary challenges and issues, a well-written narrative review could be considered. Alternatively, a scoping review will identify and map available evidence, providing an overview of the topic area.

What is the Overall Study Design?

Once you decide the paper is relevant to your needs, the next step is to understand the study design and level of evidence provided. It is often tempting to skip past careful consideration of **methodology**, particularly if you do not feel confident about research. Be careful with this temptation. Regardless of whether a study addresses an important question or presents applicable or statistically significant findings, you need to be mindful that if it is poorly designed, its usefulness is limited (Greenhalgh et al 2020).

Is the Study Design Appropriate for the Research Question and Study Objectives?

Table 5.2 illustrates the types of questions that can be addressed through different study designs. In evidence-based practice, certain research designs are given greater value than others. This value is made explicit through a hierarchy of evidence, as outlined by the Oxford Centre for Evidence-Based Medicine (OCEBM 2011) levels of evidence. In this hierarchy (Fig. 5.1), the randomised controlled clinical trial (RCT) is considered the gold standard of **primary research**, with a meta-analysis of RCTs thought to offer the best available evidence. Health professionals are more likely to change practice based on the results of RCTs than on other research designs that fall lower on the hierarchy given their rigorous approach. Even so, it is important to recognise that questions of effectiveness, appropriateness, meaningfulness and feasibility require different types of study designs (Jordan et al 2019). Reflecting a more nuanced hierarchy of evidence model, JBI has developed a model of evidence types, suited to answering particular types of questions. If you are unfamiliar with the hierarchy of evidence model, the Additional resources at the end of this chapter provides a link to JBI resources (see Chapter 3 and 4 for more detail).

Generally, the evidence will be stronger when the design chosen is at the higher end of the hierarchy of evidence. If it is towards the lower end, you need to consider why the authors have chosen this design and how this might impact implementation of the findings. Do not automatically dismiss a study that sits towards the lower end of the spectrum, as these studies can be best suited to answer certain questions. Although RCTs sit towards the top of the evidence hierarchy, they are not necessarily best suited to answering all clinical questions, such as those focused on experience or description. For example, Frazer and colleagues' 2016 Cochrane review presenting evidence of the impact of legislative smoking bans internationally demonstrates the use of non-RCT designs. Moreover, in clinical settings, it is not always feasible to use blind treatment allocation or to randomise patients (an essential element of the randomised trial design).

TABLE 5.2

Examples of Different Question Types and the Hierarchy of Study Designs Suited to Answer the Question

Type of Question	Hierarchy of Suitable Study Types
Effectiveness In patients with type 2 diabetes and obesity, is a structured exercise program more effective than standard medical treatment in improving diabetic control?	Meta-analysis > RCT > prospective cohort study > retrospective cohort study > case control > case series > qualitative study
What are the effects of legislative smoking bans on: 1. morbidity and mortality from exposure to second-hand smoke; and 2. smoking prevalence and tobacco consumption?	Narrative synthesis > interrupted time series > cohort or case control > cross-sectional study
Experience of Treatment How do patients with type 2 diabetes and obesity experience participation in a group exercise program?	Qualitative systematic review > in-depth qualitative interview > case study
Aetiology, Prognosis or Causality What are the potential predictors of mortality in patients with COVID-19?	Meta-analysis > prospective cohort study > retrospective cohort study
What were the characteristics of illness presentation among children diagnosed with measles during a specific outbreak?	Meta-analysis > retrospective case series > case study
Is tachypnoea a strong predictor of clinical deterioration in adult emergency department patients?	Prospective cohort study > retrospective cohort study > cross-sectional study > case study

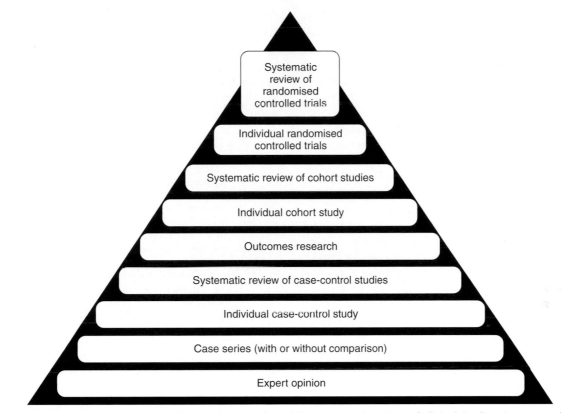

Fig. 5.1 ■ **Illustrative hierarchy of evidence.** (Source: Adapted from National Institute of Clinical Studies. Emergency department stroke and transient ischaemic attack care bundle: information and implementation guide. Melbourne, 2009, National Health and Medical Research Council. https://www.nhmrc.gov.au/sites/default/files/images/appendix-f-levels-of-evidence.pdf.)

Therefore, an RCT (either the option of a single-blinded RCT or a double-blinded RCT) is not possible. RCTs are also more suited to interventions, such as drug therapy. It is also important to consider that like all research designs, RCTs can have varying degrees of quality, and so quality appraisal is necessary when considering the evidence derived from any designs.

Furthermore, nurses and midwives often seek to answer highly contextualised questions that are well suited to exploratory study designs (Jordan et al 2019). It is important to understand that when little is known about a problem or issue, feasibility studies are often more descriptive and at the 'lower' end of the evidence spectrum. As the body of knowledge grows, so does the capacity to refine a more tightly structured and rigorous design. Importantly, experience and meaning cannot be revealed through purely quantitative study designs such as RCTs; rather, qualitative exploratory approaches are required (Green & Thorogood 2018).

What is Patient and Public Involvement in Research?

Patient and public involvement in research is an essential criterion to improve the relevance, design and quality of research (Bagley et al 2016). The National Institute for Health and Care Research (2022) states that patients and the public are interested in being part of and getting involved with health and social care research for a variety of reasons. Most of all, not only are they hopeful of benefiting from more treatments but they also want to help others who are experiencing the same condition as them. Increasingly, researchers are engaging with patients and consumers as partners in the research design and processes, focusing on what matters most to them and identifying their priorities and preferred outcomes (Rosario et al 2020). According to Smits and colleagues:

> *Patients and public possess unique knowledge and specific experiences. They have ideas about relevant research questions, about research designs and research procedures that are acceptable to them, and they provide a complementary perspective on findings and their interpretation.*
>
> **(Smits et al 2020, p. 3)**

In considering the hierarchy of evidence, it is important to consider patient or consumer engagement in the research process as a criterion for assessing the quality of evidence. Arnstein's ladder of engagement (1969), and adaptation of it (Ocloo & Matthews 2016), are used as frameworks to describe the level of involvement. Patient and public involvement may range from consultation to shared partnership (Arnstein 1969, Ocloo & Matthews 2016). The GRIPP2-LF and GRIPP2-SF (Staniszewska et al 2017) are tools that may be used to evaluate the quality, transparency and consistency of patient and public involvement in studies.

CASE STUDY 5.1

Jamie is working through the literature on the experiences and support needs of people with learning disabilities adjusting to life with type 1 diabetes. As Jamie becomes more familiar with the literature, it appears that the literature is focused on people in the 40 to 60 years age group, whereas Jamie's case study is focused on a teenager. What are the implications of this for Jamie? How can Jamie assess the value or use of this literature for a younger population?

THE DETAILED APPRAISAL

Even if a paper reports statistically significant findings or the authors mount a convincing argument to substantiate their results and the integrity and application of the methods, appraising the evidence requires a little detective work to ensure validity and **reliability** and that the findings drawn are relevant and credible.

Assessing Methodological Quality

When performing a more detailed appraisal of methodological quality, careful consideration needs to be given to assessing features such as the sample and approach to recruitment, as well as issues of internal validity and reliability in quantitative research or rigour in qualitative research (see Box 5.2).

BOX 5.2
QUESTIONS TO ASK WHEN APPRAISING METHODOLOGY

1. For quantitative studies, is the sample size adequate and does it have sufficient power? What was the response rate?
2. For qualitative studies, are participants the most appropriate to provide access to the type of information sought?
3. Are details provided on how ethical principles were maintained and was ethics approval granted by a Human Research Ethics Committee?
4. What was the source of the sample or participants and are they representative of the broader population to whom the research might apply?
5. Is sufficient detail provided on recruitment and inclusion/exclusion criteria for the study?
6. For quantitative studies, what was the sampling method? How were participants selected? Could the sampling method have introduced bias?
7. For quantitative studies, are the groups identical except for difference in exposure to the treatment or variable under investigation?
8. For experimental designs, are participants and investigators 'blinded' to treatment allocation?
9. Is there a clear description of how data were collected?
10. For quantitative studies, are the data collection methods and tools valid and reliable? Was the instrument used previously validated?
11. For qualitative studies, how do the researchers account for their own presence in the data collection and analysis? Have the authors provided detail as to how trustworthiness was achieved?
12. Were there any distorting, extraneous or contaminating factors that might have influenced the data collected? If methods change during the study, are these adequately accounted for?
13. What level of public and patient involvement is reported (consider GRIPP2) (Staniszewska et al 2017).

Sample Size and Design

For quantitative studies, the first consideration is the size of the sample and whether it has sufficient power to detect differences or establish causal relationships (LoBiondo-Wood & Haber 2018). Establish whether the authors have reported power—usually, a power of 90% will give you confidence in the sample size (LoBiondo-Wood & Haber 2018). Also, check that the sample size at the end of the study, and in all groups, is sufficient to meet the initial power calculations. For research to apply to other similar study populations, it is also important to establish whether participants are representative of the group from which they are drawn and the wider population to whom the findings might be applied (Liamputtong 2017). The authors should also provide sufficient detail for you to be confident that the treatments of comparison groups are similar.

The sample size for qualitative studies can be more difficult to appraise as often these studies are exploratory in nature, are focused on subjective experience and do not aim to be generalisable. Qualitative studies will often continue to recruit and collect data from participants until analysis of the data is not producing any 'newer' knowledge or themes (**data saturation**). Therefore, qualitative studies often have a smaller number of participants as exploring and elucidating phenomena is the primary aim. Similar to quantitative studies, it is also important to determine whether the sample was representative in answering the research question.

Representation in Qualitative Research

As previously stated, in qualitative studies rigour is described and determined by trustworthiness. **Trustworthiness** refers to the extent to which the data captures participants' experiences and encapsulates the concepts of credibility (that the results are credible and accurately represent the data), transferability (the ability of the results to be transferred or generalised to other settings), confirmability, the extent to which the results can be confirmed by others (Amankwaa 2016) and dependability (could the study be replicated and the same conclusions drawn?) (Forero et al 2018). To determine rigour when critically appraising qualitative research, it is important to ask questions such as the following.

- Have the researchers developed an audit trail for the study to be replicated?
- Is there a clear description of the study participants?

- Are participants' voices presented in the findings to reflect credibility?
- How many researchers were involved in data analysis?
- Were findings confirmed by more than one researcher?
- Could these findings be relevant to other participants in other healthcare contexts?

Measurement in Quantitative Research

In considering **validity**, you are aiming to establish the extent to which the measurement undertaken is accurate and measures what it intends to (Hickman & Disler 2019). Some forms of measurement are particularly inaccurate and introduce 'bias'; for example, asking people to recall events over extended periods. You should also be mindful of whether or not the measurement tool employed is reliable, which means that it can consistently measure a construct with repeated use (Hickman & Disler 2019). Both the validity and the reliability of the measurement tool should be reported. In addition, if multiple individuals are collecting data, it is important to establish whether the results would be the same between these people and what steps are taken to ensure consistency in the results. To improve confidence in the reliability, studies may test for reliability between assessors (inter-rater reliability), calibrate instruments between measurements or perform random spot checks to identify any errors or inconsistencies in data collection (LoBiondo-Wood & Haber 2018).

CASE STUDY 5.2

Martha is reading research about maintaining nutritional status in people living with dementia. As she reads through the papers, she realises that the research is largely based on the needs and experiences of people from the dominant white culture and that issues of cultural diversity and ethnicity are not addressed. The literature does not recognise the role or symbolism of food in cultural life and identity. How might Martha incorporate these findings into Mrs Patel's care plan given her cultural background?

Identifying Bias in Quantitative Research

As you read a paper, you also need to think about whether there is evidence of **bias** in participant selection, data analysis and/or data collection methods that may influence the results (LoBiondo-Wood & Haber 2018). Bias can occur when there are differences between study participants or study groups that are poorly controlled or not accounted for in the analysis. In many studies, randomisation, stratification of the sample and **blinding** of treatment and allocation to groups are common strategies to limit bias (Higgins et al 2011). Missing data is another factor that should be considered when you review study findings for bias. A study may commence with a balanced design, or the same number of subjects in each arm of the study, and due to loss of subjects to follow up or incomplete data (missing data), bias can be introduced into the study (Liamputtong 2017). In cohort studies or controlled trials, deaths and study participants leaving the study ('dropouts') can occur. You need to consider how many participants dropped out, and whether there are any clues to bias in the reasons for this happening.

Equality, Diversity and Inclusion

It is essential to appraise research in terms of inclusion and diversity to ensure that outcomes are appropriate and applicable in real-world care settings. These characteristics may include sex/gender, race, ethnicity or disability. Ní Shé and colleagues (2019) identify multiple program theories that warrant review in thinking about which populations are excluded from research, including marginalised and seldom-heard groups. If a study is focused on minority communities or populations, it is also important to consider the level of involvement from members of that community or population in the design and conduct of the research. These issues are considered in more depth in Chapter 11.

Data Analysis and Findings

The next step in the appraisal is to establish whether the data analysis methods or statistical tests are appropriate for the data and whether the conclusions drawn are relevant to the findings presented (Box 5.3). Having worked through the questions on the method, you will have a good understanding of why and how the study was performed, making the results easier to understand and evaluate.

Data Analysis Methods

Qualitative studies collect narrative data rather than numbers. When appraising qualitative research

---

BOX 5.3
QUESTIONS TO ASK WHEN APPRAISING DATA ANALYSIS AND FINDINGS

1. Is the type of analysis appropriate for the type of data collected?
2. For qualitative studies, is there sufficient in-depth description of the analysis method?
3. Are the data clearly presented?
4. Are dropout or missing data accounted for sufficiently?
5. For qualitative studies, are the results credible and trustworthy?
6. Are measures of clinical significance presented?
7. Are the conclusions drawn relevant to the findings?

---

findings, it is important to assess the data collection methods and analysis techniques used to determine whether these were congruent with the research methodology and design (see Chapter 8 for more on qualitative design). For example, if the research used a grounded theory approach, analysis is performed through comparisons between collected data to generate theory. Or, if the study was ethnographic, data collection methods should include direct involvement of the researcher with the researched population and culture through observation and interviews (Aspers & Corte 2019). Although qualitative research does not generally use the term 'significant' as reported in quantitative research, findings from qualitative studies should be new and of use and/or importance to the target audience.

When reporting quantitative data analysis, the authors should report the tests used and the results. For example, were paired t-tests used to analyse and compare two measurements of a dependent variable, was a measure of variance such as ANOVA (analysis of variance) used to compare differences among more three or more groups or were correlation coefficients determined to report the association and strength of the relationships between two variables (LoBiondo-Wood & Haber 2018)?

Identifying Statistical and Clinical Significance

When you read the results of statistical analysis, you can be confident the findings are significant (not due to chance) when the *p*-value is below 0.05 (LoBiondo-Wood & Haber 2018). The lower the *p*-value, the more confident you can be that chance has not influenced the results. To understand the clinical benefit of a study, it is important to look beyond **statistical significance** and establish **clinical significance**, as the *p*-value does not necessarily provide evidence of clinical benefit (Ohl & Schelly 2017) (see Box 5.4). For more information on the *p*-value, see Chapter 7. Clinical significance refers to findings that represent a change that makes sufficient difference to a clinical outcome.

In clinical trials, measures of clinical significance are often calculated in terms of effect size. A commonly reported measure of effect is the confidence interval (CI). This measure provides the limits for the true effect size of the treatment or intervention in the population of interest. The CI is expressed as a range between two numbers, with the true but unknown effect value falling within this range. A 95% CI means that you can be 95% certain the level of effect for the study population falls within the calculated range (Liamputtong 2017). The CI also provides insight into how precise the study results are and whether the same results would occur if the study was replicated. When appraising a study, look for a CI value of 95% or above and a small gap in the interval. A wide gap between the upper and lower CIs (e.g. 0.48–0.93) indicates poor precision (LoBiondo-Wood & Haber 2018). Another important aspect of the CI is whether the range contains the value for 'no effect' for the test performed, indicating a non-significant result.

BOX 5.1
EXAMPLES OF QUESTIONS RELEVANT TO ESTABLISHING THE CLINICAL SIGNIFICANCE

- How confident am I that I could use this treatment or intervention in practice?
- How many patients would need to be treated for one to benefit?
- What are the odds a patient will benefit?
- Might there be a risk of harm associated with the treatment?
- How many patients might be treated before one is harmed?

Other measures of clinical significance include ratios of hazard or risk, measures of risk reduction and the number needed to treat (NNT) to gain a benefit. For absolute measures of clinical significance, such as NNT and measures of risk reduction, the value for no effect is 0, while for ratio measures (such as the odds ratio or relative risk), the value for no effect is 1. Therefore, a CI range of 0.8–2.1 for a test of relative risk is not statistically significant, as the value for no effect (1) lies within the CI range (Greenhalgh et al 2020). It is possible to calculate many of these measures from the data reported in a paper.

PUTTING IT ALL TOGETHER: TWO APPRAISAL EXAMPLES

To help you put the appraisal checklist outlined into practice, the following section provides two worked examples of an appraisal. Once you have read these through, you should find it relatively straightforward to start using the checklist to conduct your appraisals.

Example Appraisal for a Mixed Methods Study

In this first example (Hughes et al 2020), the authors employed a feasibility RCT design to compare a sexual health promotion intervention (three individual 1-hour sessions with a practitioner) to treatment as usual for people living with a serious mental illness (see Box 5.5). The study included a nested or embedded qualitative component. This design is appropriate for establishing the feasibility and acceptability of the evidence-based intervention to promote sexual health and identify the key parameters to inform a future RCT. (Refer back to Table 5.2.) From the initial screening of the abstract, the study appears to be well designed and the results presented are important in considering the feasibility of the methods in a realist study context.

Using a feasibility design the authors present the challenges of recruiting for a study about a topic that receives less attention in mental healthcare settings. The authors reported retention rates within the study, and evidence indicating the acceptability of the study design, methods of recruitment, information and the intervention for the target population.

BOX 5.5
RESULTS OF PRELIMINARY APPRAISAL

AIM

To establish the acceptability and feasibility of a trial of a sexual health promotion intervention for people with serious mental illness (SMI).

DESIGN

Randomised controlled open feasibility trial. A nested qualitative study was embedded in the design.

ETHICS

No detail is provided in the abstract. This does not necessarily mean ethical approval was not gained. One would read further to establish the point. The study was registered with the International Standard Randomised Controlled Trials Number (ISRCTN) registry, an international registry enabling and promoting transparency in clinical trials.

SAMPLE AND SETTING

Targeted sample of 100 participants was not achieved over the 12 months of the study; 72 people were enrolled. Intervention group at 3 months = 28, treatment-as-usual group at 3 months = 29; 22 participants completed qualitative interviews.

INTERVENTION/OUTCOME

Three individual sessions (health promotion intervention) each of 1-hour duration.

RELEVANCE OF RESULTS AND CONCLUSION

Improvements in sexual health outcomes in the intervention group were reported. Qualitative data identified acceptable study methods. The study manual was developed including patient and public involvement (PPI).

CONCLUSION DRAWN

Effective methods ensuring retention rates, both groups indicated acceptability and feasibility of the study for people with SMI. A powered RCT is required to establish effectiveness of the intervention in adopting safer sex practices.

STUDENT CHALLENGE

Research Participant Perspectives

Refer back to Table 5.2.

In the study by Hughes and colleagues (2020), what is the value in completing a feasibility study? Consider the challenges in recruitment from a seldom-heard population. Consider the value of patient and public involvement (PPI) in developing research.

Example Appraisal for a Qualitative Study

In this second example, Facchinetti and colleagues (2021) aimed to explore the experiences of older

BOX 5.6
RESULTS OF PRELIMINARY APPRAISAL

AIM

Explore the experiences of older patients with chronic disease when discharged from hospital.

DESIGN

Multicentre descriptive qualitative study

IS THE STUDY DESIGN APPROPRIATE FOR THE RESEARCH QUESTION AND STUDY OBJECTIVES?

The qualitative research design was suited for the data collection methods of semi-structured individual interviews and inductive content analysis data analysis method.

DID THE STUDY MEET EXPECTED STANDARDS OF ETHICS?

The relevant ethics committee granted ethics approval.

SAMPLE AND SETTING

Two Italian hospitals, recruiting 65 older patients with chronic disease.

OUTCOME

Six main categories of experience emerged from the analysis. These highlighted positive and negative emotions about discharge, the need for further information and support, feelings of fragility, the need for trusting and stable healthcare relationships and home as a caring place.

RELEVANCE OF RESULTS AND CONCLUSION

The findings of this study contribute to understanding discharge as a transition period. At this point of transfer of care, frail elderly patients felt vulnerable, with this vulnerability reduced through trusting relationships with health professionals and the provision of information.

CONCLUSION DRAWN

Discharge can be a period of conflicting emotions for older patients. For older patients with chronic disease, discharge requires personalised planning and providing them with the tools and knowledge to better manage their chronic disease. Reframing discharge as a point of transition highlights the importance of ensuring continued support and continuous relationships with trusting health professionals.

---

people with chronic illness at discharge from the hospital. The study employed individual semi-structured interviews, with the interview transcripts analysed using thematic analysis. The preliminary screening (see Box 5.6) indicated that the aim of this study was clear and the research design was congruent with the analysis and data collection methods. The findings of the study were relevant to how health professionals can better understand and plan for the needs of this group of older people at hospital discharge.

However, on further appraisal, some challenges the authors faced can be identified, along with the strategies they employed to address these issues. As summarised in Box 5.7, this study was undertaken at the time of discharge. The authors report this led to challenges in data collection as time pressures meant that participants' answers were often brief. To address this issue, the authors continued collecting data until no new themes emerged during the interviews. This study took place in Italy. This raises the issue of whether the findings adequately represent the cultural context in which your practice takes place, which may impact the transferability of the research. (See Chapter 7 for further discussion on credibility and trustworthiness in qualitative research.)

STUDENT CHALLENGE

Consider the Context of Research

In the study reported by Facchinetti and colleagues (2021), the participants were older Italian people with chronic disease being discharged from hospital. Participants reported an awareness that their chronic disease was long term and would accompany them through life, making the support of trusted healthcare professionals important to their ongoing care. Based on the information provided, what steps would you take to ensure older people are discharged with appropriate support?

Qualitative research can provide the opportunity for in-depth exploration of the perspective of people directly affected by an experience, like caring for an older person with a chronic disease. When you think about planning a discharge, reflect on whether this process is informed by evidence about the types of support older people require.

CONCLUSION

This chapter has provided an introduction to how to critically appraise research. As a clinician, it may be daunting at first to apply a critical lens to published research. When you have had a little practice at using the checklists provided in this chapter, you will find it is only a short step to reading and considering the utility of research for practice regularly.

BOX 5.7
RESULTS OF DETAILED APPRAISAL

1. SAMPLE AND RECRUITMENT

What was the source of the sample or participants, and are they representative of the broader population to whom the research might apply? Participants were recruited from two hospitals prior to discharge. The study focused on the experiences of these older people.

What was the sampling method? Purposive sampling was employed, based on the presence of chronic disease at time of discharge. This sampling method is suitable for qualitative studies. Inclusion and exclusion criteria were provided. Data were collected while patients were waiting to be collected from the hospital.

2. CREDIBILITY AND TRUSTWORTHINESS

Is there a clear description of how data were collected? Yes, there is description of pilot interviews through which the interview guide was developed and how the interviews were conducted.

For qualitative studies, how does the researcher(s) account for their own presence in the data collection and analysis? While the authors do not explicitly account for their presence, they do provide detail on strategies to ensure credibility, dependability and authenticity of the analysis.

3. DATA ANALYSIS METHODS

Are the data analysis methods appropriate for the type of data being measured? Data collected from the interviews underwent inductive content analysis, an appropriate data analysis method used in qualitative research.

For qualitative studies, is there sufficient in-depth description of the analysis method chosen? Yes, the authors included the coding process and outlined the emergent categories and subcategories. The data analysis was independently peer reviewed by the authors, followed by panel discussion.

4. FINDINGS PRESENTED

Are the data clearly presented? Findings from this study are clearly identified through categories with excerpts of data to provide examples.

For qualitative studies, are the results credible and trustworthy? Yes, peer review was undertaken during the data analysis and other strategies detailed for trustworthiness. Detail was provided on how categories were derived.

5. CONCLUSIONS DRAWN

Are the conclusions drawn relevant to the findings? The conclusions drawn from this study are relevant to the findings and may be useful in determining how better to individually plan discharge for elderly patients with chronic disease.

ADDITIONAL RESOURCES

Agency for Healthcare Research and Quality: http://www.ahrq.gov

Nesta: https://www.nesta.org.uk/project/evidence-and-experimentation/

Cochrane Library: https://www.cochranelibrary.com/

Critical Appraisal Skills Programme (CASP): http://www.casp-uk.net

JBI Critical Appraisal Tools: https://jbi.global/critical-appraisal-tools

JBI Levels of Evidence: https://jbi.global/sites/default/files/2019-05/JBI-Levels-of-evidence_2014_0.pdf

Mixed Methods Assessment Tool: Hong QN, Fàbregues S, Bartlett G, et al: The mixed methods appraisal tool (MMAT) version 2018 for information professionals and researchers, Education for Information 34, 285–291, 2018. https://doi.org/10.3233/EFI-180221

NHMRC Evidence Hierarchy https://www.mja.com.au/sites/default/files/NHMRC.levels.of.evidence.2008-09.pdf

The University of Oxford: Centre for Evidence-Based Medicine: https://www.cebm.ox.ac.uk/resources/ebm-tools/critical-appraisal-tools

REFERENCES

Amankwaa L: Creating protocols for trustworthiness in qualitative research, Journal of Cultural Diversity 23(3):121–127, 2016.

Arnstein SR: A ladder of citizen participation, Journal of the American Planning Association 35:216–224, 1969. https://doi.org/10.1080/01944366908977225.

Aspers P, Corte U: What is qualitative in qualitative research, Qualitative Sociology 42(2):139–160, 2019. https://doi.org/10.1007/s11133-019-9413-7.

Bagley HJ, Short H, Harman NL, et al: A patient and public involvement (PPI) toolkit for meaningful and flexible involvement in clinical trials—a work in progress, Research Involvement and Engagement 27(2):15, 2016. https://doi.org/10.1186/s40900-016-0029-8.

Bauer MS, Damschroder L, Hagedorn H, et al: An introduction to implementation science for the non-specialist, BMC Psychology 3(1):32, 2015. https://doi.org/10.1186/s40359-015-0089-9.

Critical Appraisal Skills Programme (CASP): Critical appraisal, n.d. https://casp-uk.net/glossary/critical-appraisal/.

Delves-Yates C: Beginner's guide to reflective practice in nursing, London, 2021, SAGE.

Duncome DC: A multi-institutional study of the perceived barriers and facilitators to implementing evidence-based practice, Journal of Clinical Nursing 27:5-6;1216–1226, 2018. doi: 10.1111/jocn.14168.

Facchinetti G, Albanesi B, Piredda M, et al: 'The light at the end of the tunnel'. Discharge experiences of older patients with chronic diseases: a multi-centre qualitative study, Journal of Advanced Nursing 77(5):2417–2428, 2021. doi: 10.1111/jan.14790.

Forero R, Nahidi S, De Costa J, et al: Application of four-dimension criteria to assess rigour of qualitative research in emergency medicine, BMC Health Services Research 18:120, 2018. https://doi.org/10.1186/s12913-018-2915-2.

Frazer K, Callinan JE, McHugh J, et al: Legislative smoking bans for reducing harms from secondhand smoke exposure, smoking prevalence and tobacco consumption, Cochrane Database Systematic Review 4 Feb, 2(2), 2016. https://doi.org/10.1002/14651858.CD005992.pub3.

Green J, Thorogood N: Qualitative methods for health research, ed 4, London, 2018, SAGE.

Greenhalgh TM, Bidewell J, Warland J, et al: Quantitative research. In Understanding research methods for evidence-based practice in health, ed 2, Queensland 2020, John Wiley & Sons.

Hickman L, Disler R: Quantitative research. In Borbasi S, Jackson D, East L (eds), Navigating the maze of research: enhancing nursing and midwifery practice, ed 5, Sydney, 2019, Elsevier, pp. 109–147.

Higgins JP, Altman DG, Gotzsche PC, et al: The Cochrane Collaboration's tool for assessing risk of bias in randomised trials. BMJ 343:d5928, 2011. https://doi.org/10.1136/bmj.d5928.

Hong QN, Fàbregues S, Bartlett G, et al: The mixed methods appraisal tool (MMAT) version 2018 for information professionals and researchers, Education for Information 34:285–291, 2018. https://doi.org/10.3233/EFI-180221.

Hughes E, Mitchell N, Gascoyne S, et al: The RESPECT study: a feasibility randomised controlled trial of a sexual health promotion intervention for people with serious mental illness in community mental health services in the UK, BMC Public Health 20:1736, 2020. https://doi.org/10.1186/s12889-020-09661-x.

Jordan Z, Lockwood C, Munn Z, Aromataris E: The updated Joanna Briggs Institute model of evidence-based healthcare, International Journal of Evidence-Based Healthcare 17(1):58–71, 2019. https://doi.org/10.1097/XEB.0000000000000155.

Liamputtong P: Research methods in health: foundations for evidence-based practice, ed 3, South Melbourne, 2017, Oxford University Press.

LoBiondo-Wood G, Haber J: Reliability and validity. In Nursing research: methods and critical appraisal for evidence-based practice, ed 9, St Louis, 2018, Elsevier Mosby, pp. 262–280.

Morris ZS, Wooding S, Grant J: The answer is 17 years, what is the question: understanding time lags in translational research, Journal of the Royal Society of Medicine 104(12):510–520, 2011. https://doi.org/10.1258/jrsm.2011.110180.

National Institute for Health and Care Research: Involve patients. National Institute for Health and Care Research, 2022. https://www.nihr.ac.uk/health-and-care-professionals/engagement-and-participation-in-research/involve-patients.htm.

Ní Shé É, Morton S, Lambert V, et al: Clarifying the mechanisms and resources that enable the reciprocal involvement of seldom-heard groups in health and social care research: A collaborative rapid realist review process, Health Expectations 22(3):298–306, 2019. https://doi.org/10.1111/hex.12865.

OCEBM. The Oxford Levels of Evidence 2. Oxford Centre for Evidence-Based Medicine. 2011. https://www.cebm.ox.ac.uk/resources/levels-of-evidence/ocebm-levels-of-evidence.

Ocloo J, Matthews R: From tokenism to empowerment: progressing patient and public involvement in healthcare improvement, BMJ Quality & Safety 25:626–632, 2016. http://dx.doi.org/10.1136/bmjqs-2015-004839.

Ohl A, Schelly D: Beyond p-values: a case for clinical relevance, British Journal of Occupational Therapy 80(12):752–755, 2017. https://doi.org/10.1177/0308022617735048.

Parker S: Becoming a critical thinker. In Daly J, Speedy S, Jackson D (eds), Contexts of nursing: an introduction, ed 5, Sydney, 2017, Elsevier, pp. 93–109.

Robinson R, Haviland JS: Understanding statistical significance and avoiding common pitfalls. Clinical Oncology Dec;33(12):804–806, 2021. http://doi.org/10.1016/j.clon.2021.06.008.

Rogers L, De Brún A, McAuliffe E: Defining and assessing context in healthcare implementation studies: a systematic review, BMC Health Services Research 20:591, 2020. https://doi.org/10.1186/s12913-020-05212 7.

Rosario MK, Hebert MA, Sahota BK, Eurich D: Capacity development in patient-oriented research: programme evaluation and impact analysis, Health Research Policy and Systems 18: 89, 2020. https://doi.org/10.1186/s12961-020-00606-9.

Rosenfeld P: How strong is the evidence? A primer on appraising the evidence and quality of research journal articles, World Council of Enterostomal Therapists Journal 37(1):12–15, 2017.

Saunders H, Gallagher-Ford L, Kvist T, Vehviläinen-Julkunen K: Practicing healthcare professionals' evidence-based practice competencies: an overview of systematic reviews, Worldviews on Evidence-Based Nursing 16(3):176–185, 2019. doi: 10.1111/wvn.12363.

Smits DW, van Meeteren K, Klem M, et al: Designing a tool to support patient and public involvement in research projects: the Involvement Matrix, Research Involvement and Engagement 6:30, 2020. https://doi.org/10.1186/s40900-020-00188-4.

Staniszewska S, Brett J, Simera I, et al: GRIPP2 reporting checklists: tools to improve reporting of patient and public involvement in research, BMJ 358:j3453, 2017. http://doi.org/10.1136/bmj.j3453.

6

NAVIGATING ETHICS

ANDREA DONALDSON ■ LESLIE GELLING

LEARNING OBJECTIVES

*After reading this chapter and following critical reflection, readers
should be able to:*

■ identify the rights of human participants in research

■ describe the ethical issues related to research

■ discuss what constitutes vulnerable participants

■ understand the relationship between the risks and
  benefits of research

■ describe how to obtain ethical approval.

KEY TERMS

autonomy

beneficence

confidentiality

consent

ethical principles

ethics

fidelity

human rights

informed consent

justice

non-maleficence

nursing ethics

privacy

research ethics

risk

veracity

ABSTRACT

Research undertaken by nurses and midwives, or about the practice of nursing and midwifery, is often undertaken either directly or indirectly with human participants. When planning and conducting such research, researchers must consider important ethical principles which seek to ensure that the research is conducted in an ethical manner. Importantly, the research should have the potential for benefit (beneficence) through improvements to available care and treatment, by improved knowledge and understanding, and by minimising the risks (non-maleficence) to those participating in the research. Above all other considerations, researchers need to ensure that all those participating in their research have freely given informed consent (autonomy) before participating. These and other ethical principles have evolved in response to harmful events in the history of health research. Now there is a societal expectation that all health researchers adhere to these principles. Planning and conducting research can be complex and time-consuming but researchers must include consideration of ethical principles during all stages of the research process.

STUDENT QUOTE

Considering the ethical principles while planning a research project helped me work out what was important, both about what I was trying to do and what I was expecting from participants.

INTRODUCTION

Nurses and midwives must be confident that the evidence they use in their practice was generated through the appropriate scientific methods. People who participate in research must do so willingly and have faith in the integrity of the researchers. This chapter is designed to help you understand the issues related to human participation in research and navigate the processes involved in undertaking an ethical research project. Any research you conduct or any research you draw on to inform your practice must conform to ethical codes of practice.

ETHICAL CODES OF PRACTICE

The word **ethics** is derived from the Greek word *ethos*, which means 'custom habit' or guiding beliefs (Kumari

& Kamala 2017). **Nursing ethics** is defined as 'the examination of all kinds of ethical and bioethical issues from the perspective of nursing theory and practice' (Johnstone 2019, p. 17). Healthcare ethics can be traced back to the late 19th century (Epstein & Turner 2015). At that time, it was thought that ethics involved virtues such as physician loyalty, high moral character and obedience (Epstein & Turner 2015). In 1953 the International Nursing Code of Ethics was developed by the International Council of Nurses (ICN). Now, most individual countries have produced their own version adopted from this code. Nursing codes of ethics have been revised to represent advances in technology, societal changes, cultural influences, advanced nursing practice roles, research, education and health policy.

Nursing codes of ethics help to guide nurses in their daily professional practice and set out the primary goals and values for the profession. Ethical dilemmas arise as nurses care for people and communities and as they interact with other nurses and stakeholders. These dilemmas may, at times, conflict with the code of ethics or with the nurse's individual ethical values. Therefore, nurses must find a balance between advocating and supporting the patient's needs while delivering professional patient care that does not cause harm.

There are seven main **ethical principles** that guide all nursing and midwifery practice.

- **Autonomy**: the right to self-determination. This assumes that the individual or a group of people have the wisdom to make the best choice for themselves.
- **Beneficence**: the concept of doing good. This assumes the performance of actions leading to the potential for benefit through improvements to available care and treatment or through improved knowledge and understanding outcomes that would be regarded as worthwhile.
- **Non-maleficence**: the concept of avoiding harm. This can vary according to context, and influences what we think and do to prevent harm to others.
- **Justice**: the concept that society has a responsibility to treat people fairly. This concept is considered in three categories: fair distribution of resources, respect for people's rights and respect for morally acceptable laws.

- **Confidentiality**: the privacy of written/spoken information or observed behaviour acquired through privileged access.
- **Veracity**: When one's actions, speech and behaviour between individuals and groups of people are truthful and honest.
- **Fidelity**: The obligation to remain faithful to one's commitments to others, particularly promises given in confidence.

PRACTICE VALUES AND ETHICS

Values are the beliefs that members of a group agree with in terms of what is imperative, has merit, is decent or is not immoral. They set standards and the criteria for judging behaviour. Nursing and midwifery research comprises both values and **ethics**. For example, as nurses and midwives, we value evidence. We, therefore, pursue such evidence through research. Ethically, we must obtain the evidence in a way that ensures human participants are fully informed about a study and freely **consent** to the activities involved in research participation.

Ethical behaviour in research is necessary to:
1. uphold the broad aims of research such as information, truth and preventing mistakes
2. endorse the values that are necessary for collaborative research such as trust, responsibility, respect and fairness
3. be accountable to the public that funds and supports research activities
4. ensure high-quality research that is ethical and has integrity in both its conduct and the dissemination of findings
5. adhere to other relevant social values such as human rights, animal welfare, compliance with the law and public safety (Resnik 2020).

The design that researchers choose for their study should be the one best suited to answering the research question while meeting ethical standards. Studies can be either invasive or non-invasive, low risk or high risk, therapeutic or non-therapeutic, and comparative or non-comparative. A study's features and design, and the context in which it is carried out, all factor into the ethical considerations that researchers must make.

STUDENT CHALLENGE

Understanding and Applying Ethics and Values in Practice

1. How might nurses and midwives demonstrate and uphold ethics in research?
2. In what types of situations might nursing values and ethics clash in research?

CASE STUDY 6.1

In reading the literature on maintaining the nutritional status of people with dementia, what ethical issues might Martha (Case study 5.2) expect to see? Remember that the population of interest is older people with cognitive impairment, and some studies report on people living in residential care. What impacts might these factors have on ethical practices such as consent?

BASIC HUMAN RIGHTS IN RESEARCH

Human rights are rights inherent to everyone regardless of our background, where we live, sex, race, religion, language or any other status. They are based on the principles of dignity, equality and mutual respect. Everyone is equally entitled to be free from discrimination. Governments are required to protect people's rights *and so protections are often embedded in law, such as treaties. International human rights law lays down the responsibilities of Governments to act in certain ways or to refrain from certain acts, to promote and protect human rights and the fundamental freedoms of people.*

(**United Nations 2021**)

Four rights must be observed when conducting research. They relate to the right not to be harmed (physically, mentally, emotionally and/or spiritually), the right to treatment, the right to self-determination and autonomy, and the right to **privacy**.

1. *The right not to be harmed* relates to ensuring that people involved in research will have their physical, spiritual, emotional and mental health protected and their dignity preserved. Possible

harm can occur where research interventions pose greater exposure than normal, such as in the case of drug trials, or when the nature of the research causes distress to participants, such as interviewing people following a disaster or traumatic experience. Any procedure conducted in a study must maintain the person's self-respect and self-esteem. This right is related to the principle of beneficence and 'doing good'.

2. *The right to treatment* is a fundamental right in healthcare. In some instances when a person presents for treatment, a researcher might offer an alternative treatment option as part of an experimental trial. Any alternative treatment must be matched by the traditional treatment so that participants are not denied a service that is known to be effective to address their health needs. This right is linked to the principle of justice, where all participants must be treated fairly.

3. *The right to self-determination and autonomy* is related to the principle of respect and includes informed and voluntary consent to participate and the right to refuse to participate or to withdraw at any time without disadvantage. The researcher must make this known to the participant and address any worries they might have about the consequences of declining to participate. While participants may be reimbursed for their participation or offered an incentive to participate, researchers must not induce participation with promises of money or free care.

If a participant decides to withdraw from a project, the researcher must accept that decision. If data have been collected from that participant, those data must be destroyed if they are identifiable or have not already been aggregated into the findings of the project as a whole.

Informed consent relates to participants having full knowledge of the project including:
- the identity and credentials of the researchers
- its purpose and significance
- how they were selected to participate
- everything they will be asked to do, including the amount of time it will take
- any potential risks, discomforts, distress and benefits

- how the data collected will be used and who will have access to it
- how their privacy, confidentiality and anonymity will be maintained and any mandatory reporting requirements
- that consent is voluntary and they may withdraw at any time (as long as their data is identifiable)
- any reimbursements for expenses/time or incentives to participate
- the contact details of the researchers.

Informed consent means that the disclosures made to the participants are kept on file and participants will not be deceived in any way. The participants' dignity and self-respect will be upheld at all times. Informed consent must be given without coercion or influence of any kind. Where a researcher has a relationship with a participant, such as in the case of a university lecturer and students, that researcher must provide the opportunity for the participant to give consent to another member of the research team.

Box 6.1 provides an example of a Participant Information Sheet (sometimes called the Plain Language Statement) and Box 6.2 provides an example of a consent form.

4. *The right to privacy* is taken very seriously and there is privacy legislation to ensure it is maintained. Privacy is also associated with respect.

Any data collection method that could be construed as invading privacy, such as the use of digital recorders and taking photographs or video recordings, must be disclosed to the participant. All data that are collected must be stored safely so that only the research team has access to it. After the research has been completed and after the required period of storage (in most cases between 5 and 10 years), all data are permanently destroyed using the appropriate means: recordings are erased, computer files deleted and paper records shredded.

Any participant identifiers (names or codes) must be kept separate from the research data, and where data are shared between research teams, they must have unique codes so they cannot be linked to the participant by anyone other than the

BOX 6.1
PARTICIPANT INFORMATION SHEET

Participant information [name of organisation]
Full project title:
Principal researcher:
Student researcher:

1. **Introduction**

    You are invited to take part in this research project. This is because you *[reason for selecting the participant]*. This Participant Information Sheet tells you about the research project. It explains what is involved to help you decide if you want to take part.

    Please read this information carefully. Ask questions about anything that you don't understand or want to know more about. Before deciding whether or not to take part, you might want to talk about it with a relative, friend or your local health worker.

    Participation in this research is voluntary. If you don't wish to take part, you don't have to.

    If you decide you want to take part in the research project, you will be asked to sign the consent section. By signing it you are telling us that you:

    ■ understand what you have read
    ■ consent to take part in the research project
    ■ consent to be involved in the procedures described
    ■ consent to the use of your personal and/or health information as described.

    You will be given a copy of this Participant Information Sheet to keep.

2. **What is the purpose of this research project?**

    The aims of the project are to:

    [include the information about the study and its significance]

3. **What does participation in this research project involve?**

    [include everything the participant is required to do]

    All information collected will be de-identified.

    You will not be paid for your participation in this research.

4. **What are the possible benefits?**

    It is anticipated that the outcomes of this research will assist to *[add the anticipated benefits]*.

    There is likely to be no direct benefit to individuals involved in the research.

5. **What are the possible risks?**

    It is unlikely that this research will present any risks to you as an individual. All data collected will be de-identified and recorded in terms of themes. Notes about a particular individual will not be taken.

    If you become upset or distressed as a result of your participation in the research, the researcher will arrange for counselling or other appropriate support. Any counselling or support will be provided by professionals who are not members of the research team.

6. **Do I have to take part in this research project?**

    Participation in this research project is voluntary. If you do not wish to take part, you do not have to.

    You are also free to 'opt out' at any time during the project. You may choose to 'opt out' completely for the duration of the research project, or just 'opt out' for a particular time period.

    If you decide to 'opt out', please notify a member of the research team, so that you can be excluded from further data collection. If you decide to leave the project part-way through, the researchers might be unable to destroy any data, especially if the data already collected has been de-identified.

    Your decision whether or not to take part, or to take part and then withdraw, will not affect your relationship with *[add organisation here]*.

7. **How will I be informed of the final results of this research project?**

    At the completion of the study, a summary report will be made available via … Also, a copy of any publications that are produced from this research will also be made available via …

8. **What will happen to information about me?**

    All hard-copy and electronic data will be stored in a locked filing cabinet in the locked office of the researcher, and will be accessible only to the researchers named on this project. The data associated with this research will be stored for seven (7) years in accordance with the National Statement on Ethical Conduct in Research Involving Humans. Seven years after the completion of this study, all electronic files will be deleted and all paper records will be shredded.

    Data collected in this study will not be included in any other research projects.

    This research does not involve the establishment of a data bank.

    In any publication and/or presentation, information will be provided in such a way that you cannot be identified.

9. **Can I access research information kept about me?**

    In accordance with relevant privacy and other laws, you have the right to access the information collected and stored by the researchers about you; however, all information collected as part of this study will be de-identified, so it is not possible to identify which information relates specifically to you. Please contact one of the researchers named at the end of this document if you would like further information.

BOX 6.1
PARTICIPANT INFORMATION SHEET—cont'd

10. **Is this research project approved?**

The ethical aspects of this research project have been approved by the Human Research Ethics Committee of [*insert name of organisation*].

This project will be carried out according to the National Statement on Ethical Conduct in Human Research (2007) produced by the NHMRC of Australia. This statement has been developed to protect the interests of people who agree to participate in human research studies.

11. **Who can I contact?**
For further information:

If you want any further information concerning this project or if you have any problems that may

be related to your involvement in the project (for example, feelings of distress), you can contact the researcher: [*supply name and contact details*].

For complaints:

If you have any complaints about any aspect of the project, the way it is being conducted or any questions about being a research participant in general, then you may contact:

[*supply name and contact details of ethics complaints officer for your organisation*].

BOX 6.2
PARTICIPANT CONSENT FORM

Project title:
This research project is undertaken by: [*insert name of researcher*]

1. I have read the Participant Information Sheet for this study and have had details of the study explained to me.
2. My questions about the study have been answered to my satisfaction, and I understand that I may ask further questions at any time.
3. I also understand that I am free to decline to answer any particular questions in the study.
4. I agree to provide information to the researchers under the conditions of confidentiality set out on the information sheet.
5. I wish to participate in this study under the conditions set out in the Information Sheet.
6. I understand that my participation is voluntary and I may withdraw at any time.

Contact details: [*insert researcher's contact details*]
Participant Name:
Participant Signature: _____
Date: / /
Researcher Name: _____
Researcher Signature: _____
Date: / /

research team. You should not be able to identify any participant in a research report (anonymity). Therefore, all data are pooled and reported as an aggregate (group information). In the case of interview transcripts, pseudonyms or participant

coding are often used. Any information the participant discloses must not be reported elsewhere except in the case of mandatory reporting requirements, such as suspected child abuse or poor professional practice. In this situation, the requirement for mandatory reporting must be disclosed to the participant before consent is obtained.

HUMAN RIGHTS AND THE VIOLATIONS

We must protect the rights of human participants and there are abundant examples from the past when these rights were violated. In particular, the atrocities of World War II committed by the Nazis, the Milgram (1963) behavioural experiment on student obedience, the Tuskegee syphilis study with African-American men (Brandt 1978), the Willowbrook State School hepatitis study (Krugman 1971), the Porton Down nerve agent experiments (Schmidt 2006) and the New Zealand experiment on women with cervical cancer (Cartwright 1988). Table 6.1 provides a summary of these studies. Nurses were involved in these studies and, while they were not the chief investigators, they were complicit in the unethical treatment of human beings. Nurses and midwives have a responsibility to raise awareness of the ethical conduct of research and to report incidents where research is unethical.

Unethical research might occur in other ways. Researchers themselves might not be ethical in their

TABLE 6.1		
Examples of Unethical Research		
Example	**Description**	**Ethical Issues**
Nazi experiments	Medical experiments performed on concentration camp inmates such as exposing them to freezing temperatures, malaria, poisons and incendiary bombs, among other things, without their consent and with blatant indifference to the suffering of the human participants by the researchers. Many inmates died, were disabled or were disfigured.	Do no harm Right to self-determination Informed consent
Milgram study	An experiment of compliance with authority where student participants thought they were inflicting progressively stronger electric shocks to other participants. The authority figure (experimenter) urged and reassured participants there would be no damage to the person receiving the shocks. However, participants were clearly psychologically distressed at being urged to inflict pain on another person. The associated deception and the requirements of the study caused the participants embarrassment and distress.	Do no harm Right to self-determination Deception Withdrawal of consent
Tuskegee syphilis study	A 40-year study by the United States Public Health Service (1932–1972) where poor rural African-American men with a diagnosis of syphilis were denied treatment (penicillin) so researchers could study the progression of the disease. In addition, they were not told of their diagnosis and were recruited into the study with promises of free healthcare and other inducements.	Right to treatment Right to self-determination Do no harm
Willowbrook State School	Admission of severely disabled children to Willowbrook State School in the United States was granted on the proviso the children enter the hepatitis study. These children were placed in the isolation area and deliberately exposed to hepatitis. The parents of these children were previously told that there were no vaccines at the school.	Right to self-determination Do no harm Vulnerable groups Coercion and inducement
The Porton Down chemical experiments	In the 1950s and 1960s, at the height of the Cold War, British scientists at Porton Down experimented with nerve gases, including sarin, on 1500 military personnel. One participant died, leading to an extensive investigation, but it is unclear how many others had adverse outcomes.	Right to self-determination Do no harm Vulnerable groups
New Zealand cervical cancer study	Commenced in 1966, 948 women with cervical cancer in situ (CIS) were denied active treatment. By 1988, it was determined that these women were four times as likely to develop invasive cancer. It is unclear how many women died as a result of the study. Many were compensated following an inquiry in 1988.	Right to treatment Informed consent

conduct during research. Researchers must act with integrity and honesty while conducting the study and in reporting the findings of their research. For example, there have been fraudulent studies where the research was never actually undertaken; there were faked trials and methods (Martin 1989); or results have been falsified or fabricated (Debaets 2006, Yong, Ledford & Van Noorden 2013). The researchers found to be unethical in these examples were subject to research law. This law is drawn from the laws of consent,

contract, negligence and intellectual property. In addition, laws govern human rights, patents, privacy and data protection, and discrimination (Largent 2016), which all directly influence research activity.

According to Gupta (2013), fraud includes forgery, distortion and stealing of data. Fabrication means that data or results are made up or records are altered. Documents, such as informed consent forms and participant diaries, can also be falsified. It includes the deliberate misrepresentation or exclusion of undesired data or results.

Students will be familiar with the meaning of plagiarism, which is the unacknowledged use of the work and ideas of someone else. Dishonesty in research is using another person's ideas, theories, rhetorical strategies and interpretations, including purposefully ambiguous statements in research proposals or other documents and taking illegitimate credit for that work (Awan, Naureen & Ali 2021).

Much research is supported with funds from various organisations such as government agencies and departments, charities, pharmaceutical and other companies, professional bodies and philanthropic trusts. These funds enable the development and evaluation of programs, the testing of products, the examination of the impact of a policy, or analysis of interest. Consequently, these funding bodies may exert various controls on the research team, including determining whether certain research designs be used or placing restrictions on the publication of the research findings. An acknowledgment of the funding source should be included in the research report. However, any imposition placed on the research process that impedes the collection and dissemination of accurate data and its interpretation is unethical. The Australian National Health and Medical Research Council states:

A conflict of interest may compromise the research process itself and/or the institutional processes governing research and may lead researchers or institutions to base decisions about the research on factors outside the research requirements.

(NHMRC 2007, p. 79)

In the United Kingdom (UK), the UK Research Integrity Office states in its Code of Practice for research that:

Researchers should comply with their organisation's policy for addressing conflicts of interest, as well as any external requirements relating to conflicts of interest, such as those of funding bodies. This should include declaring any potential or actual conflicts of interest relating to their research to: their manager or other appropriate person as identified by their organisation; any ethics committee which reviews their research; and when reporting their findings

at meetings or in publications. Conflicts of interest should be disclosed as soon as researchers become aware of them.

(UK Research Integrity Office 2009)

ETHICAL CODES OF CONDUCT

As the knowledge of those early experiments and breaches of integrity became public, inquiries were undertaken and codes of ethics were developed. The most notable is the Nuremberg Code of 1949 (US National Institutes of Health 2014). In Nuremberg, Germany, Nazis were tried for crimes against humanity, including the unethical treatment of people in research (Box 6.3). Following that, the World Medical Association (WMA) was formed and, by 1964, the Declaration of Helsinki was ratified (WMA 2014), building on the Nuremberg Code. The Declaration of Helsinki has been revised numerous times and now includes reference to:

- the duty of researchers to protect human rights
- scientifically defensible research
- research being reviewed by an independent human ethics committee

BOX 6.3
CRITERIA IN THE NUREMBERG CODE

- Researchers must inform participants about their studies and obtain voluntary consent.
- Research must be for the good of the society.
- Where possible animals should be used for experiments rather than humans.
- Researchers must avoid harming participants.
- No study must be undertaken where serious injury or death might occur.
- The degree of risk must not outweigh the benefit of the study.
- Proper facilities and preparation must be made to protect participants from harm.
- Researchers must be qualified to undertake research.
- Participants can stop the research if problems arise.
- Researchers must cease the study if they believe that an unacceptable risk to participants has arisen.

Source: US Government Printing Office: Trials of war criminals before the Nuremberg Military Tribunals under Control Council Law 10(2):181–182. Washington, 1949.

- research that is lawful
- special protections for children and other vulnerable groups
- research reports that are accurate and include both positive and negative results.

A Code of Ethics for nurses was first adopted by the ICN in 1953. It was not until 1988 that the New Zealand Nurses Organisation produced a Code of Ethics specific to Aotearoa (NZNO 2019). In New Zealand, the Code of Ethics includes consideration of Māori values. In Australia, the NHMRC provides clear guidelines and codes regarding what constitutes ethical research (NHMRC 2018b). New Zealand's National Ethics Advisory Committee, also known as Kāhui Matatika o te Motu, has published the National Ethical Standards for Health and Disability Research and Quality Improvement (NEAC 2019). These guidelines are also used by Health and Disability Ethics Committees (HDECs) that review research study proposals to check that each study meets the ethical standards set out in NEAC's guidelines.

The UK Research Integrity Office (2009) has published a Code of Practice for Research. In the United States (US), the National Institutes of Health published Guiding Principles for Ethical Research (2016). It is imperative that any research plan has accounted for the ethical considerations. When you are reading research reports, you will note that authors clearly outline how they managed any ethical dilemmas they anticipated or encountered.

VULNERABLE GROUPS

Several groups that are of interest to nursing and midwifery researchers are considered to be vulnerable because they have diminished capacity to give informed consent or are considered to be vulnerable populations as they are not completely free to give consent.

Children, fetuses, people living with mental illness or intellectual disabilities, and those with impaired consciousness or cognition are considered not to have the capacity to deliberate the risks and benefits of a research project. Therefore, they have limited capacity to give informed consent to participate. While, increasingly, these people may be involved in the consent process, informed consent to undertake research with these groups often will need to be obtained from the parent or legal guardian. In the case of minors between 10 and 18 years of age, it is wise to provide them with the information about the study as they have the right to assent to participate so that a parent or guardian knows and understands the wishes of the minor before consenting for their child to participate.

People with life-limiting illnesses might also be considered vulnerable as their consent to participate may be predicated on the hope that they will be cured of their illness. In their desire for a cure, such individuals might agree to research procedures or treatments that could be harmful.

Persons who are incarcerated are also considered vulnerable because they are not really 'free' to give consent. They might believe that agreeing to participate could lessen their sentence. In addition, ordinary financial compensation could be seen as a very large sum by people with limited earning capacity, which may place them in a precarious position in relation to other prisoners.

Members of the armed services are considered vulnerable as they might not question the researcher's intent or the procedures, and they may agree to participate because it is customary for them to obey without question. They might not see that they can refuse to participate or can withdraw without penalty because they are trained to obey orders.

Other groups that might feel compelled to participate include students and employees. Both these groups could have a dependent or unequal relationship with the researcher, especially if the researcher is the student's teacher or an employee's manager. Even if the research is being undertaken by another student or employee, the recruitment of these participants must be undertaken from classes or workplaces where the researcher has little or no involvement. In that way, participants will be free to consent or not, without feeling they have been coerced or influenced.

Lastly, we must also be sensitive to the cultural background of potential research participants. In some cultures, it is seen as polite to agree to a request to participate, especially if that request is made by someone who is deemed to be an authority. Therefore, consent may be given even if the person is unclear or hesitant about the research. All information provided to people from culturally and linguistically diverse (CALD) backgrounds must be in a language they can understand,

and they must be given an opportunity to ask questions in the appropriate language. Unfortunately, many researchers make the requirement to speak English an inclusion criterion for their research. While this may be due to resource constraints, this eliminates a potential source of rich data from people whose primary language is not English.

It is also important to recognise the special needs of Indigenous people. For example, there is great diversity across the many Indigenous cultures and societies; research involving these groups requires special consideration and is governed by discrete guidelines (NEAC 2019, NHMRC 2018a). For more detailed discussion on Indigenous issues in research, refer to Chapter 10.

In New Zealand, the National Ethical Standards for Health and Disability Research and Quality Improvement standards (NEAC 2019) reflect the principles of the Te Tiriti O Waitangi (founding document of Aotearoa, New Zealand) by incorporating Te Ara Tika, which is a set of Māori ethical principles that draw on the foundation of tikanga (Māori protocols and practices). Te Ara Tika means 'to follow the right path' and is used as a generic set of principles commonly shared by many generations and communities of Māori; however, they apply to all people in Aotearoa New Zealand (Hudson et al 2010). In addition, the standards have a separate section dedicated to research involving Māori. It is expected that all health and disability researchers in New Zealand are aware of these standards and that they implement these when undertaking any health and disability research.

The NHMRC's Guidelines for Ethical Conduct in Aboriginal and Torres Strait Islander Research are based on six core values identified as being important to Aboriginal and Torres Strait Islander peoples. The use of these core values, and other cultural and local language conventions, should be decided by the Aboriginal and Torres Strait Islander communities or groups involved in the research (NHMRC 2018a). The six core values are:

1. reciprocity
2. respect
3. equality
4. responsibility
5. survival and protection
6. spirit and integrity.

For further information related to Indigenous people, please refer to Chapter 10 of this book.

Care must be taken to consider the needs of vulnerable groups, as simply excluding them from research can serve to perpetuate inequities and be unethical as it does not allow their voice to be heard through research. Chapter 11 provides further insight into ensuring diversity of participants that can include strategies to engage vulnerable groups.

CASE STUDY 6.2

While studying the literature on people with learning disabilities who are living with type 1 diabetes, Jamie notices that most of the research is focused on the perspectives and views of carers and health professionals. There are several papers on carer burden, but no papers on the burden to the person with the learning disability and diabetes. Many papers cite ethical issues for excluding recruitment of people with learning disabilities as they are not able to give consent. What is your view on that? How might this omission influence what is known about the issues for this population?

UNDERSTANDING THE RISKS AND BENEFITS OF RESEARCH

Risk is the potential for people to be harmed through participation in a study. All researchers must balance the potential for harm against the overall benefits of the research to both the participant and the broader community. There are risks associated with data collection methods, special groups, the relationship between the researcher and the participant, confidentiality and privacy, incentives and inducements, the reporting of the outcomes of the research and where the study is located. The researcher needs to assess each of these risks and mitigate each one so that the rights of participants are not violated. Sometimes an adverse outcome cannot be predicted or was considered highly unlikely to occur. However, should this occur, the researcher must manage the outcome appropriately and notify the proper authority. When you read a research report, you will see the rationale for the

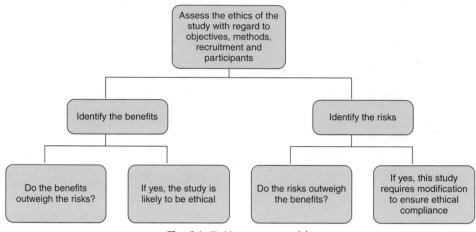

Fig. 6.1 ■ How to assess risk.

project. This usually outlines the benefits of the study and any risks that might be involved.

Fig. 6.1 shows how to assess risk.

HUMAN RESEARCH ETHICS COMMITTEES

All institutions involved in research must convene an institutional ethics committee. While in Australia they are commonly called a Human Research Ethics Committee (HREC) (NHMRC 2018b), in the UK, they are called Research Ethics Committees (RECs) (UK NHS Health Research Authority 2021) and in the US they are known as Institutional Review Boards (IRBs) (US Food & Drug Administration 2019). Ethics committees are often composed of both lay people and experts. Members may include researchers, statisticians, lawyers, clergy and consumers. Each member assesses the research project according to the rules that govern such committees and according to their individual expertise and interest. All research requiring human participants must secure ethical approval from a Human Research Ethics Committee before recruiting any participants or collecting any data.

Ethics committees have two functions: to assess the scientific merit of a project and to assess the risk to participants that the project poses. Some have argued that as an ethics committee, their remit is to judge the ethical and not the scientific issues within a proposal and that these scientific issues should be left to another

body. However, research that is not scientifically rigorous is also not ethical as it is inappropriate to expose participants to research that is poorly constructed and would have no clear contribution to knowledge generation (Dingwall et al 2017). The methods sections of research reports should describe the design, methods, procedures and analysis to be undertaken clearly so that the scientific aspects of the project can be scrutinised. Authors should also include any limitations of the project to explain aspects where the credibility of the research must be evaluated.

In Australia, institutional ethics committees require the researcher to apply for ethics review and may require the use of an application form that is produced by that institution or the use of the NHMRC Human Research Ethics Application (HREA) (available at https://www. nhmrc.gov.au) or both. The HREA is designed for projects that involve multiple committees and is intended to reduce the effort by researchers in completing multiple forms. However, it is generally the case that the researcher is required to submit the HREA as well as the local form.

In New Zealand, two types of ethics committees conduct ethical reviews. The Health and Disability Ethics Committees (HDECs), which are ministerial committees, and institutional ethics committees (IEC). As a general guide, research originating in a tertiary educational institution will normally be reviewed by an ethics committee of that institution (an IEC). HDECs requires the researcher to apply for ethics review (HDEC forms available at https://ethics.health.

govt.nz/guides-templates-and-forms/) if it involves one of the following: consumers or relatives of health or disability support services including for clinical trials, use of human tissue and the use of or disclosure of health information. Approval is given if the study meets the ethical standards as determined by the NEAC Kāhui Matatika o te Motu.

In the UK, applications for ethical approval which involve accessing participants through the NHS are made through the Integrated Research Application System (IRAS) via the NHS Health Research Authority (available at https://www.myresearchproject.org.uk). Similar to the HREA, the IRAS is a one-step procedure for applying for ethical approval for health research and enables the researcher to enter information about a project once, rather than reproduce the information in multiple application forms. There are different requirements for ethical approval if your research participants are staff or students.

It is the responsibility of the researcher to identify all the ethical issues and risks and state how each will be addressed. When the ethics committee is satisfied the research is sound methodologically and ethically, approval is given. The approval is for a defined period and the researcher must provide interim and final reports to the committee. Any unforeseen consequences of the research must be reported to the committee immediately and any modification to the research plan must also be approved. You will note when you read research articles that the researchers often state that ethical approval has been granted and cite the approval number.

PUBLISHING YOUR RESEARCH

Part of the ethical conduct of research is to make the results widely known. Ethics committees will seek confirmation that dissemination of the results will be undertaken in a range of ways. For example, the results may be published in peer-reviewed journal articles, conference presentations, summary sheets provided to research participants and reports to funding agencies. There are important guidelines for ethical publication of research.

The ICMJE (International Committee of Medical Journal Editors) has compiled a guide for authors. Importantly, to be an author you must have made a substantial contribution to the conception or design of the work or the acquisition, analysis or interpretation of data for the work; AND drafted the paper or revised it critically for important intellectual content; AND agreed to final approval of the version to be published; AND agreed to be accountable for all aspects of the work in ensuring that questions related to the accuracy or integrity of any part of the work are appropriately investigated and resolved.

(ICMJE 2022)

Furthermore, it is deemed highly unethical to:
- submit or publish the same paper in more than one journal without informing the editors
- not inform a collaborator that you intend to publish the research
- include a colleague as an author if that person did not contribute significantly to the paper
- discuss confidential material from a paper that you are peer reviewing
- use data, ideas or methods from a paper that you are peer reviewing
- manipulate data without discussing how and why this was done in your paper (Resnik 2020).

STUDENT CHALLENGE
Navigating the Ethics and Etiquette of Researcher Collaboration

Ahmed, the undergraduate student you have met previously, is planning a qualitative study in which he will explore the experiences of patients who have chronic health problems while they care for others. Ahmed plans to interview people who have chronic health problems and care for others in their own homes, such as the 87-year-old man with chronic heart failure and newly diagnosed COPD, who also has carer responsibilities for his 85-year-old wife living with dementia.

Ahmed is considering the issues he will need to consider when applying for research ethics approval.
1. What research ethical principles might inform Ahmed's thinking when planning this research?
2. What issues might most concern the research ethics committee about interviewing participants who have both chronic conditions and are caring for others?
3. To what risks will Ahmed be exposed in this research and how might the risks be minimised?
4. What issues will Ahmed need to consider when planning his dissemination strategy, including sharing findings with research participants?

CONCLUSION

This chapter has provided an overview of navigating the issues related to the ethics of research and the process of obtaining ethical approval to undertake research. We have examined: the relationship between ethics and values; the basic rights of humans and vulnerable and special groups; how studies have been conducted that have not been ethical; and the process for achieving ethical approval for research. Finally, we have addressed the issues related to ethical publishing of research. As you read research reports, you should be able to identify the ethical issues that were addressed by the researchers. Scientific methods and ethics are fundamental to good research. They are inseparable, and while navigating the ethics approval process might seem like a hindrance to undertaking your research, it is essential to protect the rights of both the participant and the researcher.

ADDITIONAL RESOURCES

The following websites are helpful to understand your ethical responsibilities in conducting research projects.

Australia: *Privacy Act 1988*: https://www.oaic.gov. au/privacy-law/privacy-act

Health & Disability Commissioner, Code of Health and Disability Consumer's Rights: https://www. hdc.org.nz/your-rights/about-the-code/code-of-health-and-disability-services-consumers-rights

Health Research Authority, Research Ethics Committees overview: https://www.hra.nhs. uk/about-us/committees-and-services/res-and-recs/research-ethics-committees-overview

National Health and Medical Research Council, Australian Code for the Responsible Conduct of Research: https://www.nhmrc.gov.au/about-us/publications/australian-code-responsible-conduct-research-2018

National Health and Medical Research Council, National Statement on Ethical Conduct in Human Research: https://nhmrc.gov.au/about-us/publications/national-statement-ethical-conduct-human-research-2007-updated-2018

National Institutes of Health, Guiding Principles for Ethical Research: https://www.nih.gov/health-information/nih-clinical-research-trials-you/guiding-principles-ethical-research

New Zealand Nurses Organisation, Guideline—Code of Ethics, 2019: https://www.nzno.org. nz/Portals/0/publications/Guideline%20-%20Code%20of%20Ethics%202019.pdf?ver=19LQpYx8wspprjbTNt9pWw%3d%3d.

New Zealand: *Privacy Act 2020*: https://www. legislation.govt.nz/act/public/2020/0031/latest/LMS23223.html

UK Research Integrity Office, Promoting good practice and preventing misconduct 2009: http://ukrio.org/publications/code-of-practice-for-research

REFERENCES

Awan R, Naureen G, Ali G: Academic dishonesty among youth: faculty and students' perceptions about plagiarism in research work, Research Journal of Social Sciences and Economics Review 2(2):436–443, 2021. https://ojs.rjsser.org.pk/index.php/rjsser/article/view/372.

Brandt AM: Racism and research: the case of the Tuskegee syphilis study, Hastings Centre Report 8(6):21–29, 1978.

Cartwright S: The report of the committee of inquiry into allegations concerning the treatment of cervical cancer at National Women's Hospital and into other related matters, Auckland, 1988, Government Printing Office.

Debaets AM: Korean cloning scandal and scientific fraud, Ethics and Medicine 22(1):61–62, 2006.

Dingwall R, Iphofen R, Lewis J, et al: Towards common principles for social science research ethics: a discussion document for the academy of social sciences. In Iphofen R (ed), Finding common ground: consensus in research ethics across the social sciences, Advances in research ethics and integrity, 1, Bingley, 2017, Emerald Publishing Limited, pp. 111–123.

Epstein B, Turner M: The nursing code of ethics: its value, its history, Online Journal of Issues in Nursing 31 May;20(2):4, 2015.

Gupta A: Fraud and misconduct in clinical research: a concern, Perspectives in Clinical Research 4(2):144–147, 2013.

Hudson M, Smith B, Milne M, et al: Te Ara Tika: Guidelines for Māori research ethics: a framework for researchers and ethics committee members, Auckland, 2010, Health Research Council of New Zealand. https://www.hrc.govt.nz/resources/te-ara-tika-guidelines-maori-research-ethics-0.

International Committee of Medical Journal Editors: Defining the role of authors and contributors, ICMJE, 2022. https://www.icmje.org/recommendations/browse/roles-and-responsibilities/defining-the-role-of-authors-and-contributors.html.

Johnstone MJ: Bioethics: a nursing perspective, ed 7, Melbourne, 2019, Elsevier.

Krugman S: Experiments at the Willowbrook State School, Lancet 8 May;1(7706):966–967, 1971. http://doi.org/10.1016/s0140-6736(71)91462-0.

Kumari DN, Kamla SM: Core human values and professional ethics, International Journal of Multidisciplinary Educational Research 6(4):94–104, 2017.

Largent E: Recently proposed changes to legal and ethical guidelines governing human subjects research, Journal of Law and the Biosciences 3(1):206–216, 2016.

Martin B: Fraud and Australian academics, Thought and Action 5(2):95–102, 1989.

Milgram S: Behavioural study of obedience, Journal of Abnormal and Social Psychology 67(4):371–378, 1963.

National Ethics Advisory Committee (NEAC): National ethical standards for health and disability research and quality improvement, Wellington, 2019, Ministry of Health. https://neac.health.govt.nz/publications-and-resources/neac-publications/national-ethical-standards-for-health-and-disability-research-and-quality-improvement/.

National Health and Medical Research Council (NHMRC): National statement on ethical conduct in human research, 2007. https://nhmrc.gov.au/research-policy/ethics/national-statement-ethical-conduct-human-research.

National Health and Medical Research Council (NHMRC): Guidelines for ethical conduct in Aboriginal and Torres Strait Islander research, 2018a. https://nhmrc.gov.au/research-policy/ethics/ethical-guidelines-research-aboriginal-and-torres-strait-islander-peoples.

National Health and Medical Research Council (NHMRC): Australian code for the responsible conduct of research, 2018b. https://nhmrc.gov.au/about-us/publications/australian-code-responsible-conduct-research-2018.

National Institutes of Health (NIH): Guiding principles for ethical research, 2016. https://www.nih.gov/health-information/nih-clinical-research-trials-you/guiding-principles-ethical-research.

New Zealand Nurses Organisation (NZNO): Guideline—Code of Ethics, 2019, Wellington, NZNO, 2019. https://www.nzno.org.nz/Portals/0/publications/Guideline%20-%20Code%20of%20Ethics%202019.pdf?ver=19LQpYx8wspprjbTNt9pWw%3d%3d.

Resnik D: What is ethics in research & why is it important? National Institute of Environmental and Health Sciences 23 Dec, 2020. https://www.niehs.nih.gov/research/resources/bioethics/whatis/index.cfm.

Schmidt U: Cold War at Porton Down: informed consent in Britain's biological and chemical warfare experiments, Cambridge Quarterly of Healthcare Ethics 15(4):366–380, 2006.

UK NHS Health Research Authority: 2022. https://www.hra.nhs.uk.

UK Research Integrity Office: Code of practice for research: promoting good practice and preventing misconduct, Croydon, 2009, UK Research Integrity Office.

United Nations: Office of the High Commissioner for Human Rights: what are human rights? 2021. https://www.ohchr.org/en/what-are-human-rights.

US Food & Drug Administration: Institutional review boards (IRBs) and protection of human subjects in clinical trials, 2012. https://www.fda.gov/about-fda/center-drug-evaluation-and-research-cder/institutional-review-boards-irbs-and-protection-human-subjects-clinical-trials.

US National Institutes of Health: Nuremberg Code, 2014. https://history.nih.gov/research/downloads/nuremberg.pdf.

World Medical Association: Declaration of Helsinki, 2014. https://www.wma.net/publications/wma-doh-1964-2014/.

Yong E, Ledford H, Van Noorden R: Research ethics: 3 ways to blow the whistle, Nature 503(7477):454–457, 2013.

7 QUANTITATIVE RESEARCH

ROCHELLE WYNNE ■ EAMON MERRICK ■ JOANNE BROOKE

CHAPTER OUTLINE

LEARNING OBJECTIVES

After reading this chapter and following critical reflection, readers should be able to:

■ define quantitative research

■ describe quantitative research classifications

■ discuss the phases of the research process as they relate to quantitative research

■ describe how a quantitative study is designed

■ describe the steps involved in conducting a quantitative study

■ describe the process of analysing quantitative data

■ describe how quantitative results are applied in practice

■ discuss the relationships among phases of the research process using a quantitative method

■ cite examples of steps and phases of the research process using a quantitative method.

KEY TERMS

alternative hypothesis
blinding
concurrent validity
confidence interval
control group
correlation
data
dependent variable
descriptive statistics
distribution
directional hypothesis
extraneous variables
face validity
generalisation
hypothesis
independent variable
inferential statistics
instrument
non-experimental research

normal distribution
null hypothesis
power analysis
predictive validity
probability
problem statement
p-value
quantitative research
quasi-experimental research
randomisation
reliability
research design
research process
type 1 error
type 2 error
validity
variable

ABSTRACT

Quantitative research approaches follow systematic logical processes to answer questions about measurable concepts. Quantitative research projects are classified as experimental or descriptive (non-experimental) and enable the researcher to solve a problem using numeric data to evaluate an intervention or describe a situation. The type of quantitative design chosen will be determined by the project aims, the variables to be measured and the researcher's capacity to control or manipulate variables during the research process.

The research process is comprised of five phases from the formulation and development of researchable questions to confirmation of probable answers.

1. *Conceptualising the study*: thinking about the problem and how this relates to existing research and theory, and stating a research question.
2. *Designing the study*: a plan is developed that specifies a research design, the subject or participants to be studied, the instruments that will be used to take measurements and how the data will be analysed.
3. *Conducting the study*: the study plan is implemented and data is collected.
4. *Analysing study data*: data analysis is completed, ensuring that the research questions are answered and placed within context.
5. *Using the study*: the results are examined for their relevance to clinical practice and future research.

Results are compared to existing evidence and placed within the context of what is already known. Recommendations are suggested for practice, education and future research. These recommendations are communicated to clinicians, policymakers, researchers, higher education institutes and the wider public.

STUDENT QUOTE

To answer interesting questions, you need to collect data and then explain it. Quantitative research is a bit like cooking: the study design or recipe has the type of ingredients or variables you need, and how they should be combined or measured and analysed to achieve a tasty end-product or reliable results. If you can follow a recipe or the design of a study, you can bake a cake or competently complete a quantitative study.

INTRODUCTION

In this chapter, different types of quantitative **research designs** and quantitative research processes are defined, described and discussed. Quantitative research language can be challenging to read and understand at first. This is to be expected when you are learning a new way of thinking about things. The more you read about and reflect on the new terms, the more familiar they will become. Quantitative research underpins evidence-based practice. The ability to appraise evidence is a lifelong skill that begins with understanding quantitative concepts. It is important to remember not everything that can be counted counts, and not everything that counts can be counted! At the end of this chapter, you will understand what is needed to critically read, consider and use quantitative research to inform practice.

WHAT IS QUANTITATIVE RESEARCH?

Quantitative research is a systematic, objective process used to gather and analyse numeric information. Experimental quantitative methods can be used to generate and test theories, describe relationships or examine relationships between cause and effect. In contrast, descriptive (non-experimental) quantitative methods provide a detailed insight into a group of people, a particular situation or context. Quantitative methods take a systematic and logical approach to finding answers. In a specific study, variables come from the concepts identified in the problem statement and are specified in the research questions or hypotheses. The population to be studied is also specified in the research questions or hypotheses. Box 7.1 provides examples of research questions and hypotheses derived from problem statements.

Hypotheses

Hypotheses are required in all experimental quantitative studies. All hypotheses contain at least one independent variable and at least one dependent variable. Simple hypotheses contain one independent and one dependent variable. Other hypotheses are called complex hypotheses because they contain more than one independent and/or dependent variable. Example 3 in

---

BOX 7.1
SAMPLE PROBLEM STATEMENTS, RESEARCH QUESTIONS
AND HYPOTHESES*

PROBLEM STATEMENTS

1. Common characteristics possessed by older individuals who seek care in an emergency department.
2. The effect of parental presence on anxiety and behaviour of young children undergoing suture repair of a laceration.
3. There may be a relationship between implementation of a stimulation protocol on oxygenation of premature infants.
4. Effect of meat-eating on serum cholesterol in healthy men aged 55 to 60 years.

QUESTIONS/HYPOTHESES

1. What percentage of total emergency department visits are by older individuals over the age of 65? What are the chief presenting complaints of older people? Is use affected by time of day, season of year, availability of general practitioner, public or private status, gender or age of the person? (research questions)
2. Will there be a difference between the anxiety levels and disruptive behaviours of young children whose parents are present during laceration repair versus those with no parental presence? (research question)
3. Premature infants who receive extra tactile stimulation will have higher pO_2 levels than those who do not. (directional hypothesis)
4. There will be no difference in serum cholesterol in healthy meat-eating and non-meat-eating males aged 55 to 60 years. (null hypothesis)

---

*Examples are taken from student theses.

Box 7.1 shows a hypothesis that predicts one group of infants will be better oxygenated than another group. The independent variable in this hypothesis is the presence or absence of extra tactile stimulation and the dependent variable is pO_2 level. The population is premature infants. Hypotheses can also be further classified; (Box 7.1) a **null hypothesis** predicts there will be no relationship between the independent and dependent variables in a specified population. An **alternative hypothesis** predicts a particular relationship between the independent and dependent variables. A **directional hypothesis** specifies the direction of the predicted relationship between the independent and dependent variables.

A **hypothesis** is an 'educated guess' about the relationships between variables and the expected outcomes of the study. It is a statement about the nature of the relationship(s) between variables. The results of the study will either support or refute the hypothesis. The researcher will state both the hypothesis and the opposite (or null) hypothesis. A null hypothesis is usually a negative statement that assumes the intervention or variable of interest will have no effect. For example, if the hypothesis states there is a relationship, then the null will state there is not a relationship. The hypothesis and null hypothesis support the researcher to consider two important errors that can occur,

namely: type 1 and type 2 errors (Banerjee et al 2009). In a **type 1 error**, the researcher believes that there is an effect, when in fact there is not, and incorrectly rejects the null hypothesis. In a **type 2 error**, the researcher believes there is no effect, when in fact there has been an effect, and incorrectly accepts the null hypothesis. To test the hypothesis, answer your research question or solve your problem, you need to define the *variables* you want to measure and the *data* you will collect.

Variables

Most problems, questions and hypotheses are described using a proposed cause and a proposed outcome or effect. **Variables** are identified concepts or traits that are measured, manipulated or controlled in an experimental quantitative study. A variable is a concept or trait that varies. The variable thought to be the cause is known as the predictor or **independent variable** because it does not depend on other variables. The outcome or effect is called the **dependent variable** because it depends on the cause (independent variable). In experimental research, researchers will try to manipulate the independent variable to test the effect it has on the dependent variable, or they will assess the effect of the predictor variable on the outcome. For example, a researcher may be interested in finding the optimal dose of an antiemetic medication (independent variable) to reduce the frequency and/or severity of nausea and vomiting in pregnant women (dependent variable).

However, it is also important to think about other things that may affect this relationship. **Extraneous variables** can affect the dependent variable and interfere with the relationship between the independent and dependent variables. There are many types of extraneous variables and they may be associated with the sample, the researcher or the environment. Some extraneous variables can be expected to play a role in the relationship between the independent and dependent variables. These expected variables can moderate and/or mediate the expected relationship between the independent and dependent variables (these are referred to as moderating and mediating variables). If a researcher was exploring the impact of a pressure-relieving mattress (independent) on sleep quality (dependent), some extraneous variables might be the room temperature, noise levels and/or the comfort of clothing worn. Researchers try to identify all potential extraneous variables so they can control them and keep them from interfering with the relationship between the independent and dependent variables. If they cannot be controlled, then researchers will try to measure them so the size of the effect can be calculated. Sampling and statistical techniques are used to help the researcher exert control over extraneous variables. An extraneous variable that impacts the outcome of the study is called a confounding variable.

Levels of Measurement

Variables can be measured on scales that range from categorical to continuous. Categorical variables have categories that in their simplest form contain just two categories, which are called binary or dichotomous variables (e.g. dead or alive, pregnant or non-pregnant). If there are more than two options then the variable is nominal (e.g. red hair, blonde hair, black hair, brown hair). If these options travel in a specific direction, they are called ordinal (e.g. low, medium, high).

Continuous variables reflect any value on the measurement scale being used. Data measured on the interval level has the same difference between each unit of measurement, equal intervals represent equal differences. Data measured on the ratio level have the same interval, but the scale has to begin with zero and

scores have to make sense (e.g. 200 grams of chocolate is twice as much as 100 grams and half of 400 grams). Data measured on a discrete level can only have certain values (e.g. a 5-point scale, which only has values of 1 to 5).

The measurement of data is undertaken using an instrument. **Instruments**, such as questionnaires, sphygmomanometers or pulse oximeters, are used to capture measures and collect numerical information. Instruments need to be valid and measure what they set out to measure and reliable in that they measure what they set out to measure consistently. Data are valid when instrument measurements are the same as objective criteria (criterion validity). When a new instrument provides the same measurement outcomes as an old instrument, it has **concurrent validity**, and if an instrument can be used to predict observations again later, it has **predictive validity**. It does not matter what types of quantitative research you do, the level of measurement and instrument validity will underpin how reliable the results are.

TYPES OF QUANTITATIVE RESEARCH METHODS

The spectrum of healthcare research is sometimes described in terms of bringing evidence from 'the bench to the bedside'. Basic research or bench-based research is often undertaken in a laboratory to generate hypotheses. This type of research can be done without necessarily thinking about the practical use of the research results. Research that happens in the clinical context is called applied research and is designed to test hypotheses and solve practical problems for, and often with, the people who will benefit. Nursing and midwifery are practice-based professions and so most of the research undertaken within these disciplines is applied. Basic and applied research reflect either end of the spectrum that is used to generate evidence. The overarching methods of quantitative research can be used in both basic and applied research. Quantitative research can be categorised as either experimental or descriptive (**non-experimental research**) depending on the nature of the research question.

Experimental Methods

Experimental designs are characterised by three factors, namely: manipulation of a variable; use of a

control group; and random assignment of participants. These three factors give the researcher greater control over the experiment and reduce the chances that changes in the dependent variable are caused by extraneous variables.

Experimental studies are designed to test cause and effect by manipulating variables and comparing outcomes between a treatment/intervention group and the control group/usual care. By manipulating the independent variable, the researchers can measure how this variable (often a treatment) will change or affect the dependent variable (outcome).

A control group is essential to ensure the change in the dependent variable is due to the manipulation of the independent variable (the treatment) and not some other extraneous variable. The researcher will allocate some of the participants into the control group and some participants into a treatment group. Participants allocated into the control group receive the 'usual' or 'normal' treatment. The control group is used to compare outcomes to those who receive the treatment (experimental group). If the dependent variable changes for the treatment group and does not change for the control group, and there is no evidence of extraneous variables, then it can be concluded that the treatment is probably causing the change.

Randomisation means that there is an equal chance of each participant being allocated into either the experimental or the control group. The allocation is done in a random way so that the researcher cannot influence or bias who is allocated into each group. In some research, each group has an equal chance of being designated as the treatment group (cluster randomisation). Additionally, in some studies, even the researchers do not know which group is receiving the treatment. This is referred to as **blinding**. In example 3 in Box 7.1, the infants were randomly assigned to group 1 and group 2 using a table of random numbers (Table 7.1). The treatment group was then selected by placing two pieces of paper with the words 'group 1' and 'group 2' in a hat. One piece of paper was drawn and that group was designated as the treatment group.

The **Randomised Controlled Trial** (RCT) is the traditional and most rigorous form of experimental research. Findings from a well-designed RCT are Level II evidence as defined by the National Health and Medical Research Council (NHMRC). The most common type of RCT is a parallel study where participants

TABLE 7.1									
Sample of a Section of a Table of Random Numbers									
77	51	30	38	20	19	50	23	71	74
21	81	85	93	13	51	47	46	64	99
99	55	96	83	31	86	83	42	99	01
69	97	92	02	88	93	27	88	17	57
68	10	72	36	21	62	53	52	41	70

are randomised to treatment or control; there can be different types of treatment, but participants stay in the group to which they have been allocated for the duration of the trial. In crossover RCTs, participants have treatment A then crossover to treatment B and vice versa. In this kind of study, each participant serves as their own control. There are also cluster RCTs where randomisation is not at the subject level but by group, for example, by hospital or ward. Cluster RCTs are often used to avoid the intervention and control groups from influencing or contaminating each other and potentially changing the outcomes of the trial. For example, patients who attend the same practitioner may discuss the steps involved in a smoking cessation trial in the waiting room and consequently change their behaviour. Randomising at a cluster level will prevent this contamination. There may also be practical reasons for using a cluster RCT design, for example, it would be impractical to allocate half of the nurses or midwives in one department to 12-hour shifts and the other half to 8-hour shifts. It would, however, be feasible to compare two different intensive care units with similar staff and patient profiles, with randomly allocated 12- or 8-hour shift schedules.

Clinical trials also have phases (Box 7.2) that align with ensuring safety during testing. Look at example 3 in Box 7.1. This is an experimental study. The researcher had two groups of premature infants. The treatment group received the extra tactile stimulation treatment (manipulation). The control group received the usual care given by the nurses in the neonatal intensive care unit (NICU). Oxygen (pO_2) levels (dependent variable) were measured for both groups. The researcher was observing to see if there was a difference in pO_2 for the treatment group compared to the control group.

lower doses and had better compliance with their insulin. While quasi-experimental designs are often used, the data is not as strong as that gained from experimental studies as it is more vulnerable to threats to **validity** and **reliability**.

Observational Methods

Research Questions

In experimental research, we test hypotheses and manipulate variables. When a study contains independent and dependent variables and the independent variable cannot be manipulated, it may be because all outcome events have already occurred, or it would be morally or ethically wrong to manipulate these variables. When hypothesis testing is not possible or desirable, researchers will ask a research question to describe or explore the problem. Research questions in observational, non-experimental or descriptive quantitative research use an interrogative format to identify the variables to be studied and possible relationships or differences between those variables. Example 1 in Box 7.3 is from a descriptive study and shows a question used to identify and describe the variables

Quasi-experimental research designs involve the comparison of outcomes between a treatment and control group but without randomisation. This type of quantitative study is also sometimes called a non-equivalent control group, a pre-test/post-test study or a time-series study. Randomisation enables a researcher to control for variability caused by unknown factors or unsystematic variation. In quasi-experimental research, researchers do their best to control for unsystematic variation. Quasi-experimental studies are one of the most popular designs used in quantitative nursing and midwifery research, as it is often not possible to blind or randomly allocate participants to groups. For example, Huang and colleagues (2022) tested the effect of nurse-led online education for patients with type 2 diabetes mellitus (T2DM). In their quasi-experimental study, participants were divided into two groups according to the time in which they were prescribed insulin rather than being randomised. The treatment group received systematic online health education and the control group usual care involving education and medical follow-up. The results demonstrated that patients in the treatment group required (number of emergency department [ED] visits, chief complaints, time of day, season of year, ED category, payment method, gender and age) and the population (older adults using the ED). The second example is from an exploratory study and shows a question used to ask about differences in two dependent variables (anxiety levels and disruptive behaviours) for two different groups of people (children with and without parental presence). Parental presence/absence is the independent variable and young children with lacerations are the population. Research questions serve as queries about variables and how they might interact with one another.

Correlational Research

When we explore data to solve a problem, we try and find relationships or **correlations** between variables. For example, Milesky, Baptiste and Shelton (2017) explored how the provision of education, mentoring and real-time feedback to motivated staff may lead to improvements in handover communication methods, yielding positive patient outcomes. In another study, Slater, Stanik-Hutt and Davidson (2017) explored the potential of cerebral oximetry monitoring to identify adult patients at risk of neurological complications after surgery. When the research is focused on a particular disease or condition, we might match *cases to controls* or follow groups of participants, known as a *cohort*, from exposure to outcome. For example, Curtis and colleagues (2021) examined the impact of implementing an evidence-based guideline for care for patients who had experienced blunt chest trauma. They identified that the intervention was associated with a reduction in unplanned intensive care admissions and the use of mechanical ventilation. Observational studies that involve repeated measures, over time, are called *longitudinal* studies.

Correlational studies can be used to describe the direction (positive or negative) and strength of a relationship or an association. Rao and colleagues (2015) showed that adult women who use prayer or spiritual healing experienced improved health symptoms and health-seeking behaviours, which could support the need for prayer or spiritual healing

practices within healthcare settings. Correlational information can be used to build models to predict the effect of variables and determine what factors are likely to increase the **probability** of an outcome or situation occurring, therefore generating hypotheses to test in future research.

For example, Phillips and colleagues (2017) tested the impact of an online, evidence-based educational intervention on cancer nurses' pain assessment capabilities and adherence to pain screening and assessment guidelines. Implementing evidence-based educational interventions offers the potential for changing clinical practice. Using an online learning platform allows for the delivery of learning content that mimics clinical decision-making and offers the potential of changing entrenched clinical practices.

Descriptive Research

When descriptive research is undertaken, the researcher describes participants based on naturally occurring variables or characteristics. It commonly looks at the prevalence, magnitude and/or characteristics of a particular concept or various factors. An example of a descriptive nursing study can be found in the work of Skela-Savič and colleagues (2020). This study aimed to describe the presence, characteristics and content of courses focused on evidence-based practice in nursing programs in six European countries. It concluded that evidence-based practice was still not sufficiently embedded in the nursing curricula. Another example can be found in the work of Wilson, Avery and Slack (2020). This study aimed to explore student nurses' perceptions, knowledge and beliefs about immunisations and vaccination hesitancy through a survey. The study identified that current nursing curricula did not prepare nursing students to be able to effectively educate parents and patients regarding immunisations.

Observational data can be gathered by using a variety of instruments, including surveys/questionnaires, observations, physical measurements/tests or via medical record data. Using surveys allows for easy distribution across a wide geographical area not necessarily accessible if data collection relied on face-to-face data collection.

WHAT IS THE RESEARCH PROCESS?

The **research process** is an orderly series of phases and steps that guide the researcher from identifying a problem to finding an answer. The answer, in turn, suggests new questions for future research. Thus, research can be envisaged as a circular process, as illustrated in Fig. 7.1. Although the phases and steps occur in the general order indicated by Fig. 7.1, the order may vary, steps may overlap and the researcher may shift back and forth between various steps or phases. In some studies, certain steps are unnecessary and may be omitted. However, we can use these phases and steps as a guide to how a quantitative study will be conducted. This will help you understand how a researcher develops and conducts a study.

Phase 1: Conceive the Study

The first task for any researcher is to decide what to study. The activities in this phase involve reading previous research and theory, thinking about your area of interest and conceptualising (theorising) how the problem could be solved. The steps of problem identification, literature review and thinking about how to solve the problem (theorising) often occur simultaneously. These steps lead to the formulation of research hypotheses and research questions.

Identify the Problem

The **problem statement** describes the focus or intent of the study. It identifies what concepts will be researched and is commonly undertaken using a Problem/Patient group, Intervention or Exposure, Comparison, Outcome and Timeframe—PI(E)CO(T)—framework. The purpose of the study (intent or goal) is also described and limits are drawn to ensure the study is both relevant and achievable. Many research studies include more than one problem statement or statement of purpose. However, this may increase the complexity of the study. Whether the researcher uses a problem statement or a statement of purpose, or both, the intent is the same. These statements guide and focus the research (see Box 7.3 for examples of problem statements) and inform whether the study is likely to be experimental or observational.

Why Should the Problem be Solved?

It is important to consider the potential impact of your problem. Consider why the problem should be solved, and who the solution would benefit. This can help to refine the problem statement or question. Often this step follows the development of a conceptual framework or theory. Considering the potential outcomes is an essential part of the research process and is useful for crafting an impactful question, designing the study, considering the ethical conduct of the study and communicating the results.

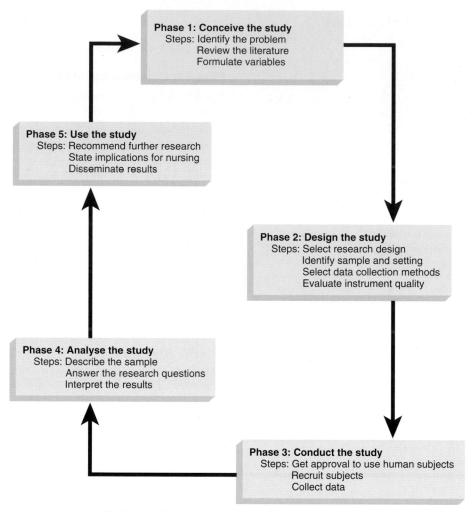

Fig. 7.1 ■ The phases and steps of the research process.

Review the Literature

The literature review is an essential component to inform the design and methods of a quantitative study. As you discovered in Chapter 3, the literature tells us what is currently known about the area under study, identifies opportunities to replicate existing research, if there is a knowledge gap, and how your study fits into the larger picture. The literature review may provide information about the best way to design the study or the best way to measure the appropriate variables.

Identify Variables

Variables are material objects, forces, concepts or traits that can be measured, manipulated or controlled. Once

variables are identified in your study design, they must be defined. Variables are defined in two ways. The first is a conceptual definition, which is a definition you can find in a dictionary. This definition explains what the word means in a given context. At this stage, it is important to think about how and why the variable is an accurate representation of what you are trying to measure. Doing so will help establish '**face validity**' (does it appear that the measurement represents the intended variable?). The second definition is an operational definition. This definition states how the variable will be measured. For example, the variable 'anxiety' might be conceptually defined as 'uneasiness or apprehension about an impending event'. The operational definition might state 'anxiety will be measured using the Clinical Anxiety Rating Scale'. Operational definitions are often decided in phase 2 of the study. It is useful to identify how previous researchers have measured the variable, as selecting an accepted measurement supports the establishment of face validity.

Variables come from the concepts identified in the problem statement and are specified in the form of research questions or hypotheses. The population to be studied is also specified in the research questions or hypotheses (we discuss populations in the next phase of the research process). Box 7.1 provides examples of research questions and hypotheses as derived from the problem statement.

Phase 1 can be thought of as the conceptualisation phase. This is when the foundations of the study are laid. A strong foundation will ensure all elements of the study are robust and will support the reliability of the results. Now you have read about phase 1, try the next student challenge.

STUDENT CHALLENGE

Perusing Phase 1

Select one of the case studies presented earlier in this book.

Select several quantitative research papers related to Ahmed's, Martha's or Jamie's research topics and answer the questions below.

1. Find the problem statement. Can you find examples of the interrogative form and the declarative form? Did the studies label it as a problem statement? If not, look for a statement such as 'the purpose of the study was …' or examine the title or the abstract.
2. Was a literature review provided? Did it help you understand the context of the study better?
3. Can you identify the study design?
4. Can you identify the variables being studied?
5. Can you find the hypotheses or research questions? Can you identify independent and dependent variables? What about extraneous variables? (Look for phrases such as '… was controlled using …'.)

Did the researcher state how the variables were defined?

6. What sort of hypotheses are used? Did they identify the null hypothesis or were the hypotheses alternative or directional?
7. Were different elements easier to spot in some studies than in others? Were some elements obvious in all the studies? Were any elements missing in all the studies you looked at?

Now, take a moment to think about your area of practice. Have you performed a procedure, administered medication or encountered a situation that you were unfamiliar with? The best research questions often come from common clinical practice, which is seldom questioned, and the best people to ask these questions are clinicians. Thinking about this moment of clinical practice, try to write a PICO(T) statement in the box below.

	Elements of PI(E)CO(T)	Example	Your PI(E)CO(T)
Population	Who is your study about? It is important to consider who your study will exclude. For example, some comorbidities are likely to alter your outcome (e.g. patients with pneumonia and COPD are likely to take longer to recover)	Patients older than 65 years with a diagnosis of pneumonia (excluding respiratory comorbidities)	
Intervention/ Exposure	What will be done to the population? (Often this is your independent variable.) A lot of research does not actively intervene but looks back in time to examine the outcomes of an exposure	Nurse encouraged and facilitated time sitting in an upright (Fowler's) position	
Comparison	To evaluate the effect of the intervention, it is important to have a similar population who did not experience the intervention or exposure	No intervention, patients able to position themselves as desired	
Outcome	Select an outcome that could logically be impacted by the intervention or exposure	Length of stay and destination on discharge	
Timeframe	Whether you are looking for the outcomes of an intervention or exposure, it is important to select enough time to see a change	Patients admitted to a medical facility between 2021 and 2022	

Phase 2: Design the Study

In phase 2 of a study, the researcher makes decisions about how to conduct the study. The research question determines the research design. It is very important to achieve coherence between the aims, research question, hypotheses and study design. When designing a study, the researcher selects the sample, determines the appropriate setting, operationally defines the variables, selects and evaluates the instruments and outlines procedures for data collection. These decisions have implications for the credibility of the study findings. If the research design is flawed or inappropriate, then the results will be limited.

Let's examine each step involved in making decisions about the study design. The order of the steps may vary slightly when making decisions, but all the steps are crucial in the design process.

Select a Research Design

The research protocol is the overall plan that guides how the study is designed, conducted and analysed; that is, the recipe. As described earlier, there are two major types of quantitative research design: experimental or quasi-experimental and descriptive (non-experimental). There is one important distinction between experimental/quasi-experimental and non-experimental designs. The researcher is an active agent in an experimental or quasi-experimental study, deliberately manipulating the independent variable to change the dependent variable. This manipulation is often labelled as a treatment or intervention. In a non-experimental study, the researcher is an observer and recorder, and there is no manipulation or treatment.

Identify Sample and Setting

Once the research design has been selected, the participants and setting for the study must be considered. The setting is the physical location for the study and the conditions under which the study takes place. It is important to consider whether the site is appropriate for the intervention and whether the site will enable an appropriate sample to be recruited. For example, the study in example 2 in Box 7.1 investigates children receiving suture repair (population) and measures their anxiety level and behaviour (dependent variable) depending on the presence or absence of their parents (intervention and independent variable). This study

took place in the suture room of an ED in one children's hospital (site). Similarly, the study involving premature infants (population) and stimulation (intervention and independent variable), in example 3 in Box 7.1, took place in a single NICU of a large teaching hospital (site). The location of this study is important as the NICU has computerised equipment capable of continuously monitoring pO_2 levels. It is also a tertiary referral hospital from the surrounding suburbs and will therefore be an appropriate location for both the intervention and the study population.

The participants of interest for a quantitative study are known as a population. These participants possess certain common characteristics or traits that make them appropriate for inclusion in the study. For example, young children with lacerations that require sutures are the participants of interest in example 2 in Box 7.1. Study participants need not be human; they might be animals such as mice or bacterial colonies in petri dishes. Populations are usually large, and it is not necessarily feasible to study every individual in that population. To overcome this, the researcher chooses a representative sample or subset of a population (Fig 7.2). Participants are selected from the population using a process known as sampling.

When selecting the sample, researchers try to make sure the included sample has characteristics that resemble the overall population characteristics as closely as possible. A sample that represents the larger population allows the study results to be applied to the whole population. This is known as **generalisation**. For example, if the children in the laceration study were less anxious during the suturing process when a parent was present, it is helpful if this result can be applied in many EDs and to all children receiving

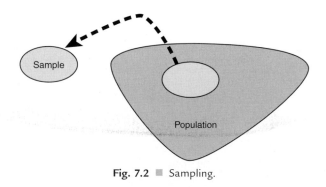

Fig. 7.2 ■ Sampling.

BOX 7.4
CATEGORIES OF SAMPLES

PROBABILITY SAMPLING—RANDOM SELECTION

1. A simple random sample is the most basic form of probability sampling in which all subjects in a population are numbered and a sample is selected randomly using a lottery or table of random numbers.
2. A stratified random sample is subdivided into groups according to some characteristic (e.g. gender—males and females; or ethnicity—those from an English-speaking background, those from a non-English-speaking background, Torres Strait Islander or Aboriginal). The subsets are then randomly sampled.
3. A cluster sample is a multistage sampling in which larger clusters (groups) are randomly selected first (e.g. hospitals) and then smaller clusters are randomly chosen (e.g. patients).
4. A systematic sample selects every kth (e.g. every fifth or seventh or twentieth) subject from a randomised list.

NON-PROBABILITY SAMPLING—NO RANDOM SELECTION

1. A convenience sample selects the most convenient subjects at hand.
2. A quota sample is conveniently selected according to pre-specified characteristic(s) (e.g. gender or ethnicity). A specific number from each characteristic is chosen.
3. A purposive sample uses subjects that are hand-picked by the researcher, based on a set of defined criteria.
4. A non-random systematic sample selects every kth (e.g. every fifth or seventh or twentieth) subject from a non-randomised list or every kth subject as they become available (e.g. every third patient admitted to the unit).

---

sutures for lacerations. The ability for results to be generalised from the sample to the broader population is determined by the sampling process.

There are two major categories of samples: probability and non-probability. Box 7.4 presents and defines sample categories and subcategories. Review these so you can recognise the vocabulary used to describe sampling in a research article and can distinguish between probability and non-probability types of samples.

In a probability sample, the participants are chosen at random. Each subject in the population has an equal chance of being selected to participate. Probability samples ensure a mathematical representation of the population and a high degree of certainty in their results. Therefore, when researchers choose probability sampling techniques, they ensure the results of the study can be generalised to the population and can tell whether their results occurred by chance.

Participants in a non-probability sample are not chosen at random. There is no way to assess whether they are representative of the whole population. Therefore, the results can only be applied to the sample and cannot be generalised to the wider population. You need to note the sampling method used when you read research papers because it tells you whether you can confidently apply the results directly to your clinical situation.

At this point you may be asking, 'If probability samples are so much better than non-probability samples, why would a researcher ever use a non-probability sample?' Good question! Non-probability sampling may be preferable for several reasons—it is less expensive and requires less time and fewer resources. Sometimes, generating a probability sample is not possible. For example, it may not be possible to generate a list of people in the population because no comprehensive source exists. At other times, generating such a list can be prohibitive in terms of time and expense. Think about compiling and numbering a list of 1000 or 10,000 or 100,000 participants in a population. Access to certain participants in a population may also be cost-prohibitive (e.g. participants in another city, state or country). Access to certain participants may be denied by the institutions or by the participants themselves. Some populations are also hidden and/or hard to access (e.g. stigmatised populations, such as sex workers). You will find that many nursing and midwifery research studies take a pragmatic approach and use non-probability sampling techniques. Our ability to identify whole populations may change with the increases in population databases and research funding and support for nursing and midwifery research.

The size of the sample is also important in ensuring that the sample is representative of the population. As a general rule of thumb, the larger the sample, the more representative it is of the population. The researcher considers several factors when selecting a sample size. These include the size of the overall population, the availability of the population, the variation in characteristics of the population, the cost and time expended per subject and the number of participants (power analysis) required to make sure the results can demonstrate significance. The size of the sample also affects the statistical techniques that can be used. Statistics used to analyse several variables simultaneously (multivariate statistics) require larger sample sizes. When you read a quantitative paper, check the sample size. If a sample is small (under 30 participants), particularly if it is a non-probability sample, the statistical strength of the study is limited, and you should only use the study results with caution.

Calculation of sample sizes to allow for the statistical testing of hypotheses in experimental studies is called 'power analysis'. Many research reports do not provide adequate justification for sample size; instead, it may seem that an arbitrary number is selected. Studies that provide a power analysis will justify their sample size and ensure the size is neither too low nor too high. Low power is caused by having too few participants in a study and where statistical analyses are limited. Low-powered studies are not able to provide decisive results and the results may be viewed as imprecise. High power enhances the level of statistical testing and also the accuracy and probability of obtaining significant results. However, there is still the risk of having too many participants in a sample. Large sample sizes require increased resources and are more likely to detect small differences in the results, purely because of how many participants are enrolled in the study. Power analysis will vary between studies and can be calculated according to the individual circumstances of each study. There are computer software packages and online interactive sites that can assist with undertaking power analysis.

There are also ethical implications associated with conducting studies with power that is either too low or too high. Research should only be undertaken if the results are going to be relevant and applicable; using too small a sample or too large a sample influences the accuracy of the results.

Use experimental quantitative study results with caution when the sample is small, as there is no power calculation and there is non-probability sampling.

Select Data Collection Methods

To examine the proposed research questions or hypotheses, the researcher must be able to collect measurable information on the variables. These measurable bits of information are known as **data**. Quantitative data are collected using instruments. These instruments are classified by the type of data they are designed to collect and are generally physiological, behavioural or psychological. Physiological data (for physiological variables) are generally measured using specialised biophysical instruments and specialised expertise by the user. You would be familiar with several of the biophysical measurements used in healthcare and healthcare research. For example, sphygmomanometers, thermometers, pulse oximeters, electrocardiograph machines, electroencephalograph machines and so on. We regularly use these instruments in clinical practice.

Behavioural data (observable actions of the subject) are generally collected through observation. In quantitative research, these observations are evaluated and assigned numerical values. For example, the degree of uncooperative behaviour (Box 7.1) was observed and rated in the study of young children who were being sutured for a laceration. The nurse observed the child's behaviour and assigned ratings at several predetermined intervals during the suturing procedure (the scale is presented in Table 7.2).

Psychological measurements are used to collect data about knowledge, feelings and attitudes. As these variables cannot be directly observed, an instrument is used that asks the subject to self-report on these variables. Such instruments include questionnaires and interviews. Questionnaires pose a series of questions for the participants to answer. In a quantitative study, the questions are usually closed-ended. This means that the subject is asked to select from a range of choices. Box 7.5 contains an example of closed-ended questions. Questionnaires: are easy to administer; are relatively inexpensive; can be distributed to a large, widely dispersed sample; and offer confidentiality to the respondent.

Tools (such as surveys or questionnaires) used in research generally contain some type of scale designed

	TABLE 7.2		
	Uncooperative Behaviour Scale		
Score	**Behaviour**		
0	No crying or physical protest		
1	Mild verbal protest (e.g. ouch) or quiet crying		
2	More prominent verbal protest/crying with movement of body parts; still complies with physician's request		
3	Protest and movement make the procedure difficult		
4	Protest stops the procedure and behaviour is addressed before procedure can be reinitiated		
5	General prolonged verbal protest and body movement with no compliance		

Source: Adapted from Venham LL, Gaulin-Kramer E, Munster E, et al: Interval rating scales for children's dental anxiety and uncooperative behaviour, Pediatric Dentistry 2(3):195–202, 1980.

BOX 7.5
SAMPLE QUESTIONS ON A QUESTIONNAIRE

Please circle the answer that best describes you.
1. Are you:
   - male
   - female
   - prefer not to say
2. Are you currently:
   - single (never married)
   - married
   - separated
   - divorced
   - widowed
   - co-habiting

---

to measure a certain psychological variable (e.g. stress or social support). These psychological or social variables are usually referred to as *constructs*. Scales are instruments that assign numerical values to a set of responses to a series of questions or statements. These numbers are then added together to calculate a score. This score is used as a measurement of the variable. The most common scale type is the Likert scale. Participants are given a series of statements and several ranges to choose from regarding their level of agreement (agree through to strongly disagree with statements), frequency (very frequently through to never or not at all), importance (very important through to unimportant) or quality (high-quality through to low-quality). Box 7.6 gives an example of a few items from a Likert scale measuring attitudes to continuing education for nurses and midwives. The response to each item is assigned a number and the numbers from all the items are added to reflect the overall degree of agreement with the concept being measured.

One factor that will influence the efficacy of a questionnaire is the response rate. Many mailed questionnaires have a low response rate, meaning that a lot of money can be wasted on postage and printing if the questionnaire is not filled in accurately and returned. For this reason, it is very important to ensure optimal questionnaire design. An effective questionnaire is well laid out, easy to read with appropriate colours and font, not too onerous (not too long or too many questions), in plain language and accompanied by accurate instructions in a language that is simple and easy to understand. Another issue to consider when mailing out questionnaires is that there is no guarantee the respondent will be the intended target. For example, a questionnaire about a women's health issue could be mailed out with the intent that a woman will complete it. However, the woman's partner could fill it out and the researcher would have no way of knowing this. Nor would the researcher be aware of group answers, where a person answers the questions a certain way after being pressured or influenced by others; for example, a group of teenagers completing a questionnaire in a magazine.

Interviews used to collect data in a quantitative study usually consist of a series of highly structured questions with the responses assigned numbers for statistical

---

BOX 7.6
SAMPLE LIKERT SCALE

SA	Strongly agree	D	Disagree
A	Agree	SD	Strongly disagree
U	Uncertain		

Please circle your degree of agreement or disagreement with the following statements:

1. Continuing education should be compulsory for nurses and midwives.

   SA   A   U   D   SD

2. Nurses and midwives should be able to demonstrate their clinical competency every year.

   SA   A   U   D   SD

3. Nurses and midwives should be encouraged to undertake postgraduate studies.

   SA   A   U   D   SD

4. Continuing education is only necessary for nurses and midwives if they are seeking promotion.

   SA   A   U   D   SD

5. Continuing education should be part of career planning for every nurse and midwife.

   SA   A   U   D   SD

---

analysis. A structured interview is much like an oral questionnaire in which the investigator reads the questions and asks the respondent to provide their chosen response. Interviews do offer the advantage of allowing the interviewer to clarify responses and to ensure that all questions are answered. It also ensures the person who answers the questions is the one for whom the question was intended and that they understand the meaning of the question. The key disadvantages are the added time and expense involved in the interview process.

Appropriate instruments must be selected to measure each variable being studied. This includes desired descriptive variables (e.g. gender, education level and marital status), independent and dependent variables and important extraneous variables (e.g. variables that must be controlled using statistics). Choices are made based on criteria such as the category of data (e.g. physiological, behavioural, psychological), cost, availability and the skill required to administer the instrument. It is important that the instrument chosen is appropriate for the data category and research question and is the best-quality instrument the researcher can access.

Evaluating Instrument Quality

Instrument quality plays a big role in the selection of an appropriate instrument. The researcher is looking for 'good' instruments to measure the variables in the study. What is a 'good' instrument? A good instrument is valid and reliable—validity and reliability are important concepts. A valid instrument measures what it is supposed to measure. A reliable instrument measures the variable consistently, dependably and accurately, across settings and with repeated use by different people. If an instrument is not reliable, it cannot be considered valid, because you cannot rely on the accuracy of the results. There are various ways that researchers can establish the validity and reliability of instruments. Box 7.7 lists some frequently used ways of establishing validity and reliability. Familiarise yourself with these terms.

Instruments used in research should be evaluated for reliability and validity before use. When you are reading research papers, look for comments from the authors concerning how they have ensured the validity and reliability of the instruments they have used.

Biophysical measurements are generally accepted as valid measures of the variable; that is, we accept that they measure what they say they measure. However, reliability is an issue; that is, how consistently, dependably and accurately these measures can be taken across different settings by different people. Reliability can be addressed by ensuring instruments are calibrated and that the operators have sufficient and equivalent expertise.

Now we have covered what is involved in phase 2 of a study, take some time to complete the following student challenge.

BOX 7.7
TYPES OF VALIDITY AND RELIABILITY

VALIDITY

Validity is the extent to which an instrument measures what it says it measures.

CONTENT VALIDITY

Content validity is assessed by a logical evaluation and judgment of whether the instrument adequately reflects the content of the concept. A blueprint may be used to construct the instrument or a panel of judges may be asked to evaluate the instrument. This is a weak form of validity.

CRITERION VALIDITY

Criterion validity is assessed using statistical measures. Instrument scores are correlated to scores on measures of selected external criteria. Also called concurrent or predictive validity, this is a stronger form of validity.

CONSTRUCT VALIDITY

Construct validity is assessed using a combination of logic and statistical measures. It looks for the underlying meaning of the construct being measured. This is the strongest form of validity.

RELIABILITY

Reliability is the degree of consistency or dependability of an instrument.

INTERNAL CONSISTENCY

Internal consistency uses correlation statistics (e.g. Spearman's, Cronbach's alpha or Kuder–Richardson) to measure whether the subparts of an instrument all measure the same thing. Reliability values range from 0 to 1. The closer the value gets to 1, the more reliable the instrument.

EQUIVALENCE

Equivalence correlates two different forms of the same instrument (also called parallel forms) or the scores of two or more raters (also called interrater reliability). Reliability is reported as an r-value, with values ranging from 0 to 1. The closer the value gets to 1, the more reliable the instrument.

STABILITY

Stability correlates the scores obtained when an instrument is administered twice to the same group of subjects over a period of time. Reliability or r-values range from 0 to 1. The closer the value gets to 1, the more reliable the instrument.

INTERRATER RELIABILITY

Interrater reliability refers to the degree to which two or more raters independently score the same ratings or values for the feature that is being observed or measured.

STUDENT CHALLENGE

Scrutinising Phase 2

Look again at the quantitative research papers you examined for phase 1. Scan these papers and see if you can identify each of the elements we have discussed in phase 2.

1. Can you identify if the research design is experimental or non-experimental? Remember that experimental studies use terms such as experimental, quasi-experimental, treatment group, control group, treatment, intervention or random assignment. Non-experimental studies use terms or phrases such as retrospective, ex post facto, correlational, 'purpose is to describe ...' or 'purpose is to explore ...'
2. Can you identify the sample? Can you determine what the population was? (This is harder because it is often inferred rather than directly stated.)

3. Can you determine whether a probability or non-probability sampling technique was used? Look for cue words such as 'random' for probability samples and words such as 'convenience' for non-probability samples. If the technique is not specified, the chances are it is a non-probability sample. What was the size of the sample in the studies you chose? Was power analysis discussed to determine the sample size?
4. Was the setting described?
5. What instruments were used to measure the variables? Could you tell if the instruments were reliable and valid?

Once all the decisions have been made concerning the study protocol, it is important to develop a realistic timeline. Some elements of a research project take longer than others. For example, gaining ethics approval can take a long time, so it is best to begin the ethics process as soon as possible. Other elements such as the gathering of literature may continue throughout the life of the project. When applying for research funding and ethics approval, researchers are asked to indicate a timeframe for the study; an example of a timeframe is provided in Table 7.3.

	Jan.	Feb.	Mar.	Apr.	May	June	July	Aug.	Sept.	Oct.	Nov.	Dec.
TABLE 7.3 Timeframe Table (sometimes referred to as a GANTT Chart)												
Design study	X	X										
Literature review			X	X								
Ethics approvals					X							
Recruit participants						X						
Collect data							X	X				
Analyse data									X	X		
Preparation of report and dissemination of results											X	X

Developing a Budget or Costing a Study?

Research is a labour-intensive activity that requires adequate resources. Increasingly stretched funding for healthcare and healthcare research requires researchers to provide clear and strong justification for all budget items. Potential funders will scrutinise the budget closely and will reject an application if the budget is inflated or unrealistically low. Identifying the resources required and designing the budget is a crucial part of a research proposal, and attention to detail and accuracy is essential. Research budgets are organised into five main sections.

1. Personnel: this part of the budget should cover costs such as research assistants, statistical support and transcription/data entry costs.
2. Equipment: the budget can cover essential equipment including recording equipment and measuring devices (if, for example, a researcher wanted to measure blood sugar level, glucometers would be essential), the printing of questionnaires or data collection forms, and also cover computer hardware and software; however, this is increasingly the assumed responsibility of the investigating institution.
3. Consumables: including items such as photocopying, postage and stationery; sometimes you may have to pay a licence fee to use a validated questionnaire.
4. Travel: this may be required for multisite projects and in the dissemination of research at conferences.

5. Cost for patient and public involvement and engagement (PPIE): it is important to pay for PPIE support for a research project; there are national guidelines to support this within research (e.g. in the UK at https://www.nihr.ac.uk/documents/payment-guidance-for-researchers-and-professionals/27392).

Phase 3: Conduct the Study

Once the study question and methods have been decided and the research proposal is written, the planning phases are complete and the research team is ready to conduct the study. They will now implement the study as outlined in the research protocol and collect the data using the designated instruments and procedures. This is often an exciting time in the research process.

Ethics Approval

When any research involves people, the researchers are bound by law to protect them from harm, and this process involves gaining the necessary ethical approvals before the recruitment of the first participant. The first step in conducting a study is to obtain approval from an institutional Human Resources Ethics Committee (HREC); refer to Chapter 6, where this has been discussed in detail.

Collect Data

Once all the necessary ethical approvals have been obtained, the research can commence. The first step in this process is participant recruitment, followed by the administration of data collection tools, treatments and the generation of data. All of these processes need to be completed exactly the way they have been outlined in the research proposal and ethics application. If you need to make any changes to how you are conducting your research, you will need to amend the research proposal and ethics application and seek approval for the change from the relevant ethics committee. Once all the participants have been recruited and the data has been collected, the researcher now turns their attention to organising their data into an appropriate form for analysis and phase 3 is concluded.

Phase 4: Analyse the Study

Researchers must analyse and summarise the data so others can understand and appreciate significant elements within it. Research students are often apprehensive and uncertain about statistical analysis and interpretation of the data. However, like many things in research, there is a clear systematic approach to analysing quantitative data. Statistical analysis is just another approach to understanding the meaning of the data and is something you will develop greater skills in as you get more involved in research. Quantitative research uses a combination of descriptive and inferential statistics. While **descriptive statistics** describe the participants or research topic, **inferential statistics** analyse the relationships between variables. Statistics allows the researcher to draw a numerical picture of the data collected, to look at how the variables are alike or different, to make decisions about whether variables are related or different or to determine whether one variable causes another to react in a certain way.

Describe the Sample

When analysing the data, the researcher wants to build a picture to describe the sample. There are four common ways to describe data using statistics: frequencies; measures of central tendency; measures of spread (distribution of the data); and measures of shape.

Frequency and Central Tendency. One simple thing we can do is to count the number of times (frequency) something occurs for a particular variable. Frequency counts can then be turned into percentages (number in a category divided by the number for the variable).

Table 7.4 presents sample frequencies and percentages taken from a sample of 90 nursing students. We can see from this example that most students in this sample were females who were single and aged between 22 and 27, and most were satisfied with the school. Frequencies are most useful when reporting nominal and ordinal data as you can group several scores together and report the frequency and percentage of the groups, as we did with the variable 'age' in Table 7.4. Frequencies for interval and ratio data can also be plotted on a graph to form a frequency **distribution** (Fig 7.3).

Measures of central tendency are statistical tests that describe how data for a variable tend to cluster together in a distribution. Central tendency is most commonly described using mode, median and/or mean. The measure you use is determined by the level of measurement. Mode and median are used for

TABLE 7.4		
Frequencies and Percentages (n = 90)		
Variable	Frequency (n)	Percentage (%)
Gender		
Female	82	91
Male	8	9
Current marital status		
Single	46	51%
Married	34	38%
Separated	2	2%
Divorced	8	9%
Satisfaction with school		
Very dissatisfied	2	2%
Dissatisfied	9	10%
Uncertain	18	20%
Satisfied	45	50%
Very satisfied	16	18%
Age		
19–21	16	18%
22–24	27	30%
25–27	36	40%
28–30	11	12%

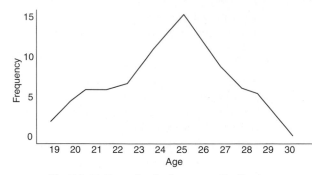

Fig. 7.3 ■ Example of a frequency distribution.

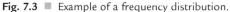

BOX 7.8
DESCRIPTIVE STATISTICAL MEASURES

Measures of central tendency are statistical tests that describe how data for a variable tend to cluster together in a distribution.

1. Mode (Mo) is the numerical value that occurs most often for a particular variable.
2. Median (Md) is the middle value in a frequency distribution of numbers.
3. Mean (M, X) is the average of all the scores.

Measures of dispersion are statistical tests that describe how data for a variable tend to spread out in a distribution.

1. Range is the distance between the highest and lowest scores for a variable.
2. Variance (V, s^2) is the average area of spread under a frequency distribution curve.
3. Standard deviation (SD, s) is the average distance of spread in a frequency distribution. It tells us how much, on average, the scores are spread out from the mean.
4. Confidence interval (CI) is the range within which the supported value is expected to lie within a given degree of certainty.

Measures of shape are statistical tests that describe the shape of the distribution for a variable.

1. Normal is where the curve or shape is bell-like.
2. Skewness reflects the degree of symmetry or asymmetry of the distribution curve (e.g. is the distribution symmetrical or asymmetrical?).
3. Kurtosis is the height of the distribution (e.g. how tall or flat is the distribution curve?).

nominal and ordinal data, while mean (average) is used for interval and ratio data (Box 7.8).

Measures of Spread and Shape. We can also use statistics to describe how data are distributed. We can describe how data clump or cluster together, how they spread apart and what shape the frequency distribution forms. These statistics are defined in Box 7.8. All these statistics let us reduce large amounts of data about a variable down to a manageable description, where the meaning is commonly understood. Imagine if you tried to make sense of the reported ages for 5000 participants if you had no precise way to count them, group them or discuss how much the participants were alike or different in age.

Most studies are conducted on a sample of participants that is selected from a population. Therefore, any statistics reported on that sample are estimates of the true population value (e.g. this could be a mean or proportion) and there will be some degree of error in the estimate. The **confidence interval** describes the range within which the supported value (i.e. the size of the effect of exposure) is expected to lie within a given degree of certainty (95% or 99%). Most health research uses a 95% confidence interval. Confidence intervals represent the probability of random errors, but not systematic errors (bias).

Answer the Research Questions

Once the researcher has described the sample, the next step is to analyse the data to answer the original research questions the study set out to answer or to see whether the hypothesis was supported.

Descriptive Analysis. In a descriptive study, the researcher can use the same descriptive statistics outlined above to describe the results from the variables set out in the research question: frequency, central tendency, spread and shape (or distribution). The research questions in example 1 in Box 7.1 regarding older people attending the ED were answered using descriptive statistics. The question, 'What percentage of total emergency department visits are by older individuals over the age of 65?' was answered using frequencies and percentages. The question, 'What are the primary presenting complaints of older people?' was answered by categorising all the primary reasons for presentation to an ED, then reporting frequencies and percentages of each category.

Analysis of relationships or differences between variables: if the study asked questions or stated hypotheses that looked at the relationships or differences between variables, then the researchers need to use statistics that enable an analysis of these relationships or differences. A wide variety of inferential statistical tests are available for such analysis. The choice of test depends on the number of variables, the level of data collected and the questions being asked. Many common statistical tests will only work if the data has a **normal distribution**. Increased access to computers and sophisticated statistical software has led to more-complex statistical tests. Many studies now identify and examine greater numbers of variables because analysis of multiple variables is now readily available. This means that reports of statistical analysis and study are increasingly complicated, making reading and understanding the results section of many papers difficult. At this stage, it is not expected that you would recognise or understand why particular statistics were selected or the precise meaning of the numbers generated by those tests. Most hospitals and universities have statisticians who can help you to understand statistical issues if you are undertaking a research project. As a clinician, you will need a basic understanding of core concepts so that you can understand the researchers' interpretation of their results.

The following strategies and information will help you with this.

- Different statistical tests have different requirements for use. Selection of the appropriate statistical test is based on several factors, including the number of variables to be analysed, the level of measurement of the variables, the nature of the question asked (e.g. testing relationships or differences), the distribution (or shape) of the data, and the sampling procedure used.
- Research hypotheses may be translated into statistical hypotheses. This is merely a restatement of the research hypothesis in symbol form and is used to help researchers with decision-making.
- The results of statistical tests are reported as a number (e.g. $t = 4.26$, $F = 3.98$, $r = 0.68$). The letter gives a clue about the statistical test used (e.g. t is a t-test, F is an analysis of variance [ANOVA] test, r indicates a correlation). Many multivariate statistics generate a series of numbers that tell the researcher about several variables and how they vary as part of a multiple variable set.
- The results from statistical tests (the numbers) are either significant or not significant. Significance is reported using a **p-value** (e.g. $p = 0.17$,

$p = 0.03$, $p = 0.01$). A p-value of < 0.05 is generally considered statistically significant. Some researchers use a p-value of < 0.01 to decide if a value is statistically significant. Sometimes, non-significance is reported by using the letters NS.
- A significant p-value ($p < 0.05$) means there is a less than 5% possibility that the relationship or difference found between variables was caused by chance. In other words, you can have a high degree of certainty, 95% certain, that a difference or real relationship (correlation) exists between the variables tested. The lower the p-value, the more significant the result and the decreased likelihood of the result occurring by chance.
- Statistical results are often displayed in table form.

When you read the results section, do not panic over the numbers and the discussion of those numbers. The researcher should explain and summarise the statistical results in the text at some point in the presentation of results or the discussion. Look for this summary as you read and see if it answers the research questions or hypotheses that were first discussed. You are looking for information as to whether the variables are related or whether a particular group had different results from another group.

In example 2 in Box 7.1, the research question is: 'Will there be a difference between the anxiety levels and disruptive behaviours of young children whose parents are present during laceration repair versus those with no parental presence?' Hotelling's t-squared test was used and the test found there was no significant difference (p-value was > 0.05) in behaviour or anxiety in those children who had their parents present when compared to those children whose parents were not present.

Remember, we noted that the effects of extraneous variables (influences from sources outside the study) were sometimes controlled using statistics. In the study of children's anxiety and behaviour, age was identified as an extraneous variable that might influence whether parental presence made a difference. Another statistical test (analysis of covariance: ANCOVA) was used to look at differences between anxiety and behaviour when the age of the children was controlled as an outside influence (extraneous variable). Using this test, the researchers could see that if looking at younger children only, there was a significant difference in both behaviour and anxiety when parents were present, with younger children being less anxious and more cooperative. As children became older, parental presence did not affect anxiety or behaviour. Researchers often look at the influence of particular aspects of a population to make sure they have not missed anything by analysing the group altogether.

In example 3 in Box 7.1, the research hypothesis is: 'Premature infants who receive extra tactile stimulation will have higher oxygen (pO_2) levels than those who do not'. In this study, a t-test was used to compare the average (mean) pO_2 levels between those infants who received stimulation and those who did not. The resulting t value was significant ($p < 0.05$), indicating there was a statistically significant difference between the pO_2 levels in the two groups.

Interpret the Results

Once the statistical analysis has been performed and the results have been examined, the researcher must interpret the results. This means making sense of the results and how they fit into the existing literature. Results from descriptive studies are used to secure a tentative picture. There is very little to interpret because no relationships are tested among the described variables. Results from exploratory studies that ask questions about relationships or differences among variables provide a starting point for the researcher to explain why relationships or differences were or were not present.

Results from studies in which relationships or differences were predicted in the form of hypotheses allow for and require the most interpretation. An explanation of the results is straightforward if the hypothesis is supported.

- The researcher would use the theoretical evidence to make a guess about variable relationships and whether this has been supported as was anticipated.
- The study would be interpreted to lend more proof to the underlying theoretical foundations.

However, if the hypotheses are not supported, the researcher must try to explain whether the negative result was due to a problem in the theoretical structure or the design of the study. Answers to these questions are usually presented in the discussion section of a paper and lead to the final phase of the process. It is important to remember that a failure to support hypotheses is not failed study. Negative results are

critical for advancing our knowledge. Negative results tell future researchers about what does *not* work. Research is a process of trial and error, and there continues to be debate about why more negative results are not published in peer-reviewed journals.

Phase 5: Use the Study

One important phase remains after the researcher discovers the answers to the questions posed in a study. The research results must be used to make recommendations for further research, to advise on the implications of this research for current practice and to share the results with a broad audience so that others can learn from this knowledge. This phase completes the research process, demonstrates the circular nature of the research process and is an ethical obligation to the participants who made the research possible. Some journals will require authors to provide a section about the implications or recommendations, while others will include this in the discussion section.

Recommend Further Research

Once the results are stated and discussed, the researcher must decide what the results mean for future research and consider what the next study might look like. That researcher or another researcher can seek to validate results or build on the knowledge gained. This continuing process accelerates the advancement of knowledge.

The researcher should take the time to examine and discuss any problems encountered while doing the study. In peer-reviewed papers, this is often referred to as the 'limitations'. An honest discussion of limitations allows the reader to understand these issues and consider their impact on whether the data can be applied to their practice. It also allows future researchers to correct errors that might occur when repeating or extending a similar study. Examples of limitations might include uncontrolled extraneous variables that interfered with study results, difficulties in data collection or not having enough participants to complete a type of statistical analysis. In this way, future research can avoid these errors and generate more accurate and credible evidence. An honest discussion of the limitations also assures the reader that they can have confidence in the credibility of the study.

Implications for Practice

The researcher must also decide what implications, if any, the results can provide for clinical practice, policy or social discussion and debate. This assists the audience to make sense of the results and make decisions about how and in what way the results should inform practice. Stating the implications of the results for practice also helps the researcher to identify who would benefit from the findings. The researchers can then begin to communicate the findings to the desired audience.

Communicate the Results

The final obligation on the part of the research team is to communicate the results of the study. This is known as dissemination. The most common forms of communication are through peer-reviewed published papers in nursing, midwifery or specialty journals, or through presentations at conferences. Publishing research in an internationally recognised, well-read and cited journal has the most widespread impact. Publishing the results in a peer-reviewed journal gives the audience some confidence that the results are valid and meaningful; the submitted article is critically reviewed by other researchers in the field before publication. However, publication in a well-regarded peer-reviewed journal is only the beginning of the communication process. If the findings are important or have significant implications for practice or policy, the researcher will often directly contact key decision-makers, publish on social media or even communicate the results

to journalists. While health professionals must keep their practice current and evidence-based, keeping up with the latest research can be hard work. For this reason, the effective researcher makes it as easy as possible for clinicians and the public to access, understand and interpret their work.

STUDENT CHALLENGE

Entertaining the End

1. Examine your chosen research papers for future research recommendations and implications for nursing or midwifery practice.
2. Rejoice in the fact you have now worked through the entire research process.

CONCLUSION

This chapter has explored quantitative research as a systematic, objective process. The process involves the use of an instrument to gather information about variables, the analysis of data, the description of associations between variables and the testing of cause-and-effect relationships. In this chapter, we have explored various ways in which quantitative research can be classified and identified, and we have discussed the specific steps of the quantitative research process. Quantitative research that is conducted systematically and uses robust research methods to generate knowledge may be generalised to a large population. For this reason, quantitative research can quickly and meaningfully influence clinical practice. The quantitative approach does, however, have limitations. Although objectivity is prized and strict controls are imposed to limit bias, outside influences can never be entirely removed. In the context of health research, limiting the type of participant included in a study allows for safer comparisons, but can oversimplify the common complexities of a person and social context. Limiting and accounting for some of these confounding factors is possible. This can be more easily achieved if the researcher has a deep insight into the complexities of the phenomena of interest. In this way, quantitative and qualitative research are complementary and should be used to inform the other. Qualitative research designs and methods (see Chapter 8) are also commonly used in nursing and midwifery research; these are covered in the next chapter.

ADDITIONAL RESOURCES

Want to Know More About Quantitative Research?

- If you want more details and guidelines for different types of quantitative research, try looking at some established reporting guidelines that are available on the internet, such as the sites listed below.
  - STROBE, **St**rengthening the **R**eporting of **Ob**servational Studies in **E**pidemiology: http://www.equator-network.org/reporting-guidelines/strobe
  - CONSORT, **Con**solidated **S**tandards **of** **R**eporting **T**rials: http://www.equator-network.org/reporting-guidelines/consort
  - PRISMA, **P**referred **R**eporting **I**tems for **S**ystematic Reviews and **M**eta-**A**nalyses: http://www.equator-network.org/reporting-guidelines/prisma
- National Health and Medical Research Council (NHMRC): NHMRC Levels of evidence and grades for recommendations for developers of guidelines, 2009. Online. Available: https://www.nhmrc.gov.au/sites/default/filcs/images/NHMRC%20Levels%20and%20Grades%20(2009).pdf
- Check out the activities on the Evolve website http://evolve.elsevier.com/AU/Jackson/maze/ for further information.

REFERENCES

Banerjee A, Chitnis UB, Jadhav SL, et al: Hypothesis testing, type I and type II errors, Industrial Psychiatry Journal 18(2):127–131, 2009. http://doi.org/10.4103/0972-6748.62274.

Curtis K, Kourouche S, Asha S, et al: Impact of a care bundle for patients with blunt chest injury (ChIP): a multicentre controlled implementation evaluation, PLOS ONE 16(10):e0256027, 2021.

Huang W, Wei W, Want J, Lyn Y: Effectiveness of a nurse-led online educational programme based on basic insulin therapy in patients with diabetes mellitus: a quasi-experimental trial. Journal Clinical Nursing 31(15–16):2227–2239, 2022.

Milesky JL, Baptiste DL, Shelton BK: An observational study of patient handover communications among nurses on an oncology critical care unit, Contemporary Nurse 54(1):77–87, 2017.

National Health and Medical Research Council (NHMRC): NHMRC Levels of evidence and grades for recommendations for developers of guidelines, 2009. https://www.nhmrc.gov.au/sites/default/files/images/NHMRC%20Levels%20and%20Grades%20(2009).pdf.

Oxford Centre for Evidence-Based Medicine: Levels of evidence, Mar, 2009. https://www.cebm.ox.ac.uk/resources/levels-of-evidence/oxford-centre-for-evidence-based-medicine-levels-of-evidence-march-2009.

Phillips JL, Heneka N, Hickman LD, et al: Can a complex online intervention improve cancer nurses' pain screening and assessment practices? Results from a multicenter, pre-post test pilot study, Pain Management Nursing 18(2):75–89, 2017.

Rao A, Sibbritt D, Phillips JL, et al: Prayer or spiritual healing as adjuncts to conventional care: a cross-sectional analysis of prevalence and characteristics of use among women, BMJ Open 5(6):2015.

Skela-Savič B, Gotlib J, Panczyk M, et al: Teaching evidence-based practice (EBP) in nursing curricula in six European countries: a descriptive study, Nurse Education Today 94:104561, 2020.

Slater T, Stanik-Hutt J, Davidson PM: Cerebral perfusion monitoring in adult patients following cardiac surgery: an observational study, Contemporary Nurse 53(60):669–680, 2017.

Wilson KL, Avery JS, Slack J: Nursing students' perceptions and beliefs about immunizations: a descriptive study, Nursing Education Today 92:104491, 2020.

8

QUALITATIVE RESEARCH

LEAH EAST ■ STEPHEN NEVILLE ■ PARVEEN ALI ■ KAY ARANDA

CHAPTER OUTLINE

LEARNING OBJECTIVES

After reading this chapter and following critical reflection, readers should be able to:

- define qualitative research
- describe qualitative research classifications
- compare and contrast qualitative and quantitative research
- discuss the conceptualisation for various qualitative designs
- describe the processes involved in conducting a qualitative study
- identify methods used in analysing qualitative data
- describe the reporting of qualitative study findings and conclusions

KEY TERMS

case study

credibility

data immersion

ethnography

findings

focus groups

grounded theory

inductive reasoning

lifeworld

methodology

naturalistic paradigm

phenomenology

phenomenon

qualitative analysis

qualitative descriptive research

qualitative research

research design

setting/field

theoretical perspectives/ framework

triangulation

trustworthiness

ABSTRACT

To engage with the nursing and midwifery literature and effectively explore questions in these domains, an understanding of both qualitative and quantitative research approaches is necessary. This chapter defines qualitative research, compares qualitative and quantitative research approaches, explores various types of qualitative research and identifies and discusses phases of the qualitative research process. There are multiple ways to qualitatively explore health issues, using different understandings of knowledge and reality and with many purposes, which then shapes how we design and conduct research and analyse data. This chapter focuses largely on the research approaches underpinned by the interpretive paradigm and explores how these approaches can be used effectively to contribute to our understanding of the world.

STUDENT QUOTE

Qualitative research allows me to better understand the experiences and views of the participants, making the findings and conclusions meaningful.

INTRODUCTION

Qualitative research explores human experiences and situations by employing in-depth non-numerical methods of data collection and analysis. Research can be classified by the underlying theoretical perspective (e.g. interpretive, constructionist or critical paradigms), which guides researchers' understanding of how we know what we know. An interpretive approach aims to explore, describe and make meaning of phenomena. A constructionist approach subscribes to the idea that there are multiple subjective realities. In contrast, a critical approach aims to critique existing ideologies, empower research participants and challenge political and social norms.

Qualitative research can also be classified by research design and/or methodology and is dependent on and determined by the question being asked. Common qualitative methodologies include phenomenology, ethnography, grounded theory, case study and descriptive qualitative approaches. Qualitative research processes share some features (e.g. a

search for meaning that is context-rich), although these may vary across methodologies and according to the research aim. Data collection occurs predominantly through observation, interviews or focus groups. However, other methods can also be used, such as storytelling (e.g. in biographical narratives), photovoice, examination of historical records and creative methods such as poetry, drawing or photography. Analysis of qualitative data takes place using various techniques and procedures to manage, synthesise and interpret data. With some qualitative approaches (such as grounded theory), analysis even dictates the direction and course of further data collection. When undertaking data analysis, qualitative researchers search for patterns of meaning in the information collected, whether that be in the written narratives, observations or other types of data. **Findings** are presented in a descriptive or interpretive narrative format with excerpts of data used to illustrate the key patterns identified.

QUALITATIVE RESEARCH IN PRACTICE

Nurses and midwives have an interest in questions and issues that involve human experience and approaches, embrace subjectivity and are important in developing holistic understandings of people and responses to their experiences. Understanding patient and family experiences can directly lead to changes in practice, policy, education or management that improve healthcare delivery. The use of qualitative approaches provides nurses and midwives with rigorous ways to explore and draw meaning from life experiences. Qualitative researchers draw on **inductive reasoning** processes and seek to examine and understand the whole of a **phenomenon** of interest. Research undertaken in this way focuses on presenting concepts, which are attributed with meaning in a particular context, rather than on cause and effect, or measurement of the concepts and their relationships. Qualitative researchers view reality as a subjective, multifaceted experience rather than as a single, fixed, objective actuality. Therefore, even though people may experience a similar event, the meaning they attach to it and the way it affects them is nuanced and subject to individual interpretation.

Complex phenomena closely linked to the human experience or subjects about which little is known are readily understood using a qualitative approach. For example: What is it like to experience being diagnosed with diabetes or chronic obstructive pulmonary disease? What are the experiences of people caring for partners living with dementia? How does it feel to be a carer for someone living with learning disabilities? What is it like to be an international student studying nursing or midwifery at a university in another country? The information gained from investigating these research questions provides nurses and midwives with insight into how people experience events.

No Singularly Defined Scientific Approach

No singularly defined scientific approach governs qualitative research. It is driven by multiple approaches across various disciplines. Therefore, many aspects of qualitative research are not as clear-cut as those of quantitative research. While traditional quantitative research has concentrated on trying to establish cause and effect relationships, qualitative research permits multiple ways to explore the depth, richness and complexity inherent in most phenomena. Table 8.1 presents some of the differences between the two approaches.

Qualitative research methodology embraces the examination of subjective phenomena; findings are considered to be idiosyncratic to a particular situation. That means they are considered to be representative of a particular person (or people) in a particular context or setting, and not necessarily reflective of the experiences of the entire population. However, qualitative findings may be transferable to other people in similar contexts or settings. For example, understanding the experiences of refugees from West African countries could resonate with the experiences of refugees fleeing other areas of the world.

Qualitative research can be time-consuming because of the nature of recruitment, data collection, analysis and also writing up—often considered a craft in itself. Qualitative research methodologies are not

TABLE 8.1
Differences Between Quantitative and Qualitative Research

Quantitative	Qualitative
Focuses on a small number of specific concepts and their relationships and differences.	Attempts to understand the entirety or whole of a phenomenon within a prescribed context.
Set on a predefined theoretical foundation. 'Educated guesses' made about relationship of concepts and study outcomes.	No preconceived theoretical boundaries or preconceived notions about study outcomes.
Researcher controls and interprets data.	Focuses on people's interpretations of events and circumstances rather than the researcher's interpretation.
Tends to use larger samples.	Tends to use smaller samples.
Describes people in the study as 'subjects'.	Describes people in the study as 'participants', 'informants' or sometimes 'co investigators'.
Uses language in a way that implies neutrality, such as writing in the third person.	Can be written up using the first person.
Uses structured procedures and formal instruments to collect information.	Collects information without formal structured instruments.
Collects information under conditions of control and manipulation.	Doesn't attempt to control the context of research, but attempts to capture it in its entirety.
Emphasises objectivity in collection and analysis of information. Attempts to exclude all forms of subjective 'bias'.	Attempts to capitalise on the subjective as a means of understanding and interpreting human experiences. Is comfortable with the notion of 'bias'.
Uses 'objective' tools to collect data.	Researcher is the instrument of data collection.

fixed: they constantly evolve and develop. Qualitative researchers must have a good grasp of the underpinning tenets of qualitative research, as this will inform the nature of inquiry and methods used to collect and analyse data. Qualitative research may be classified by theoretical perspective or by research design and/or methodology (see Box 8.1).

Theoretical Perspective (Paradigm)

When **theoretical perspectives** are used to classify qualitative research, they indicate the underlying belief system that informs the research (Creswell & Poth 2018). For example, the interpretive tradition generally seeks understanding of the world through the perspective of people who have lived a particular phenomenon (e.g. individuals living with type 1 diabetes or women who have experienced a caesarean birth) or who have a particular way of being in the world (such as those from a particular cultural or social background). On the other hand, critical theorists are agents of change. They are interested in the social construction of experience and the material resources, power dynamics and ideologies of societies, and they use research to develop transformative knowledge (knowledge to effect positive and empowering change) (Denzin & Lincoln 2018). Poststructural and postmodern studies may also be concerned with concepts such as culture, gender, power and oppression, and how these are

constructed through knowledge or expertise and come to circulate through language or discourse, producing understandings of everyday life (Dunn & Robinson-Lane 2020). These words or language have real-world or material effects in justifying and producing interventions, practices and relations evident in large structures or institutions such as healthcare systems, and other constructs of social governance; for example, in receiving a diagnosis or an illness label. Postmodern researchers pay attention to multiple, diverse accounts of realities. In contrast, phenomenological researchers, building on theories from 20th-century philosophy, seek to delineate lived experience and the shared aspects of human phenomena, aiming to point to the essences of experiential phenomena (Zahavi & Martiny 2019). Such phenomena include loneliness, recovery from illness, wellbeing or dignity (e.g. what makes the phenomenon of loneliness, recovery, wellbeing or dignity cohere through all its variations?). Consequently, the focus of this chapter is to highlight and unfold the methodologies that you are likely to encounter in your studies.

Research Design and Methodology

Classification by **research design** or **methodology** provides us with direction as to what a qualitative study might be about. It is important to realise that the same clinical issue can be investigated in slightly different ways by using various designs or methodologies. The researcher needs to consider how the different designs or methodologies impact the focus of the research question and therefore the answer that the research will generate. The following are some of the more common methodologies you are likely to see in the nursing and midwifery literature.

Phenomenology

Phenomenology is the study of phenomena *as experienced*, often referred to as lived experiences, to reflect an underpinning **lifeworld** orientation (Galvin et al 2020, Zahavi 2017, Zahavi & Martiny 2019). Phenomenological research seeks to describe and interpret the 'essence' of an experience as it is lived and to understand the subjective meanings of an experience in spatial, embodied, temporal and social ways; for example, through space or places, over time, as lived or felt emotions or sensed and expressed through the body, and in our shared

---

BOX 8.1
CLASSIFICATION SYSTEMS FOR QUALITATIVE RESEARCH

THEORETICAL PERSPECTIVE—PARADIGM

1. Postpositivist
2. Constructivist-interpretive
3. Critical theory
4. Poststructural/postmodern

RESEARCH DESIGN AND METHODOLOGY

1. Phenomenology
2. Ethnography, participant observation
3. Grounded theory
4. Qualitative descriptive research
5. Case study

Source: Adapted from Denzin NK, Lincoln YS: The SAGE handbook of qualitative research, ed 4, Thousand Oaks, 2011, SAGE.

lives with others. This methodology assumes that reality is perceived as subjective and unique to individuals based on their experiences. Examining the different ways people experience the phenomena of interest provides nurses and midwives with deeper insights and understandings. Phenomenology seeks to get beneath the everyday taken-for-granted assumptions that society or scientific disciplines may hold about a particular phenomenon and reveal it in a fresh light to produce new understandings.

Examples of research questions that might be asked by a phenomenological study are, 'What is the lived experience of anorexia?', 'What are women's experiences of assisted reproductive technology?' or 'What are the experiences of accessing healthcare for non-binary or queer people?'

Sources of data include in-depth, often unstructured interviews that aim to explore the complexity of the lived experience. A phenomenological interview often begins with a broad question to open up the topic. Following this opening question, phenomenological researchers may use more specific questioning to probe and clarify aspects of the experience. Analysis occurs by transforming the data into units of meaning, searching the data for patterns that connect the variations and descriptions of the essential features or characteristics of the phenomenon. This process is reflective and uses established phenomenological procedures to help the researcher give primacy to the phenomenon and not their pre-understandings, or the assumptions we all hold that frequently drive our interest in a research topic. This is often because, in choosing this area to focus on, the researcher may have similar lived experience, or have a passion for the area, or a commitment to understand it more deeply. Reflections are drawn on to point to the meanings inherent in the whole of the experience. Useful examples of published phenomenological studies can be found in research undertaken by Toft, Hörberg and Rasmussen (2021) who explored how people with severe obesity experience healthy lifestyle interventions, or Suddick and colleagues (2021), who explored the lived experience of being on an acute stroke unit and the role of this area as both a holding and a transitional space. Another example can be found in a paper reported by van der Meide and colleagues (2018) who explored the lived experience of the body when living with multiple sclerosis.

If done well, phenomenology can be an extremely powerful vehicle for portraying the human experience. Since phenomenology is founded on deep philosophical assumptions, at first its concepts can be hard to grasp, but several writers have developed approaches that are faithful to the philosophical foundations. For example, the work of United Kingdom academic Linda Finlay (2011) makes phenomenology more accessible for health professions (www.lindafinlay.co.uk/phenomenology). Max van Manen's Phenomenology Online is also a good starting point (www.phenomenologyonline.com).

STUDENT CHALLENGE

Developing a Question

In considering Jamie's case study, which focused on the care required for a 14-year-old woman living with learning disabilities and a new diagnosis of type 1 diabetes, formulate a question that could explore this topic using a phenomenological approach.

Also formulate a phenomenological research question focused on Ahmed's topic (care provision for an 87-year-old man with newly diagnosed COPD who is also the carer for his wife who has dementia).

Ethnography

Ethnography has its roots in anthropology and is the study of cultures and the everyday lives of people living in those cultural groups. 'Culture' is a broad term, the meaning of which could range from a study focused on a community in Western Samoa to an examination of a neighbourhood in Melbourne, Auckland or London, or an investigation of the culture of a hospital or ward. Ethnography focuses on the study of the symbols, rituals and customs of the cultural group and provides a picture of that identified group through observation and documentation of interactions in their daily lives.

The ethnographic research question focuses on issues such as:

- What procedures does a person follow that make that person part of a group?
- What practices do group members engage in that result in a particular end product?
- What type of work do members engage in to accomplish the goals of the group?

- What are the everyday rituals, norms and patterns of behaviour within a specified social setting?

Ethnography focuses on group interactions and activities rather than on individual behaviours. Researchers immerse themselves in the culture or group to be studied. Data are gathered through observation and interview and are analysed for cultural patterns to grasp the lifeways of a particular group in a specific environment.

Madeleine Leininger was a prominent nurse ethnographer who conducted a lifetime of ethnographic studies to examine the phenomenon of 'caring' from various cultural perspectives. She viewed caring as the central and unifying theme for the practice of nursing (McFarland & Wehbe-Alamah 2019). Recent examples of ethnographic studies include a study by Kvarnstrom, Jangland and Dahlgren (2018) who used ethnographic techniques to describe how interprofessional practice was enhanced when nurse practitioners were included in the team. A study by Featherstone, Northcott and Bridges (2019) used ethnography to explore the care of people with dementia, finding that routine resistance to care was perpetuated by ward cultures of timetabled rounds or mealtimes. In a further study, Wright, Pincombe and McKellar (2018) used ethnography to explore how woman-centred care is applied and practised in antenatal care consultations. As is the case with other qualitative methodologies, the philosophical, paradigmatic and theoretical aspects of ethnography are in a continuous cycle of deconstruction and reconstruction.

STUDENT CHALLENGE

Using Ethnography as a Research Approach

Reflecting on the case studies and the use of an ethnographic approach, what type of question could be formulated for Jamie's assessment, which focused on the care needs of a 14-year-old woman living with learning disabilities and who has a history of self-harm? What type of question could be formulated for Ahmed's research project associated with caring for a family member who has dementia?

Grounded Theory

In **grounded theory** research, data are collected, analysed and used to develop a theoretical explanation and to generate hypotheses for further research. Thus, the theory is generated from and 'grounded' in the data. Grounded theory is used to examine embedded social processes that occur in a given context or phenomenon. Core concepts and dominant processes occurring in interactions are often identified and the researcher endeavours to discover explanations for these concepts and processes.

Research questions revolve around the chief concern or problem of individuals in a defined area. Examples of research questions that might be asked in a grounded theory study are:

- How do people prepare themselves emotionally for surgery?
- How do patients with a cancer diagnosis achieve hopefulness?
- How do individuals in an abusive relationship develop resilience?

When undertaking a grounded theory study, a theoretical sampling strategy is used. This means participants are purposively or deliberately sought and recruited to provide the researcher with the information they need. A process of collecting and analysing data simultaneously occurs (Conlon et al 2020). Data are usually collected using observational and interview techniques. Coding helps the researcher conceptualise the underlying patterns within the data as it is collected. Categories of data are then developed. A form of analysis known as constant comparison analysis is used, whereby each new piece of data is compared to data that has already been collected. Concepts are developed as data are blended into larger categories and relationships between concepts are examined and linked into a conceptual framework. The literature is then consulted to determine whether any similar associations have already been uncovered.

A grounded theory approach has been used to explore managers' and health professionals' perceptions of midwives' work (Hansson et al 2018). Ali, O'Cathain and Croot (2019) also used this approach to develop a theory of the meaning and process of intimate partner violence from the perspective of Pakistani men and women living within and outside Pakistan. In their study, to describe young people's experiences of transitioning to independent self-care when living with asthma, Velsor-Friedrich and Hogan (2021) found that the core social process is that of 'being unprepared'.

Case Study

A **case study** is an in-depth examination of a particular phenomenon, issue or event within a real-life context. A case study can be used as a methodology, design or method. If a case study is to be used as a methodology, it needs to have a clear epistemological position (such as postpositivism or social constructionism) (Berthelsen & Hølge-Hazelton 2018). Case studies can also take a purely qualitative or quantitative approach, or use a combination of qualitative and quantitative data (mixed methods) (see Chapter 9). This approach is widely used across a variety of disciplines, including nursing and midwifery.

The types of research questions a case study can answer include those asking 'how' and 'why' to explore, describe or explain the occurrence of a particular phenomenon. Multiple data sources are used to answer the research question and can include policy and guideline documents and quantitative as well as qualitative data. Using multiple data sources generates comprehensive understandings of the case (Yin 2017). For example, if you study an illness and its effects on an individual, some characteristics of the illness can be quantified or measured (e.g. vital signs, frequency of signs and symptoms). However, other characteristics are better described using narratives (e.g. the feelings associated with illness). A case can be defined as an individual person, family or community, or a single site such as a ward, health service, school or hospital.

Once data have been collected and analysed, a process called **triangulation** occurs. Triangulation is where the findings from each of the data sources are synthesised to look for commonly occurring understandings about the phenomenon under investigation.

Triangulation is an essential component of case study research because it increases confidence in study findings, as well as contributing to an in-depth understanding of the case (Morgan et al 2017).

Recent examples of the use of case studies include an examination of nurses' experiences and perspectives on their role in administering medications to children (Farre et al 2017). Another example is Shannon (2021), who used a critical realist case study design to explain the process and outcomes of the transition of a group of older people with dementia from a traditional aged care facility to a dementia-friendly care village.

Complete the student challenge to enhance your understanding of these concepts. See Table 8.2 in the Additional resources for additional information.

Qualitative Descriptive Research

Qualitative researchers follow the assumptions of the **naturalistic paradigm** which values subjectivity, is exploratory, seeks to explore human experiences and associated meaning and aims to describe and interpret these rather than quantify a research problem. In addition to following the assumptions of the naturalistic paradigm, qualitative researchers use certain methodologies, as we have discussed, to conceptually guide the research. However, many researchers may not follow a specific theoretical positioning or methodology (such as constructionism, ethnography, phenomenology or grounded theory) and take a more generic approach to conducting qualitative research within the naturalistic paradigm. A common broad qualitative approach seen in nursing and midwifery literature is qualitative descriptive research.

Like all qualitative research, **qualitative descriptive research** focuses on exploring phenomena and contexts where there may be little known and describes

TABLE 8.2		
Difference Between Paradigm, Methodology and Methods		
Paradigm	Methodology	Methods
A paradigm is understood as a lens or a way of looking at the world; a worldview. It is made up of sets of beliefs/assumptions, values and practices that constitute a way of viewing reality. Different paradigms are characterised by ontological, epistemological and methodological differences in their approaches to conceptualising and conducting research. Each paradigm has specific perspectives on the nature of social reality and assumptions about human existence (ontology) and beliefs about the nature of knowledge: how we come to know things (epistemology). Realists, for example, believe there is a truth to be discovered out there in the world that we come to know objectively, whereas relativists believe there are multiple perspectives of reality and therefore multiple truths, and that we come to know the world subjectively and intersubjectively. The two dominant paradigms are qualitative (relativism/postpositivist) and quantitative (realism/positivist), but in this book, you will read about others, such as Indigenous paradigms (relativism, critical).	A methodology fits within the traditions of the chosen paradigm and is the approach or frame of reference taken by the researcher to guide how to undertake the research. It is informed by theory and has philosophical underpinnings, which constitute the assumptions held about knowledge, values, reality and logic. These principles determine how the methods are to be deployed and interpreted. Understanding and remaining true to the fundamental tenets of the methodology ensure the research is rigorously carried out. For example, while phenomenology and ethnography as methodologies both fall within the qualitative interpretive paradigm and are faithful to that mode of understanding, they are influenced by different strains of philosophical thought that influence how the research will be conducted; including what counts as data and how that data will be analysed.	Methods are determined by the methodology and are the techniques or processes used to sample, collect and analyse data, as well as to report the findings; for example, writing field notes or administering a survey. The methods need to 'fit' the methodological approach taken. In the previous chapter, you saw that an experimental study falls under the quantitative empirical paradigm and that data will usually be collected by instruments that have been carefully calibrated. On the other hand, the collection of qualitative data is usually undertaken by the researchers themselves. Open-ended interviews, for example, may well be used as methods in both ethnography and a study that draws on the principles of phenomenology. However, the types of questions asked in the interviews will be different because they stem from different methodologies.

the nature of that particular phenomenon. A distinguishing feature of qualitative descriptive research is that it describes an experience or situation rather than deeply interpreting or conceptualising the data, as would be the case, for example, within a temporal context (as with phenomenology) or to develop theoretical explanation (which would be expected when using a grounded theory methodology). Margarete Sandelowski's (2000) seminal work highlighted that qualitative descriptive research encapsulates, describes and presents findings through the use of everyday language, rather than within the context of a highly interpretive conceptual or theoretical framework.

Qualitative descriptive studies can have fluid boundaries, require researchers to explore data and can include a mix of qualitative methods and techniques (Sandelowski 2000, 2010). Common data collection methods include interviews and focus groups. Data analysis techniques vary but often include content analysis, or the analysis of words and phrases, or thematic analysis, the categorisation of data into common themes.

Cutler and colleagues (2021) used a qualitative descriptive approach to explore the experience of safety from the perspective of people admitted to an acute mental health facility. James and colleagues (2021) sought to understand the barriers and facilitators to lifestyle risk communication by registered nurses in Australian general practice. Similarly, Ashley and colleagues (2021) used a qualitative descriptive methodology to explore primary healthcare nurses' perceptions of risk during COVID-19.

TABLE 8.3
Identification of Phenomenon

Research Design/ Methodology	Identification of Phenomenon
Phenomenology	Lived experience
Ethnography	Issue(s) of interest within a defined culture
Grounded theory	Basic social process
Descriptive	Experiences, attitudes, perceptions
Case study	Broad area for case(s) selection

WHAT IS THE QUALITATIVE RESEARCH PROCESS?

As you likely have already observed, qualitative and quantitative research look different in the final written report format. The conduct of research is also different. While the same basic steps are followed, the processes of qualitative research are somewhat less segmented. This provides more scope for creative, expressive and innovative dimensions. Qualitative research deploys a dynamic process where several phases of the process frequently occur simultaneously or are revisited numerous times during the course of the research. Many of the decisions about various aspects of the research process are made or altered as data are collected and certain trends or patterns are noted. There is an artistry and responsiveness to qualitative research, with a much greater focus on writing and rewriting to create a text that is representative of the phenomenon under investigation.

The conceptualisation and design form only a broad umbrella-like structure for qualitative studies. Data collection and analysis dictate detailed study decisions. We will use the broad research phases identified in the previous chapter as we discuss the qualitative research process. You will see there are common issues to be addressed for all classifications of qualitative research.

Phase 1: Conceive the Study

Identify the Problem

As with any research, the first task a qualitative researcher faces is to decide what to study. This means identification of the phenomenon and the key issues the researcher is interested in exploring. Table 8.3 presents some specific examples by research design or methodology.

Unlike quantitative research, in qualitative research the initial identification of the phenomenon to be studied is undertaken in the broadest sense. Phenomenological studies identify a phenomenon to be explored and seek individuals with lived experiences of the phenomenon to be interviewed. Examples are parents of children in an intensive care unit or young people living with a long-term condition, or women who have experienced perinatal death. The ethnographer may choose a group of people or a field setting with a broad statement of what is to be investigated. For example, the health beliefs and practices of Vietnamese immigrants, older residents of a nursing home or same-sex parents might be selected. Grounded theorists begin with a broad area of social interest with no specific problem in mind. For example, the area of interest might be hopefulness and cancer. Although all researchers bring their own individual frame of reference and belief systems to their work, qualitative researchers acknowledge and accept the role of subjectivity and intersubjectivity. This means qualitative researchers may state their prior assumptions or ideas about the study at the outset (reflexivity), while others will attempt to 'bracket' them and set them aside during the investigation. Unlike quantitative research, a hypothesis-driven approach is not a feature of qualitative research and research questions are much broader.

Review the Literature

Most qualitative designs include a literature review at the outset of the study. The review serves various purposes depending on the focus, study classification and aim. For example, a review can be conducted to determine what is currently known about a phenomenon or to gather background information. Additionally, researchers may explore the literature to identify studies that have used certain theoretical perspectives and methodologies. Literature reviews are used to determine current and relevant literature, context, background and justification for a study. However, some qualitative approaches prefer that the researcher be naïve to the literature so that they are not biased by the existing knowledge. For further information on literature reviews, refer to Chapter 3.

Formulate the Research Aim and Questions

Once the phenomenon of interest is selected, a research aim is formulated which is then expressed in the form of a research question. The aim is generally broad and serves as a general focus or guide for the study (e.g. 'The aim of this study is to explore the lived experience of nurses who live with overweight or obesity.'). A research question is more defined; while it needs to be consistent with the aim, it is much more specific (e.g. 'What are the lived experiences of overweight primary care nurses when offering health promotion advice to patients?') Although broader than a quantitative research question, a good qualitative research question needs to be feasible, focused and finite. It often encompasses a population, patient or problem, an issue and a context or place or setting, as well as a potential outcome, and sometimes implies a notion of time, as per the PICO(T) acronym (Green & Thorogood 2018). More defined focal areas of the research often emerge as data are collected and analysed. Table 8.4 presents sample research aims for each design and/or methodology.

Undertake the following student challenge and see if you can identify the research intent of the studies.

STUDENT CHALLENGE

Reading Research Aims

Use the articles you located in the previous student challenges that focused on Ahmed's and Jamie's topics.
1. For each study, see if you can locate the research aims. Are the aims of each study clearly articulated?
2. Examine the literature review section, if present. Can you tell how these were undertaken? Are the reviews more comprehensive in some studies than in others? Is the research aim congruent with the chosen methodology?

TABLE 8.4
Sample Research Aims

Research Design/Methodology	Sample Purpose
Phenomenology	To explore Australian nurse leaders' experiences of mentoring relationships
	To explore the lived experience of a person who has hepatitis C
Ethnography	To explore the nurses' role on a medical assessment unit
	To explore how nurses care for women during early miscarriage in a hospital gynaecological unit
Grounded theory	To review the perceptions and strategies of both drug users and nurses with regard to pain management in acute care settings
	To explore the illness experiences and processes in relation to women undergoing coronary artery bypass graft surgery
Descriptive	To explore the experiences of young women who experienced hyperemesis gravidarum during pregnancy
	To determine perceptions of midwives associated with the medical management of hyperemesis gravidarum
Case study	To analyse and describe women's different perceptions and experiences of childbirth following prolonged or normal labour
	To explore the meanings that emergency department nurses ascribe to acts of violence from patients, their family and friends, and the impact of these meanings on how nurses respond to such acts

Phase 2: Design the Study

Once the phenomenon has been identified and the research aim is determined, the next phase is to decide on the design and/or methodology and plan the study accordingly. The chosen design dictates the general structure of the study and includes initial decisions about the setting, sample selection and data collection methods. Remember, the qualitative process is fluid, and sampling and data collection methods may evolve during data collection.

Setting

The **setting** in qualitative research is often referred to as the '**field**' because the study is set 'in the field'; that is, the natural setting where the phenomenon under investigation occurs. Settings vary by type of design or methodology. The selected setting assumes more importance in some methodologies than in others. The data collection method may also influence the selected setting.

Phenomenological research settings are usually chosen based on convenience for the people who are being studied. Since most of the data is collected through interviews with individual participants, the setting is secondary.

Ethnographic studies take place in a setting where the researcher can readily observe and interact with groups of people belonging to a particular culture. For example, if the culture of interest is midwives, a maternity unit would be an appropriate setting. If the culture of interest is critically ill people, the setting might be an intensive care unit. It is important that the setting in ethnographic research allows the researcher to see and interact with the people within the setting. Observation is a key ingredient when undertaking an ethnographic study.

Grounded theory research takes place in a setting that allows the researcher to identify and understand the selected social processes in action. This includes interviewing and, where appropriate, observing participants. Observing participants allows the researcher to better understand the environmental and contextual influences that support findings gained from the interview. The setting for qualitative descriptive studies is determined by the aim of the study and will vary. Table 8.5 lists possible settings for the common designs/methodologies.

Samples and Sampling

Sample sizes in qualitative research tend to be small and are selected using purposive or convenience sampling

TABLE 8.5 Examples of Research Settings	
Research Design/ Methodology	**Sample Settings**
Phenomenology	Work, home, social
Ethnography	Work, home, social
	Practice areas
Grounded theory	Practice interaction
	Hospital and community
Descriptive and interpretive	Work, home, particular environment
Case study	Labour ward/birthing clinic
	Rural health services
	Emergency department

techniques. In qualitative research, the researcher is not trying to recruit a sample that is representative of the whole population as they would be in quantitative research. The qualitative researcher seeks participants who will be what is termed 'information-rich'— people who have experienced or are experiencing the phenomenon of interest and are willing and able to articulate or communicate that experience. This means the participants can provide a powerful picture of the phenomenon under investigation. For example, if the researcher wants to understand the experiences of a family member who provides care for a loved one living with dementia, they will be seeking people who identify as carers of people living with dementia and who are willing to discuss their experiences with the researcher(s). Several other sampling techniques can be used to help provide an information-rich sample. These include snowball, extreme, intensity, maximum variety and critical case (Denzin & Lincoln 2018). Box 8.2 discusses these techniques in more detail.

Grounded theory studies use a specific sampling technique called theoretical sampling. In theoretical sampling, the researcher begins by collecting and analysing data from an initial sample. This sample is called an open sample because the sampling process is not guided by data analysis. As data are collected and analysed (coded), concepts begin to emerge that will help

BOX 8.2
QUALITATIVE SAMPLING TECHNIQUES

CONVENIENCE AND PURPOSIVE SAMPLING
As described previously, these are commonly seen in qualitative designs.
In addition, the following may be seen.

SNOWBALL SAMPLING
This method involves getting recruited participants to help identify and recruit additional participants.

INTENSITY SAMPLING
Selection of participants who are experiential experts or authorities about the selected phenomena (e.g. in a pain study, intensity sampling might choose those who have chronic pain).

MAXIMUM VARIETY SAMPLING
The deliberate selection of participants who are different, who come from different backgrounds, for the purpose of observing commonalities of experience. (This is particularly helpful when exploring abstract phenomena such as love, joy or hope.)

CRITICAL CASE SAMPLING
Selection of participants identified as demonstrating a 'critical incident' who can provide pertinent, valuable data. (Once critical cases have been identified, additional purposive sampling is conducted to find cases that confirm or refute the critical case.)

THEORETICAL SAMPLING
This technique is used in grounded theory. Sampling continues until the theory is sufficiently developed.

EXTREME OR DEVIANT CASE
Including highly unusual cases of the phenomenon of interest to make sure both the usual and the unusual are captured. Incorporating deviant accounts adds to the credibility of research findings.

phenomenological researchers aim for 'maximum variation'. For example, in a study about older people's mobility, participants might comprise older people who are housebound, as well as older people who can get out of the house independently or with assistance, so that the range of contexts for the phenomenon of mobility is included. In phenomenological research, it is recommended to use repeat interviews where possible to allow for an in-depth exploration (Giorgi, Giorgi & Morely 2017). Therefore, the quality of the description within the interviews is more important than the sample size.

Data Collection Methods

Data for qualitative studies are mainly gathered by using in-depth unstructured or semi-structured interviews, observation and/or focus groups. Observation is recommended when a researcher seeks to study behaviour, activity and sequences of interaction, or the context or environment in which these behaviours and actions take place. Observations may be classified by several features, such as structure, participation of the researcher and visibility of the researcher. Box 8.3 presents a more comprehensive description of these classifications. Ethnographic studies use an unstructured participant observation approach. Grounded theory mainly uses semi-structured interviews to gather data. However, this can be augmented with observation, which supports the information gained from the interviews. Phenomenology employs phenomenological interviews that are open-ended and aim for rich examples of how a phenomenon is manifest in human life (Zahavi & Martiny 2019). Descriptive qualitative methodologies often use semi-structured interviews and/or focus groups, while a case study may use multiple data collection methods.

Interviews. Interviews allow the researcher to explore the opinions, experiences, attitudes and belief systems of participants. Interviews can be on a continuum from structured to unstructured. In-depth semi-structured (through the use of an interview guide) and unstructured interviews are generally used in qualitative research. While semi-structured interviews will use an interview guide to provide the researcher with a small number of questions to provide some structure to the interview, an unstructured interview will

form an evolving theory. These concepts are called categories and are identified by their repeated presence or absence in the data. The researcher then recruits more participants, looking for additional data to support or refute the identified categories. The researcher continues the processes of sampling, data collection and analysis until all identified categories are fully explored or saturated.

Sampling in phenomenological research aims to access people who can provide descriptions and illustrations of the phenomenon under study. Sometimes,

STRUCTURE

1. Structured: specified behaviours are predetermined and listed on a checklist to be counted or checked off during an observation period.
2. Unstructured: behaviours are described and recorded as or after they occur using a journal, diary or field notes. A detailed descriptive picture is recorded.

PARTICIPATION OF THE RESEARCHER

1. Participant: the researcher is an active part of the activities or behaviours engaged in by the participants being observed.
2. Non-participant: the researcher is a bystander or passive participant in the activities being observed.

VISIBILITY OF THE RESEARCHER

1. Concealed: the non-participant observer is hidden from those being observed. The activities might be recorded on video for later viewing and analysis, or activities might be viewed from a concealed space such as behind a two-way mirror.
2. Non-concealed: the observer is in full view of the participants.

Focus Groups. **Focus groups** are another qualitative data collection technique. This is where groups of people with experience of the phenomenon under investigation are interviewed together. Focus group interviews allow researchers to collect data from a larger sample compared to individual interviews. They also appeal to those people who do not feel comfortable being interviewed one-on-one and generate data from participant interaction. Conversely, there is the risk that one or two members of the group may dominate the focus group interview and that responses will be provided in front of the whole group. However, this can be mitigated by an experienced researcher who will ensure all participants have the opportunity to contribute to the research. Focus groups usually comprise approximately six to eight people from a similar background who can provide information that will answer the research aim. It is recommended to include at least two focus groups for each participant type (Hennink, Kaiser & Weber 2019). For example, in a study to understand the experiences of refugees birthing in a hospital setting, focus groups might be held with two groups of refugees who had birthed in the hospital and two groups with midwives who had cared for these refugees. Groups are separated by participant background to avoid issues of power or conflict that may exist if participants were mixed in a single group.

The Researcher and Qualitative Data Collection. Undertaking qualitative research requires a knowledgeable and skilled researcher. This is because the amount, type and quality of data retrieved are due in large part to the skills and abilities of the researcher, who must be able to enter the field and gain the trust of the people in that environment. Qualitative interviewing, whether with individuals or in focus groups, requires considerable thought and care because it is often about sensitive or potentially distressing topics. Consequently, participants may be vulnerable. Narrative generated from the interview is often the primary source of data and poor interviewing skills will compromise the quality of data and, therefore, the study itself.

The researcher must have well-developed interviewing and communication skills, with a good feel for the ebb and flow of conversation, and be able to keep the interview flowing with well-placed responses and

only have a general topic area or question to begin the discussion. Both types of interviews are guided by the methodology and the general aim of the research and are largely conducted in a conversational, storytelling style. The researcher might begin with a very broad, open-ended request, such as, 'Tell me about ...'. As the person being interviewed tells their story, the interviewer will ask additional questions or use prompts to encourage elaboration on certain aspects of the story. To elicit information, the researcher needs to use open-ended questions rather than closed questions such as those that produce a 'yes' or 'no' response. Different styles of interview are used to produce the best data for answering the specific research question. For example, a grounded theory interview will differ from a phenomenological interview because the researcher is not seeking to explore the same aspects of the phenomenon. Interviews can be undertaken face-to-face, via telephone or increasingly via video conference.

cues. Interviewing requires active listening and the ability to pick up and follow up on subtle leads or clues provided by participants in the course of the interview or the focus group. The researcher must be able to put the participant(s) at ease and know how to elicit information that participants may find hard to express. Finally, the researcher must have a good grasp of self. This means being aware of and able to recognise and reflect on pre-understandings, perceptions and beliefs that may influence the data collection and analysis.

Researchers use several tools to record their observations or interviews. These include audio and video recordings and field notes. Audio and video recordings can be transcribed for closer analysis. Field notes are a written account of what the researcher sees, hears, experiences and thinks during and following data collection. Field notes can be classified into four basic types. The first is a brief description of what has occurred. Notes of this type contain key phrases and major events and are often jotted down in the field. The second type of note is an expansion of the first type. These are recorded immediately after a data collection session and expand on the brief notes, adding detail. The third type of note is a reflective journal, kept by many researchers and containing descriptions of personal thoughts, feelings and responses that occurred during the process of data collection. Finally, any insights, analyses of observations, judgments and interpretations made in the field are recorded and kept.

Qualitative researchers are concerned with the 'accuracy' and comprehensiveness of the data they collect (Morse 2018). They do not tend to speak in terms of reliability and validity but rather in terms of **trustworthiness**. Trustworthiness comprises four attributes: credibility, auditability, confirmability and transferability. **Credibility** is a term used to examine whether or not the explanation or interpretation of data reflects what has been described or recorded. Credibility may be examined and cross-checked using two techniques: member checks and audit trails (Flick 2018). Member checks are commonly used by qualitative researchers and involve having study participants review the transcripts or material once it has been analysed and interpreted. Credibility, therefore, is a question of validity. Some might call this 'truth' but in qualitative research, the notion of truth is a complex issue, as some people believe there may be many 'truths', each being grounded

in its own context and personal perspective (Creswell & Poth 2018). Data are considered confirmed when what is recorded matches what occurred. The use of audio and video recordings, excerpts of transcripts and investigator triangulation, combined with researchers independently analysing and confirming research findings, helps ensure data are confirmable. However, regarding trustworthiness, different procedures are used for each of the main qualitative approaches, and it is important to understand coherence and apply the procedures that are recommended for the specific kind of research you are undertaking, whether it is ethnographic, grounded theory, descriptive, phenomenological, and so on.

Audit trails (decision trails) ensure that adequate documentation is available about the data collection and analysis processes. Enough detail should be provided to enable another researcher to repeat the study. This is known as auditability or dependability. Transferability relates to when the findings 'fit' or can be transferred into contexts outside the study situation. It is important to understand that the notion of validity or rigour in qualitative research is a contested space and theorists are constantly extending its agenda. Additionally, these concepts differ from the definitions seen in quantitative research (Chapter 7) (Denzin & Lincoln 2018). Look for a decision trail and authenticity in any research report and you should be halfway there.

STUDENT CHALLENGE

Scrutinising Phase 2

Look again at the qualitative research studies you examined earlier that focused on Ahmed's and Jamie's research topics. Scan these studies and see if you can identify each of the elements we have discussed in phase 2.

1. Identify the settings.
2. Identify the sample and sample size.
3. What data collection methods were used?
4. Did any of the studies address the issues of trustworthiness? (Look for key terms such as rigour, credibility, member checks or audit trails.)

Phase 3: Conduct the Study

This phase receives a lot of time and attention in qualitative research. The conceptualisation and planning stages are usually preliminary and loosely defined, to lay a broad set of boundaries for data collection. As data collection begins, data analysis may occur simultaneously. Data collection and analysis can lead to ongoing conceptualisation and planning about further collection and analysis. So, we again see the fluid and repetitive (iterative) nature of the qualitative research process.

From your reading of Chapter 6, you will understand that the issues of informed consent as they apply to qualitative research differ from those of quantitative research. Like other researchers, investigators using qualitative approaches have to be able to demonstrate that the ethical principles of research are upheld at all times. This includes ensuring the benefits outweigh the risks, research integrity and participant autonomy through informed consent and voluntary participation, with participants being able to withdraw from the study at any time. Frequently, the focus of qualitative research is on issues and experiences that are intensely personal and even traumatic in nature. Participation in qualitative studies can involve participants being asked to recall (and therefore, in a way, re-live) very traumatic life events. This means there is the potential for emotional distress. Institutional ethics committees will expect to see strategies for dealing with the possibility of emotional distress in participants and potential vicarious trauma in researchers.

Informed consent is required for participation in interviews and audio or video recording of interviews. Video recording should only be used where specifically necessary as it is difficult to anonymise this data given it provides images of the participant. Issues related to keeping information about a participant confidential are part of the consent process and are of paramount importance. Examples of how confidentiality can be maintained include replacing names with pseudonyms and changing any identifying details in transcripts, publications or research reports. Consent may need to be renegotiated with participants as data collection progresses and information emerges that may send the collection process in a new direction.

People recruited to qualitative research studies are usually called participants or informants rather than subjects (as in quantitative studies). The term 'participant' or 'informant' is used to convey the sense of mutual participation and trust-building that occurs between the researcher and the people being researched and is reflective of a qualitative worldview.

Data collection is a lengthy process in most qualitative studies, which needs to be considered when planning the project. The process of data collection is often described in more detail in qualitative studies because the collection process is often used to make decisions about the credibility of the data. Complete the following student challenge.

STUDENT CHALLENGE
Study Conduct
Look again at the qualitative research studies you located focused on Ahmed's and Jamie's topics and examined for phases 1 and 2. Look for evidence of the steps in phase 3.
1. Were the rights of participants protected in these studies? What evidence did you find to support this?
2. Is there evidence of approval by an institutional ethics committee?
3. Was informed consent obtained?
4. What information was provided about data collection?

Phase 4: Analysis

Analysis of qualitative data is an inductive process and involves examining words, descriptions and processes. Analytical procedures vary according to the methodology, but all require the researcher to read and re-read field notes and transcripts or data sources, to ensure familiarity with the data. This is often called **data immersion**, dwelling with the data or 'getting a sense of the whole'. It lets the researcher get in touch with not only the content but also the feeling, tone and emphasis being communicated.

Initial analysis efforts are directed at setting up a system to make large volumes of data more manageable. A system is needed that allows the researcher to file, code and easily retrieve data. Computer programs, referred to as 'computer-assisted qualitative data analysis software' (CAQDAS), are increasingly used to assist in data management and analysis processes. Examples of these include ATLAS.ti, MAXQDA and NVivo. While this software helps to manage the data, it does not do the analysis like quantitative analysis software. Regardless of how the analysis is undertaken, the researcher searches for themes, patterns and meaning in the data and arranges this information in some way that classifies or categorises it.

Methods of Analysis

There are a variety of methods used to analyse qualitative data. Examples include thematic, narrative, content, reflective and discourse analysis. While these methods may be different and aligned to particular qualitative methodologies, they share commonalities. **Qualitative analysis** requires researchers to make sense of, delineate key characteristics from and synthesise what the participants have said; in other words, to find meaning from the data. Data are compared and contrasted, with similarities and differences noted and processes and relationships defined. Key concepts present both within and across transcripts or datasets are presented as themes. Themes form the basis of reporting qualitative research findings and must address the research aim and be developed into meanings.

As mentioned earlier, the analytical frameworks used to analyse qualitative data may vary depending on which qualitative methodology is employed. However, some frameworks are transportable and appropriate to use across several, but not all, qualitative methodologies. Examples include content analysis (see Lindgren, Lundman & Graneheim 2020) and thematic analysis (TA). Braun and Clarke's TA framework is currently being widely used across a variety of disciplines, including nursing and midwifery (Braun & Clarke 2021). This model identifies the following six-step approach to qualitative data analysis:

1. transcribing the data into written form, reading the transcripts several times noting down any first impressions
2. allocating commonly occurring ideas from the data into codes
3. collating these codes and associated data, and assigning these to what might become initial themes
4. generating a thematic map and re-checking to ensure the codes and data fit. This may require moving or deleting codes
5. refining and naming themes. This step requires ongoing analysis ensuring each data excerpt relates to the theme
6. incorporating the themes into the report. This is the final part of the analysis and is where the most compelling excerpts are selected to represent the theme. These must relate back to and address the research aim(s) (Braun & Clarke 2021).

However, it is important to note that some methodologies have prescribed analytical procedures that are coherent with the specific method. For example, both grounded theory and phenomenology follow their own distinctive procedures and do not rely on a generic analysis approach, such as the one just outlined.

Findings

The findings in most qualitative studies are presented in a way more immediately understandable to the novice reader of research than the results in most quantitative studies. This is because the language used is commonly in a descriptive narrative form. However, you will notice that many qualitative researchers have a very sophisticated use of language and you will see words used that you may not be familiar with. You will also notice many of these papers present very complex ideas that may require reading, reflection and re-reading to fully grasp their meaning. Frequently, findings are illustrated with the use of direct excerpts of participants' narratives. A good qualitative presentation of findings leaves the reader with a clear, cohesive picture of the phenomenon under study that is validated by quotes from the participants themselves.

STUDENT CHALLENGE

Analysis and Findings

Examine the analyses used and the findings of the analyses in the research studies you located focused on Ahmed's and Jamie's topics.

1. Can you identify the specific analytical methods employed?
2. Were the findings understandable? Did you get a sense of what had been uncovered in the study? Did they ring true?
3. How do you think the findings would differ in each study if a quantitative approach was employed?

Phase 5: Use the Study

Qualitative research is a powerful tool for bringing the human face of nursing or midwifery care into the public domain and reminding health professionals of the centrality of the human experience in healthcare. Qualitative research is used to raise awareness and understanding of issues related to the human experience of health and wellness. It is a powerful tool that may persuade policymakers and decision-makers to take heed of an issue. Qualitative research findings can change policy and inform practice, and should lead to better care by nurses and midwives. The increased insight and understanding of human experiences can inform nurses and midwives about how to modify their approaches to the delivery of healthcare to improve the experiences of patients and their families, or indeed the experiences of nurses and midwives delivering the care.

Consumers of research (such as you, the reader) need to be satisfied that the findings of qualitative research are credible and trustworthy. Although the notion of ensuring accuracy, also referred to as rigour, is contentious in qualitative work, qualitative researchers have developed concepts such as credibility to ensure that qualitative studies meet the criterion of scientific rigour.

The qualitative researcher is under the same obligation as the quantitative researcher to disseminate the study findings. The avenues for this dissemination are much the same for qualitative and quantitative researchers and include journal articles and conference presentations. However, qualitative studies may also be found in book form because of the length of the presentation. This format allows fuller description and use of a greater number and variety of example illustrations obtained from data collection.

STUDENT CHALLENGE

Examining the Studies You Located in Your Searches

1. What did you glean from the studies' conclusions?
2. What implications might stem from the studies that can be applied to:
   a. your professional practice?
   b. education and/or policy development?
3. How would you compare your overall experience of reading qualitative research studies with reading quantitative research studies?

CONCLUSION

This chapter has explored qualitative research in terms of design, theoretical positioning and the research process. It has highlighted common methodologies you are likely to see in nursing and midwifery research. One question students frequently raise is whether quantitative and qualitative methods can be used together. Some researchers do combine quantitative and qualitative methods to study certain phenomena. This is referred to as mixed methods research and is covered in the next chapter.

ADDITIONAL RESOURCES

Want to Know More About Qualitative Research?

Try entering 'qualitative research' as a search phrase using a search engine on the internet. A variety of interesting websites are devoted to qualitative research.

Check out the activities on the Evolve website http://evolve.elsevier.com/AU/Jackson/maze/ for further information.

REFERENCES

Ali PA, O'Cathain A, Croot E: Not managing expectations: a grounded theory of intimate partner violence from the perspective of Pakistani people, Journal of Interpersonal Violence 34(19): 4085–4113, 2019.

Ashley C, James S, Stephen C, et al: Primary health care nurses' perceptions of risk during COVID-19: a qualitative study, Journal of Nursing Scholarship 53(6):689–697, 2021. https://doi.org/10.1111/jnu.12698.

Berthelsen CB, Hølge-Hazelton B: Caught between a rock and a hard place: An intrinsic single case study of nurse researchers' experiences of the presence of a nursing research culture in clinical practice, Journal of Clinical Nursing 27(7 8):1572 1580, 2018.

Braun V, Clarke V: Thematic analysis: a practical guide, London, 2021, SAGE.

Conlon C, Timonen V, Elliot-O'Dare C, et al: Confused about theoretical sampling? Engaging theoretical sampling in diverse grounded theory studies, Qualitative Health Research 30(6): 947–959, 2020. https://doi.org/10.1177/1049732319899139.

Creswell J, Poth C: Qualitative inquiry and research design. Choosing among five approaches, ed 4, Thousand Oaks, 2018, SAGE.

Cutler N, Halcomb E, Sim J, et al: How does the environment influence consumers' perceptions of safety in acute mental health units? A qualitative study, Journal of Clinical Nursing, 30 (5–6):765–772, 2021. https://doi.org/10.1111/jocn.15614.

Denzin NK, Lincoln YS: The SAGE handbook of qualitative research, ed 5, Thousand Oaks, 2018, SAGE.

Dunn K, Robinson-Lane S: A philosophical analysis of spiritual coping, Advances in Nursing Science 43(3):239–250, 2020. https://doi.org/10.1097/ANS.0000000000000323.

Farre A, Heath G, Shaw K, et al: The role of paediatric nurses in medication safety prior to the implementation of electronic prescribing: a qualitative case study, Journal of Health Services Research & Policy 22(2):99–106, 2017. https://doi.org/10.1177/13558196686995.

Featherstone K, Northcott A, Bridges J: Routines of resistance: An ethnography of the care of people living with dementia in acute hospital wards and its consequences, International Journal of Nursing Studies 96:53–60, 2019.

Finlay L: Phenomenology for therapists: researching the lived world, Chichester, 2011, Wiley-Blackwell.

Flick U: Managing quality in qualitative research, ed 2, London, 2018, SAGE.

Galvin KT, Pound C, Cowdell F, et al: A lifeworld theory-led action research process for humanizing services: improving 'what matters' to older people to enhance humanly sensitive care, International Journal of Qualitative Studies on Health and Well-Being 15(1):2020. https://doi.org/10.1080/17482631.2020.1817275.

Giorgi A, Giorgi B, Morley J: The descriptive phenomenological psychological method. In Willig C, Rogers WS (eds): The SAGE handbook of qualitative research in psychology, 2017, SAGE Publications, pp. 176–192.

Green J, Thorogood N: Qualitative methods for health research, ed 4, London, 2018, SAGE.

Hansson M, Lundgren I, Hensing G, et al: Veiled midwifery in the baby factory—a grounded theory study, Women and Birth Feb;32(1):80–86, 2018. https://doi.org/10.1016/j.wombi.2018.04.012.

Hennink M, Kaiser B, Weber MB: What influences saturation? Estimating sample sizes in focus group research, Qualitative Health Research 29(10):1483–1496, 2019.

James S, Halcomb E, McInnes S, Desborough J: Barriers and facilitators to lifestyle risk communication by Australian general practice nurses, Australian Journal of Primary Health 27(1):30–35, 2021. https://doi.org/10.1071/PY20139.

Kvarnstrom S, Jangland E, Dahlgren MA: Introducing the nurse practitioner into the surgical ward: an ethnographic study of interprofessional teamwork practice, Scandinavian Journal of Caring Sciences 32(2):765–771, 2018. https://doi.org/10.1111/scs.12507.

Lindgren B, Lundman B, Graneheim UH: Abstraction and interpretation during the qualitative content analysis process, International Journal of Nursing Studies May;108(3):103632, 2020. https://doi.org/10.1016/j.ijnurstu.2020.103632.

McFarland M, Wehbe-Alamah, H: Leininger's theory of culture care diversity and universality: an overview with a historical retrospective and a view toward the future, Journal of Transcultural Nursing (6):540–557, 2019.

Morgan SJ, Pullon SR, Macdonald LM, et al: Case study observational research: a framework for conducting case study research where observation data are the focus, Qualitative Health Research 27(7):1060–1068, 2017.

Morse J, Reframing rigor in qualitative inquiry. In Denzin N, Lincoln Y (eds), The SAGE handbook of qualitative research book, ed 5, Thousand Oaks, 2018, SAGE, pp. 796–817.

Sandelowski M: Whatever happened to qualitative description? Research in Nursing & Health 23:334–340, 2000.

Sandelowski M: What's in a name? Qualitative description revisited, Research in Nursing & Health 33:77–84, 2010.

Shannon K: The creation of a dementia-friendly community in aged residential care: A critical realist case study. [Unpublished doctoral thesis] Auckland University of Technology, 2021.

Suddick KM, Cross V, Vuoskoski P et al: Holding space and transitional space: stroke survivors' lived experience of being on an acute stroke unit: a hermeneutic phenomenological study, Scandinavian Journal of Caring Sciences 35(1):104–114, 2021.

Toft BS, Hörberg U, Rasmussen, B: The ups and downs of lifestyle modification: An existential journey among persons with severe obesity, Scandinavian Journal of Caring Sciences 4 May:1–10, 2021. https://doi.org/10.1111/scs.12985.

van der Meide H, Teunissen T, Collard P, et al: The mindful body: a phenomenology of the body with multiple sclerosis, Qualitative Health Research 28(14):2239–2249, 2018.

Velsor-Friedrich B, Hogan NS: Being unprepared: a grounded theory of the transition of asthma self-care in college students, Journal of Pediatric Nursing 61:305–311, 2021.

Wright D, Pincombe J, McKellar L: Exploring routine hospital antenatal care consultations—an ethnographic study, Women and Birth 31(3):e162–e169, 2018. https://doi.org/10.1016/j.wombi.2017.09.010.

Yin P: Case study research and applications: design and methods, London, 2017, SAGE.

Zahavi D, Martiny KMM: Phenomenology in nursing studies: new perspectives, International Journal of Nursing Studies 93: 155–162, 2019.

Zahavi D: Phenomenology the basics, London, 2017, Routledge.

9

MIXED METHODS RESEARCH

ELIZABETH HALCOMB ■ DEBBIE MASSEY ■ NEESHA OOZAGEER GUNOWA

■ ■ ■ ■ ■ ■ ■ ■ ■ ■ ■ ■ ■ ■ ■ ■ ■ ■

CHAPTER OUTLINE

LEARNING OBJECTIVES

After reading this chapter and following critical reflection, readers should be able to:

- define mixed methods research
- outline the reasons for conducting mixed methods research
- identify and describe the various mixed methods research designs
- describe the practical considerations in undertaking mixed methods research
- discuss reliability, validity and rigour in mixed methods research.

KEY TERMS

concurrent mixed
  methods

mixed methods research

multimethod research

sequential mixed
  methods

triangulation

ABSTRACT

As a way of understanding the complexity of the world in which we live, many researchers and scholars are turning to mixed methods research. Mixed methods designs use a combination of qualitative and quantitative research in a single study. Mixed methods research seeks to build on the strengths and mitigate the limitations of both qualitative and quantitative approaches. Like qualitative and quantitative research, a mixed methods study needs to be systematically planned. While mixed methods research follows many of the steps of the research process of qualitative and quantitative research, it also has some unique considerations that need to be understood by both the researcher and the research consumer. Mixed methods designs can be classified by the sequence in which the qualitative and quantitative data are collected, the relative priority given to each method, the stage at which the qualitative and quantitative data are integrated and whether an overall theoretical perspective will be used to guide the research process. Mixed methods research also allows the researcher to go beyond predetermined designs to creatively develop a research plan that will most effectively answer the specific research question.

STUDENT QUOTE

Mixed methods research captures both the art and the science of clinical practice. It recognises that not all nursing and midwifery research problems can be reduced to numbers and that words do not always tell the complete picture either.

INTRODUCTION

Earlier in this book, you learned about two very different approaches to gathering data to answer research questions. An alternative approach to either qualitative or quantitative research is to combine both qualitative and quantitative approaches in a single study (Creswell 2021). This is called **mixed methods research**. This is different from **multimethod research**, which uses two or more data collection methods from either a qualitative approach (e.g. interviews and observations) or a quantitative approach (e.g. surveys and biometric data) in a single study (Flick 2017, Turner, Cardinal &

Burton 2017). As you discovered in the previous chapters, qualitative research is often useful for exploring the experiences of individuals, whereas quantitative research allows the researcher to form generalisable conclusions about a population or the effect of an intervention. So while a quantitative study would provide data to measure the impact of a new intervention on health outcomes (such as blood pressure, body weight or symptom severity), a qualitative study would provide insight into the individual's experience of the intervention and how it has impacted on their life. Used together, the combination of qualitative and quantitative approaches provides a broad and flexible approach to addressing complex research problems. The depth of insight into a research problem made available by mixed methods research makes it suitable for studying many of the complex problems explored in nursing and midwifery research (Bressan et al 2017, Halcomb 2019).

Despite its advantages, mixed methods research is not appropriate for providing answers to every research question. For example, a study seeking to identify the effect of a new drug on reducing weight loss due to hyperemesis gravidarum would be best answered through purely quantitative data about the woman's weight. Such a study would be much less resource-intensive and cost-effective than a mixed methods study on the same issue and would still provide adequate information to answer the research question. However, if the study also sought to capture the impact of hyperemesis gravidarum on, say, quality of life, well-being or mothering, then adding a qualitative dimension would likely be justified. Care must be taken to rationalise clearly why a mixed methods design, rather than a purely qualitative or quantitative approach, is being used in a particular study. The scope of the research question should be the primary driver in the decision to use a particular methodological approach.

When reading reports of mixed methods studies, all of the principles you have learned about qualitative and quantitative research design, data collection and reporting apply. A major difference in mixed methods research occurs in terms of 'mixing' or integrating the qualitative and quantitative components (Turner, Cardinal & Burton 2017). As you move through this chapter, you will see that a well-designed mixed methods study is more than simply combining qualitative and quantitative data collection in a single research report. The integration of qualitative and quantitative components is the key to quality mixed methods research (Creswell 2021, Tashakkori, Johnson & Teddlie 2020). Mixing can be undertaken during the problem identification, data collection, data analysis and/or reporting phases of the study (Creswell 2021, Halcomb & Hickman 2015, Tashakkori, Johnson & Teddlie 2020). This mixing involves tasks such as designing complementary data collection procedures, synthesising datasets during analysis and evaluating conflicting or confirmatory findings. Issues related to integration will be discussed throughout this chapter.

THE DEBATE OVER MIXING METHODS

The relative values of qualitative, quantitative and mixed methods research designs have long been a source of debate among scholars within and external to nursing and midwifery (Halcomb & Hickman 2015, Tashakkori, Johnson & Teddlie 2020). Some believe that, because of the different epistemology, ontology, philosophy and goals and purposes, qualitative and quantitative approaches cannot be mixed without causing a violation of these differences (Tashakkori, Johnson & Teddlie 2020). For other scholars, mixed methods research has increasingly become an accepted research approach (Flick 2017, Halcomb 2019).

It is not the purpose of this chapter to provide an in-depth analysis of the relative merits of qualitative and quantitative research. What we will do is demonstrate that a combination of qualitative and quantitative components has the potential to provide greater insight into many complex nursing and midwifery issues than could be gained from using either method in isolation (Andrew & Halcomb 2009, Halcomb & Hickman 2015).

RATIONALE FOR USING MIXED METHODS DESIGNS

Projects that use mixed methods designs should clearly articulate a rationale for the use of both approaches and demonstrate the qualitative and quantitative dimensions of the study (Halcomb 2018). The decision to use a mixed methods design should be based on balancing the value of combining the qualitative and quantitative data collection against the increased resources and skills required (Halcomb & Hickman 2015).

Given the importance of demonstrating a rationale for undertaking a mixed methods study rather than conducting a purely qualitative or quantitative investigation, it is useful to understand the goals to be achieved by using mixed methods designs. While clearly research problems where multiple perspectives will provide a more detailed understanding of the issues are most suited to mixed methods approaches, there are several purposes of using mixed methods designs. These are: confirmation/corroboration; complementarity; initiation; development; expansion; and enhancement of significant findings (Creswell 2021, Halcomb & Hickman 2015, Tashakkori, Johnson & Teddlie 2020). Researchers are not limited to one reason for conducting mixed methods research but rather may have multiple motives for using a mixed methods design in their work. Table 9.1 outlines the purposes for which mixed methods designs can be used and provides examples from the literature.

Confirmation/Corroboration

The early social science, psychology and educational researchers saw the combination of qualitative and quantitative data as a means of confirming the results of one method with those of the other (Campbell & Fiske 1959). This use of different datasets was also known as **triangulation** (Turner, Cardinal & Burton 2017). Results and conclusions from the different data collection methods were expected to converge and this was seen as a way of confirming the study findings and increasing their validity (Tashakkori, Johnson & Teddlie 2020).

Complementarity

Complementarity refers to the use of both quantitative and qualitative data to elaborate on findings, enhance the meaningfulness of findings and provide illustrations and clarification of the data from one method with the findings of the complementary method (Halcomb & Hickman 2015, McKim 2017, Tashakkori, Johnson & Teddlie 2020). In this way, the format of the mixed method uses the strengths and weaknesses of quantitative and qualitative data collection to complement each other. This can give the study more

	TABLE 9.1	
	Purposes of Mixed Methods Research	
Purpose	**Definition**	**Example**
Confirmation/ corroboration	Corroborate results using data collected through different methods	Goh and colleagues (2020) collected data concurrently via a combination of a descriptive survey and focus groups with nurses from a Singapore hospital. Data from each method were analysed separately and then triangulated to compare findings.
Complementarity	Seek elaboration, illustration or clarification of the results from one method using the data collected from the other method	Khan (2021) disseminated an online survey to all nurses currently working in adult critical care areas across England. This was followed by semi-structured interviews to gain in-depth accounts and clarify nurses' intention to leave adult critical care areas and nurses' views and experiences about their working conditions.
Initiation	One method is used to reveal the contradictions in findings from the other method	Andrew and colleagues (2011) investigated patient satisfaction using quantitative surveys and qualitative interviews. The results for the quantitative survey indicated patients were highly satisfied with their care. Data integration allowed the researchers to examine the contradictions between the quantitative and qualitative findings, as some patients had a suggestion for change even if they scored their care high on the survey.
Development	Studies with sequential designs, where the data from the initial data collection inform the development of the subsequent method	In their study of skin diversity in pressure injuries, Oozageer Gunowa and colleagues (2021b) used data collected from classroom observation and documentary analysis to inform questions for subsequent focus groups and interviews.
Expansion	Extend the depth and scope of the inquiry by using different measures to explore different inquiry components	In an evaluation of the impact and sustainability of the Care Maker program in England, an online survey was distributed to all care makers and then semi-structured interviews were conducted to expand understanding of their perspectives (Zubairu et al 2017).

Source: Adapted from Halcomb EJ, Hickman L: Mixed methods research, Nursing Standard, 29(32):42–48, 2015; Andrew S, Halcomb EJ: Mixed methods research is an effective method of enquiry for working with families and communities, Advances in Contemporary Nursing 23(2):145–153, 2006.

breadth and scope than either method could achieve if used in isolation (Hall 2020).

Initiation

Researchers undertaking mixed methods research seek to explore inconsistency and contradiction, and take new perspectives on existing frameworks (Hall 2020). This can lead to reframing the research question to explore the research problem from a variety of perspectives (Tashakkori, Johnson & Teddlie 2020). By exploring the research from different perspectives, the breadth and depth of the results and interpretations are increased (Creswell 2021). Thus, mixed methods research may reveal unique characteristics of the phenomenon being studied that may be overlooked when using either qualitative or quantitative methods alone.

Development

Findings from one method of data collection may also generate questions or a hypothesis that needs to be tested by another method (Tashakkori, Johnson & Teddlie 2020). Some common types of mixed methods investigations involving development include instrument development, sample identification and action research. To develop an instrument to measure the quality of life in people with COPD, the investigation may start with qualitative interviews or focus groups with people about their experiences of living with COPD. These findings can be used to develop a research instrument, which is then piloted by a quantitative survey (Creswell 2021, Tashakkori, Johnson & Teddlie 2020). Sometimes in-depth interviews may be conducted at the same time as the survey is administered to determine the effectiveness or clarity of the items in the instrument (this is known as cognitive interviewing). Another example relates to sampling. In this strategy, one method of data collection may be used to identify particular individuals or cases that then become the sample for the second method of data collection. For example, a survey could be used to explore health and wellbeing after an acute exacerbation of COPD. From this survey, individuals who indicate depressive symptoms could be approached to participate in interviews to explore their specific experiences.

Expansion

Studies undertaken for the purpose of expansion seek to broaden the scope of the investigation by using different methods of data collection to measure most appropriately the various components of the research problem (Creswell 2021, Hall 2020, Tashakkori, Johnson & Teddlie 2020).

Enhance Significant Findings

The final purpose of using mixed methods designs is to enhance significant findings (Creswell 2021, Halcomb & Hickman 2015). The significance of a study can be determined in terms of statistical, practical, clinical or economic significance (Wisdom et al 2012). The collection of both qualitative and quantitative data in a single study can assist in a more comprehensive evaluation of the significance of study findings in each of these areas. This may be particularly useful when an intervention may provide clinically, but not statistically, significant improvement in an outcome measure.

PHILOSOPHICAL APPROACHES TO MIXED METHODS RESEARCH

Mixed methods research has been increasingly described as the third methodological approach, in addition to the traditional qualitative and quantitative (Creswell & Creswell 2018). However, to consider mixed methods research as a methodological approach, its underlying philosophical basis must be identified and understood. A philosophical approach, sometimes described as a worldview, is the lens through which someone sees the world (Cutler, Halcomb & Sim 2021). A range of worldviews can be used to underpin mixed methods research. These can

include pragmatism, a transformative (emancipatory) worldview or, more recently, critical realism (Creswell & Creswell 2018).

Pragmatists argue the researcher should use whatever techniques work to achieve the best answer for a specific research question. They value both subjective and objective measures to reveal answers to the research question (Creswell & Plano Clark 2017). From this perspective, it is justifiable to combine qualitative and quantitative data collection methods in a single study if this is the most appropriate means to answer the research question.

In contrast to other methodological approaches, a transformative (emancipatory) approach, which seeks to recognise cultural and power differences and injustices throughout the entire research process (Garnett et al 2019), is the aim of mixed methods. Mixed methods designs provide a focused strategy by which multiple perspectives can be gathered and considered. This can help to reduce power imbalances, promote engagement in the research and illuminate the perspectives of vulnerable groups.

Critical realism accepts that considering multiple outlooks can facilitate the best understanding of reality (Halcomb & Hickman 2015). Since mixed methods research provides a framework for gathering multiple outlooks, it is well suited to a critical realist approach to research (Schoonenboom 2019).

Creswell and Plano Clark (2017) describe various models of adopting worldviews within mixed methods research that are beyond the scope of this introductory book. These models can involve employing a single or multiple worldviews within the study design. While there is no right or wrong philosophical approach for a mixed methods study, the way in which the study is designed and undertaken should be consistent with its underlying philosophical assumptions.

DECISIONS IN MIXED METHODS DESIGNS

Researchers need to make several decisions that have an impact on the design of mixed methods research. Creswell and Plano Clark (2017) propose three questions that must be addressed by the researchers during the planning stage of mixed methods research.

1. In what sequence will the qualitative and quantitative components be implemented?

2. What relative weighting will be given to the qualitative and quantitative methods?
3. At what stage of the project will the qualitative and quantitative data be integrated?

Implementation Sequence

The timing of the data collection within a mixed methods study may be simultaneous (concurrent or parallel) or sequential (Halcomb & Hickman 2015, NIH Office of Behavioral and Social Sciences 2018). In **concurrent mixed methods** studies, qualitative and quantitative data are collected at, or approximately at, the same time. Therefore, in concurrent studies, data integration must occur during either the data analysis or the interpretation phases. Concurrent studies have the advantage of being able to collect a large amount of data over a relatively short timeframe (NIH Office of Behavioral and Social Sciences 2018). **Sequential mixed methods** studies involve at least two phases of data collection, one after the other. In sequential studies, the study duration is often much longer than a single qualitative or quantitative study, as the data collected during the first phase are usually used to inform the subsequent data collection. This may be problematic when the researcher is working within set time constraints, such as during a research degree (Halcomb & Andrew 2009).

Priority

The second consideration is the relative priority given to the qualitative and quantitative methods of data collection (Halcomb 2019). This decision is guided primarily by the study aims. For example, in exploratory studies where there is limited under-standing, the qualitative method is often given higher priority to inform the researcher's understanding of the phenomenon (Creswell & Plano Clark 2017). In studies where there is unequal priority, one dataset is clearly secondary to a larger primary design (Creswell & Creswell 2018, NIH Office of Behavioral and Social Sciences 2018). Alternatively, researchers may collect comprehensive qualitative and quantitative datasets and give them equal emphasis in the analysis.

Integration

The integration of qualitative and quantitative refers to the 'point of interface' at which the researcher mixes the two datasets (Creswell & Creswell 2018,

Halcomb 2019). For obvious reasons, the researcher needs to consider the sequence in which data are collected when deciding at which point integration will occur. The purpose of integration is also to maximise the strengths of each method while at the same time minimising their weaknesses (NIH Office of Behavioral and Social Sciences 2018). Despite its importance, until recently there has been limited attention paid to this aspect of mixed methods research (Halcomb 2019, Younas, Pedersen & Tayaben 2019). In practical terms, the integration of qualitative and quantitative aspects can be undertaken at various stages throughout the research process. The three distinct approaches that have been proposed for integration are described in Table 9.2 (Creswell 2021, NIH Office of Behavioral and Social Sciences 2018, Younas, Pedersen & Tayaben 2019).

Connecting or building data involves using one data-set to inform the second data collection (Creswell 2021, NIH Office of Behavioral and Social Sciences 2018). For example, a survey may assist in identifying individuals with particular characteristics who are then interviewed. Alternatively, collecting qualitative data first can be used to inform the design of tools used to collect subsequent quantitative data (Younas, Pedersen & Tayaben 2019).

Merging data can be achieved in various ways (Creswell 2021, Halcomb & Hickman 2015). One example is when statistical survey findings are reported followed by interview quotes that either support or refute the statistical data (van de Mortel, Needham & Henderson 2021). Another example is developing a table (also known as a joint display) to compare the qualitative and quantitative findings, including where they triangulate but also where one method might add an expansion to the other method (Younas, Pedersen & Durante 2020). Finally, data can be transformed to allow comparison between datasets (e.g. counting the themes or quotes in qualitative data).

The final strategy for integrating the datasets is embedding data (Creswell 2021, NIH Office of Behavioral and Social Sciences 2018). In these designs, a secondary data collection, usually qualitative, may be undertaken to explore the experience of participants and/or providers within an experimental study (Creswell & Plano Clark 2017). This qualitative data collection provides important process evaluation data to inform the future implementation of the intervention.

During data collection, open- and closed-ended items can be included in the same survey tool, and

	TABLE 9.2	
	Models of Mixing	
Model of Mixing	**Definition**	**Example**
Connecting/ building	One approach is built on the findings of the other approach.	Halcomb and colleagues (2020) surveyed Australian primary healthcare nurses about their experiences during COVID-19. In a second phase of the study, a series of interviews with a subgroup of survey participants was conducted to explore the issues raised from the survey data (Ashley et al 2021, James et al 2021).
Merging	Qualitative and quantitative data are collected concurrently and analysed separately. Integration occurs during the interpretation.	Darwin and colleagues (2017) administered surveys and conducted interviews with women who had used a volunteer doula service in five low-income communities. The qualitative and quantitative data were analysed separately and integrated for reporting.
Embedding	The analysis of one type of data is embedded within the other. Commonly, this involves a small qualitative component nested within a quantitative study.	Zwar and colleagues (2017) conducted a pilot trial to test the uptake and effectiveness of a general-practice-nurse-led hypertension intervention. Qualitative interviews were conducted with patients, nurses and general practitioners who participated in the trial to evaluate the implementation, feasibility and acceptability of the intervention (Stephen et al 2018).

Source: Adapted from Halcomb EJ, Hickman L: Mixed methods research, Nursing Standard, 29(32):42–48, 2015; Zhang W, Creswell J: The use of 'mixing' procedure of mixed methods in health services research, Medical Care 51(8):e51–e57, 2013.

during data analysis or interpretation, qualitative and quantitative data can be compared (NIH Office of Behavioral and Social Sciences 2018).

Regardless of the nature and timing of the integration, care must be taken to ensure the two methods, datasets or findings are truly integrated (NIH Office of Behavioral and Social Sciences 2018), rather than simply using one dataset to embellish the 'real' results (Halcomb 2019).

MIXED METHODS RESEARCH DESIGNS

Mixed methods research designs allow a degree of creative freedom that is not always available with other research designs. With this in mind, the following discussion provides an overview of some of the common types of mixed methods designs. Broadly, there are three types of designs in mixed methods research: concurrent (or convergent/ parallel) designs; sequential (explanatory or exploratory) designs; and embedded (or nested) designs (NIH Office of Behavioral and Social Sciences 2018). The characteristics of each of these designs are summarised in Table 9.3 and will now be discussed.

Currently, there is no universally agreed terminology for mixed methods research designs and this

uncertainty can make it challenging for researchers to describe and apply mixed methods research. While the most popular design names have been used here, names may vary in the literature. Additionally, many authors of mixed methods research do not explicitly identify the type of mixed methods design within their research report. Moreover, some research designs do not explicitly identify themselves as being mixed methods research, although they commonly use qualitative and quantitative methods within their design.

Case study research may use qualitative and quantitative methods with the design providing a 'bridge' or link between the qualitative and quantitative data collections (Guetterman & Fetters 2018). For example, Hopkinson and colleagues (2021) used a mixed methods case study design, using a variety of methods including observation, interviews, focus groups and data extraction to identify the critical factors for resolving crises for a person with dementia living at home. This provided a more holistic view of the phenomena.

Evaluation studies may use both qualitative and quantitative methods to determine the effectiveness of clinical practice, a model of care or an educational program. To evaluate the national implementation of a

TABLE 9.3				
Types of Mixed Methods Designs				
Research Design	Process	Purpose	Level of Interaction	Priority
Convergent parallel (concurrent)	Qual Quant	To obtain different but complementary data to answer a single research question.	Data collected and analysed independently.	Equal
Sequential explanatory	QUANT → qual	Qualitative data are collected to explain the quantitative findings.	Quantitative data frames qualitative data collection.	Quantitative dominant
Sequential exploratory	QUAL → quant	Quantitative data builds on qualitative findings to provide generalisability.	Qualitative data frames quantitative data collection.	Qualitative dominant
Embedded/ nested	Qual (quant) or Quant (qual)	To obtain different data to answer a complementary research question.	Embedded dataset provides answers to a complementary research question.	Can be either qualitative or quantitative dominant

Source: Halcomb EJ, Hickman L: Mixed methods research, Nursing Standard, 29(32):42–48, 2015; reproduced with permission from Nursing Standard.

COPD management program, Strassmann and colleagues (2021) used a combination of interviews/focus groups and surveys/document analysis to assess the impact of the program on health, its acceptability and reach.

Participatory action research involves critical reflection and action with both the researcher and the study participants working together; for example, to evaluate and change clinical practice or model of care. Breimaier, Halfens and Lohrmann (2015) worked with nursing staff to reduce falls at an Austrian hospital using a participatory action research approach with a before-and-after mixed method design using questionnaires, group discussions and semi-structured interviews.

We emphasise that the research question must be the primary driver when choosing a research design, and thus the use of a particular methodological approach.

Concurrent Designs

A concurrent, convergent or parallel design is implemented when the researcher uses quantitative and qualitative methods to confirm or corroborate findings (NIH Office of Behavioral and Social Sciences 2018). As integration occurs during the data analysis phase, data are collected concurrently. The process of data analysis involves merging and comparing the two sets of data (NIH Office of Behavioral and Social Sciences 2018). Although the relative priority of the datasets is ideally equal, priority may be given to either dataset (Halcomb & Hickman 2015). For example, Baillie and Thomas

(2017) conducted a concurrent mixed method study of the impact of day-shift length on patient care in two older people's medical wards in south-east England. They combined interviews with nurses and structured observation of nurses' interactions using a measurement tool collecting patient demographics and discharge survey data. The survey results and the nurse interactions data were analysed statistically and reported in separate subsections, followed by the integrated results with overarching themes drawing on data from both qualitative and quantitative data. For example, for the theme 'How day-shift length affects patient care', they reported on both qualitative data from nursing staff about how shift length affects mealtimes and the quantitative patient survey findings about whether they received enough help with eating. This approach enabled comparisons (triangulation) between the qualitative and quantitative findings to achieve a comprehensive understanding of the topic.

Sequential Designs

Sequential designs are multiphase projects in which one data collection follows when the other is completed. While often there are two phases, larger projects may involve additional phases.

Sequential Explanatory

A sequential explanatory study involves a primarily quantitative study followed by qualitative data collection (Guetterman & Fetters 2018, Halcomb & Hickman

2015). This design is highly suitable for the detailed exploration of a problem where little is already known or to explain the results of a quantitative study (Creswell 2021, McKim 2017). The use of a sequential explanatory design can identify subjective meanings behind purely quantitative survey responses. For example, in their study about nurse education and pressure injuries among people with dark skin tones Oozageer Gunowa and colleagues (2021a) used a data collection tool to explore the inclusion of pressure injury teaching in relation to people with dark skin tones in pre-registration nurse classroom education. Subsequently, interviews and focus groups were undertaken with purposively selected students and nurse educators to gain a richer understanding of the quantitative results (Oozageer Gunowa et al 2021b).

Sequential Exploratory

Like the sequential explanatory design, the sequential exploratory design has two phases, with priority given to the initial data collection (Halcomb & Hickman 2015). However, in the sequential exploratory design, the first phase is comprised of qualitative data collection and analysis, followed by quantitative data collection and analysis (Halcomb & Hickman 2015). The most common situations where this design is used include developing and testing research instruments, identification of the prevalence of a particular phenomenon within a population or any problem where there is a need to interpret relationships (Creswell 2021, Halcomb & Hickman 2015).

An example of a sequential exploratory study can be found in the study reported by Salvador, Alqahtani and Sauce (2020), who sought to develop a tool to measure the quality of nursing care plans written by nursing students. Initially, they undertook interviews with students to explore their understandings of nursing care plans and experiences in writing these. The findings from these interviews informed the development of a survey tool which was then pilot tested before being administered to a broader sample of nursing students.

Embedded/Nested Designs

The embedded or nested design has a predominant method of data collection that guides the project and then a secondary method, of lesser priority, nested within the predominant method (Creswell 2021, Tashakkori, Johnson & Teddlie 2020). A nested approach can provide a broader perspective of the research problem by adding quantitative data to enrich the description of participants or collecting qualitative data to explore an aspect of the issue that cannot be quantified. The most common example of a nested study is the collection of qualitative data from participants or intervention providers in an experimental study to understand their experience of the intervention process (Creswell 2021, Tashakkori, Johnson & Teddlie 2020). In a nested design, mixing of the qualitative and quantitative data occurs during the analysis phase of the project (Creswell 2021, Tashakkori, Johnson & Teddlie 2020).

An example of a nested design can be seen in the pilot trial of a nurse-led hypertension intervention for primary care patients with uncontrolled hypertension conducted by Zwar and colleagues (2017). Quantitative outcomes from this trial included blood pressure, body weight, absolute cardiovascular risk and medication adherence. In addition, doctors, nurses and patients were asked to participate in interviews about the feasibility and acceptability of the intervention (Stephen et al 2018).

STUDENT CHALLENGE

Identifying Mixed Methods

Choose two journal articles that report mixed methods studies. Note that it can be challenging to locate articles reporting mixed methods designs. In addition to using 'mixed method' as a keyword in your search, it may be necessary to look for articles that contain both 'qualitative' and 'quantitative' as keywords. Remember that 'multimethod studies' is a subject heading in many databases. Although using this term will retrieve papers reporting mixed methods studies, it may also locate studies that collect data using two or more data collection methods from the same research tradition.

1. Review each of the journal articles and identify the:
   a. type of mixed methods designs used
   b. sequence in which the qualitative and quantitative data were collected
   c. relative priority given to the qualitative and quantitative data collection and analysis
   d. stage of the project at which the qualitative and quantitative data were integrated.
2. Also consider the following questions.
   a. If you were to replicate the study, would you have sufficient information about how integration was achieved by the researchers?
   b. Was it clear how the two sets of data informed the development of the study results?
   c. How does the format of these papers differ from purely qualitative and quantitative studies?

MIXED METHODS KNOWLEDGE TRANSLATION

Mixed methods research offers important opportunities for knowledge translation (KT). As illustrated in the examples in this chapter, mixed methods research allows the exploration of complex topics. The strength of the mixed methods approach is that researchers use complementary philosophical approaches, methodological frameworks and research methods to create new questions, develop new methods and promote new knowledge (Meister 2018). The opportunity to combine qualitative and quantitative components can be helpful in explaining or exploring findings in a way that can directly inform their translation into usual care.

Nurses and midwives need to incorporate KT into their clinical practice to ensure best-practice care and optimal patient outcomes. Translation of findings should be considered in the initial study design and should be a major consideration when developing the study aim(s) (Curtis et al 2017). The key to successful KT is engagement of end users throughout the research process; that is, end users are identified as users of the knowledge and are able to make informed decisions (Olson & Oudshoorn 2020). The end user can be a healthcare provider, patient or family member.

PRACTICAL CONSIDERATIONS FOR MIXED METHODS RESEARCH

Meticulous planning and justifiable rationales are as vital when planning mixed methods research as when planning purely qualitative or quantitative projects (Younas, Pedersen & Tayaben 2019). In addition to having a realistic research problem of sufficient interest and the capacity and resources needed to gather the required data, the size and scope of data collected during mixed methods research needs to be considered (Halcomb 2019). The use of two distinctly different methods of data collection requires a high level of resources and researcher time (Younas, Pedersen & Tayaben 2019). For obvious reasons, the process of data collection will likely take more time and be more expensive to conduct than a purely qualitative or quantitative study (McKim 2017).

Additionally, researchers undertaking mixed methods research require a broad range of skills in both qualitative and quantitative data collection techniques, as well as specific skills relating to the mixing of datasets (McKim 2017,

Turner, Cardinal & Burton 2017). For this reason, mixed methods research is often most effectively conducted by research teams, where several researchers can contribute different expertise to the conduct of the project (NIH Office of Behavioral and Social Sciences 2018).

The large amount of data that is often generated during a mixed methods investigation is a clear limitation. For many researchers, reporting and presenting these data in a meaningful way can be difficult (Younas, Pedersen & Tayaben 2019). Indeed, some authors choose to present their work as separate qualitative and quantitative papers rather than integrated mixed methods reports (Halcomb 2019, Younas, Pedersen & Tayaben 2019). While this may meet publication preferences, the value of integration is lost to the reader. However, the increase in the number of mixed methods papers being submitted in recent years has helped raise prominence of issues around dissemination. Wisdom and colleagues (2012) identify issues that mixed methods researchers are still faced with, including reviewers' lack of expertise, audience expectations, journal word limits and the decision-making around publishing in a mixed methods or clinical journal.

A further limitation of mixed methods research is that using two data collection methods may serve only to increase the magnitude of the inherent errors if a study has a design flaw or bias. For this reason, the use of a mixed methods approach must be clearly justified in the planning phase of the study. Additionally, consideration must be given to employing strategies to enhance the validity, reliability and rigour of the investigation (Halcomb 2018).

STUDENT CHALLENGE

The Advantages and Disadvantages of Mixed Methods Research

1. Referring to this chapter, discuss the advantages and disadvantages of using mixed methods research designs in nursing and midwifery research.
2. Considering Ahmed's assignment about exploring the best-practice care for an older man with chronic heart failure and COPD, think about the kinds of mixed methods studies that could provide evidence to support best practice. What would be some examples of research topics that might be best explored using a mixed methods approach?
3. Try writing a research question for Ahmed and Jaime's research topics that would lend itself to a mixed methods research design.

ESTABLISHING RELIABILITY, VALIDITY AND RIGOUR IN MIXED METHODS RESEARCH

Critical analysis of the validity, reliability and rigour of mixed methods studies is as important as it is in purely qualitative or quantitative investigations (Halcomb 2019). Despite advances in the literature around the use of mixed methods, many reports of mixed methods research continue to lack sufficient detail around the methods used (Bressan et al 2017). However, the restricted word limits in journals can be challenging for mixed methods researchers, who need to provide detail on several data collection methods. Broadly, any critical appraisal of mixed methods research should consider how well the work meets the qualitative and quantitative appraisal criteria as well as the specific criteria around the application of mixed methods (Halcomb 2018). In recent years, a growing number of frameworks have been proposed to guide people in critically appraising mixed methods research (Halcomb 2018, Hong et al 2018). However, to date, a consensus around what constitutes quality in mixed methods research has not been reached (Creswell 2021, Halcomb 2018). These various frameworks can look at the qualitative and quantitative components in isolation, provide broad criteria that assess both qualitative and quantitative components together, or be bespoke criteria that are designed specifically to evaluate mixed methods research (Halcomb 2018). There is significant variation across these frameworks about the considerations and their interrelationships in the evaluation of mixed methods quality. However, Box 9.1 provides an overview of the broad features that should be considered when evaluating the rigour of a mixed methods study.

CONCLUSION

Mixed methods research designs provide the nursing and midwifery researcher with means for creatively exploring the complexity of problems faced in contemporary healthcare. As researchers become increasingly skilled in the use of mixed methods techniques, a greater depth of understanding about phenomena of study will be achievable—more than would be possible through the use of either qualitative or quantitative methods in isolation. It is important to realise that a good understanding of the differences in

---

BOX 9.1
SAMPLE CRITERIA FOR CRITICAL APPRAISAL OF MIXED METHODS STUDIES

- Are there clearly stated purposes or questions that the mixed methods data collection seeks to answer?
- Are the multiple purposes or research questions matched with appropriate methods of data collection? Are both the qualitative and quantitative methods justified?
- Has the researcher followed the quality criteria for qualitative data collection?
- Has the researcher followed the quality criteria for quantitative data collection?
- Have the limitations of the various data collection methods been identified?
- Is it clear when the qualitative and quantitative data were integrated during the study? Has this integration provided a better understanding of the problem than either individual source?
- If there were conflicting results, were these adequately explained by the researcher?

the philosophical underpinnings of both approaches is essential to the successful use of mixed methods.

ADDITIONAL RESOURCES

Resources

Additional resources can be located on the internet by using keywords such as 'mixed methods' in a search engine.

Check out the activities on the Evolve website http://evolve.elsevier.com/AU/Jackson/maze/ for further information.

The *Journal of Mixed Methods Research* (SAGE Journals) is a journal devoted to publishing papers reporting mixed methods studies and methodological issues relating specifically to mixed methods research regardless of professional discipline: https://journals.sagepub.com/home/mmr

RECOMMENDED READING

Andrew S, Halcomb EJ: Mixed methods research for nursing and the health sciences, London, 2009, Wiley-Blackwell.
Creswell JW: A concise introduction to mixed methods research, ed 2, Los Angeles, 2021, SAGE Publications.

Hall R: Mixing methods in social research: qualitative, quantitative and combined methods, London, 2020, SAGE Publications.

Tashakkori A, Johnson RB, Teddlie C: Foundations of mixed methods research: integrating quantitative and qualitative approaches in the social and behavioral sciences, ed 2, Thousand Oaks, 2020, SAGE.

REFERENCES

Andrew S, Halcomb EJ (eds): Mixed methods research for nursing and the health sciences, 2009, Wiley-Blackwell. https://doi.org/10.1002/9781444316490.

Andrew S, Halcomb EJ: Mixed methods research is an effective method of enquiry for working with families and communities, Advances in Contemporary Nursing 23(2):145–153, 2006.

Andrew S, Salamonson Y, Everett B, et al: Beyond the ceiling effect: using a mixed methods approach to measure patient satisfaction, International Journal of Multiple Research Approaches 5(1):52–63, 2011.

Ashley C, James S, Halcomb E, et al: The psychological wellbeing of primary health care nurses' during COVID-19: a qualitative study, Journal of Advanced Nursing 77(9):3820–3828, 2021.

Baillie L, Thomas N: How does the length of day shift affect patient care on older people's wards? A mixed method study, International Journal of Nursing Studies, 75:154–162, 2017.

Breimaier HE, Halfens RJ, Lohrmann C: Effectiveness of multifaceted and tailored strategies to implement a fall-prevention guideline into acute care nursing practice: a before-and-after, mixed-method study using a participatory action research approach, BMC Nursing 14(1):18, 2015.

Bressan V, Bagnasco A, Aleo G, et al: Mixed-methods research in nursing—a critical review, Journal of Clinical Nursing 26 (19–20):2878–2890, 2017.

Campbell DT, Fiske DW: Convergent and discriminant validation by the multitrait-multimethod matrix, Psychological Bulletin 56(2):81, 1959.

Creswell JW: A concise introduction to mixed methods research, Thousand Oaks, 2021, SAGE.

Creswell JW, Creswell JD: Research design: qualitative, quantitative, and mixed methods approaches, ed 5, Thousand Oaks, 2018, SAGE.

Creswell JW, Plano Clark VL: Designing and conducting mixed methods research, ed 3, Thousand Oaks, 2017, SAGE.

Curtis K, Fry M, Shaban RZ, Considine J: Translating research findings to clinical nursing practice, Journal of Clinical Nursing 26 (5–6):862–872, 2017.

Cutler N, Halcomb E, Sim J: Using naturalistic inquiry to inform qualitative description, Nurse Researcher 29(3):29–33, 2021. https://doi.org/10.7748/nr.2021.e1788.

Darwin Z, Green J, McLeish J, et al: Evaluation of trained volunteer doula services for disadvantaged women in five areas in England: women's experiences, Health & Social Care in the Community, 25(2):466–477, 2017.

Flick U: Mantras and myths: the disenchantment of mixed-methods research and revisiting triangulation as a perspective, Qualitative Inquiry 23(1):46–57, 2017.

Garnett BR, Smith LC, Kervick CT, et al: The emancipatory potential of transformative mixed methods designs: informing youth participatory action research and restorative practices within a district-wide school transformation project, International Journal of Research & Method in Education 42(3):305–316, 2019.

Goh PQL, Ser TF, Cooper S, et al: Nursing teamwork in general ward settings: a mixed-methods exploratory study among enrolled and registered nurses, Journal of Clinical Nursing 29(19–20): 3802–3811, 2020.

Guetterman TC, Fetters MD: Two methodological approaches to the integration of mixed methods and case study designs: a systematic review, American Behavioral Scientist, 62(7):900–918, 2018.

Halcomb E: Appraising mixed methods research. In Liamputtong P (ed), Research methods in health social sciences, 2018, Springer Nature.

Halcomb EJ, Andrew S: Practical considerations for higher degree research students undertaking mixed methods projects, International Journal of Multiple Research Approaches 3(2):153–162, 2009.

Halcomb EJ, Hickman L: Mixed methods research, Nursing Standard 29(32):42–48, 2015.

Halcomb E, McInnes S, Williams A, et al: The experiences of primary health care nurses during the COVID-19 pandemic in Australia, Journal of Nursing Scholarship 52(5):553–563, 2020.

Halcomb EJ: Mixed methods research: the issues beyond combining methods, Journal of Advanced Nursing 75(3):499–501, 2019.

Hall R: Mixing methods in social research: qualitative, quantitative and combined methods, London, 2020, SAGE.

Hong QN, Fàbregues S, Bartlett, G, et al: The Mixed Methods Appraisal Tool (MMAT) version 2018 for information professionals and researchers, Education for Information 34(4):285–291, 2018.

Hopkinson J, King A, Young L et al: Crisis management for people with dementia at home: mixed-methods case study research to identify critical factors for successful home treatment, Health and Social Care in the Community, 29(4):1072–1082, 2021.

James S, Ashley C, Williams A, et al: Experiences of primary health care nurses in using telehealth during COVID-19: a qualitative study, BMJ Open 11, e049095, 2021.

Khan N: Factors that influence nurses' intention to leave adult critical care areas: a mixed-method sequential explanatory study. [Thesis] Oxford Brookes University, 2021.

McKim CA: The value of mixed methods research: a mixed methods study, Journal of Mixed Methods Research 11(2):202–222, 2017.

Meister L: On methodology: how mixed methods research can contribute to translation studies, Journal of Translation Studies 11(1):66–83, 2018.

NIH Office of Behavioral and Social Sciences: Best practices for mixed methods research in the health sciences, National Institutes of Health 2018.

Olson A, Oudshoorn A: Knowledge translation: a concept analysis. Nursing Forum April/June, 55(2):157–164, 2020.

Oozageer Gunowa N, Hutchinson M, Brooke J, et al: Evidencing diversity: development of a structured tool for investigating teaching of pressure injury on people with darker skin tones. Nurse Researcher 29(2):17–24, 2021a.

Oozageer Gunowa N, Hutchinson M, Brooke J, et al: Pressure injuries and skin tone diversity in undergraduate nurse education: qualitative perspectives from a mixed methods study, Journal of Advanced Nursing 77(11):4511–4524, 2021b.

Salvador JT, Alqahtani FM, Sauce BRJ: Development of student survey on writing nursing care plan: an exploratory sequential mixed-methods study, Journal of Nursing Management Jul;30(5): O23–O36, 2020.

Schoonenboom J: A performative paradigm for mixed methods research, Journal of Mixed Methods Research 13(3):284–300, 2019.

Stephen C, Hermitz O, McInnes S, et al: Feasibility and acceptability of a nurse-led hypertension management intervention in general practice, Collegian 25(1):33–38, 2018.

Strassmann A, Guler M, Steurer-Stey C, et al: Nationwide implementation of the self-management program 'Living well with COPD': process and effectiveness evaluation using a mixed-methods approach, Patient Education and Counseling 105(3):670–678, 2021.

Tashakkori A, Johnson RB, Teddlie C: Foundations of mixed methods research: integrating quantitative and qualitative approaches in the social and behavioral sciences, ed 2, Thousand Oaks, 2020, SAGE.

Turner SF, Cardinal LB, Burton RM: Research design for mixed methods: a triangulation-based framework and roadmap, Organizational Research Methods 20(2):243–267, 2017.

van de Mortel TF, Needham J, Henderson SJ: Facilitating learning on clinical placement using near-peer supervision: a mixed methods study, Nurse Education Today;102:104921, 2021.

Wisdom JP, Cavaleri MA, Onwuegbuzie AJ, Green CA: Methodological reporting in qualitative, quantitative, and mixed methods health services research articles, Health Services Research 47(2):721–745, 2012.

Younas A, Pedersen M, Durante A: Characteristics of joint displays illustrating data integration in mixed-methods nursing studies, Journal of Advanced Nursing 76(2):676–686, 2020.

Younas A, Pedersen M, Tayaben JL: Review of mixed-methods research in nursing, Nursing Research 68(6):464–472, 2019.

Zhang W, Creswell J: The use of 'mixing' procedure of mixed methods in health services research, Medical Care 51(8):e51–e57, 2013.

Zubairu K, Christiansen A, Kirkaldy A et al: An evaluation of National Health Service England's Care Maker programme: a mixed-methods analysis, Journal of Clinical Nursing 26 (23–24):4634–4645, 2017.

Zwar N, Hermitz O, Halcomb E, et al: Improving blood pressure control in general practice: Quantitative evaluation of the ImPress intervention, Australian Family Physician 46(5):306–331, 2017.

10

RESEARCH WITH INDIGENOUS PEOPLES

VANESSA HEASLIP ■ ALI DRUMMOND ■ RHONDA MARRIOTT ■ DENISE WILSON

CHAPTER OUTLINE

LEARNING OBJECTIVES

After reading this chapter and following critical reflection, readers should be able to:

■ recognise Indigenous peoples' worldviews and knowledges

■ discuss relevant ethics, values and protocols for research with Indigenous peoples

■ explain Indigenous social, historical and political contexts of health, healthcare and research

■ discuss the impacts of colonisation, current social and political contexts, and racism and discrimination on Indigenous peoples' access to determinants of health

■ discuss considerations for privileging Indigenous health realities in research using intersectionality as a framework

■ explain the principles of social justice, equity and rights as they apply to research

■ use research in a culturally safe way to inform nursing/midwifery practice with Indigenous peoples.

KEY TERMS

Aboriginal and Torres Strait Islander peoples

colonisation

culturally competent

culturally safe

discrimination

Indigenous peoples

intersectionality

Māori peoples

racism

worldview

10 ■ RESEARCH WITH INDIGENOUS PEOPLES 139

ABSTRACT

Indigenous peoples globally, while diverse, share similar colonising histories and stories of the subjugation of their knowledge forms. Understanding the historical events of imperialism and colonisation that have enforced cultural changes and negatively influenced Indigenous knowledge systems and ways of knowing is crucial when looking at research. It is especially important to use this understanding to inform research and, subsequently, clinical practice when working with Indigenous peoples. Indigenous peoples are best positioned to discover knowledge and strategies to resolve the many health challenges they face. Recently, they have been actively involved in reclaiming and developing Indigenous health knowledge. Understanding worldviews, Indigenous knowledge systems and ethical processes can reduce the risk of perpetuating colonial racialised imaginations about Indigenous peoples and their knowledge systems. It can also assist students to identify their own cultural ideologies and positions, and better evaluate research with Indigenous peoples.

The authors respectfully acknowledge the diversity of Aboriginal and Torres Strait Islander peoples across Australia, Māori across Aotearoa New Zealand, Gypsy, Roma and Traveller peoples across the United Kingdom and Europe, and other Indigenous peoples throughout the world. We pay respects to all their Elders, past, present and emerging. We use the term Indigenous peoples throughout this chapter when referring to the collective of Aboriginal and Torres Strait Islander peoples, Māori, Gypsy, Roma and Traveller peoples and other Indigenous peoples.

I am worth no more or no less than other living things; the world I inhabit has been created by ancestral beings and it is organic and alive with spirits and signs which inform my way of knowing. Thus, respect and caution frame my approach to knowledge production; the more I know the less that I know because there are other forms of knowledge that exist beyond us as humans.
(**Moreton-Robinson 2013, p. 341**)

STUDENT QUOTE

I treated all my patients the same. I now realise that equality does not mean everyone being treated the same and that Indigenous peoples experience ongoing social and health disparities.

INTRODUCTION

Indigenous peoples have established ways of viewing and understanding the world, and have been researching the world for centuries. Yet, until relatively recent times, their ways of knowing and research have been largely invisible. The quote from Moreton-Robinson (2013) highlights the holistic nature of Indigenous knowledge that is inclusive of knowledge that exists beyond the human realm, and the need for respect and caution to underpin knowledge production in cross-cultural research. Therefore, non-Indigenous researchers need to understand that Indigenous cultural realities have a different cultural orientation or **worldview**. The best possible evidence must inform nursing and midwifery practice as well as the development and provision of health services, given the health status and health inequities with which Indigenous people live. Such evidence must not only be relevant and reflective of Indigenous peoples' lives, as determined by themselves, but it must also provide an accurate interpretation of their cultural positioning, the ongoing effects of historical injustices and their sociocultural and political realities. In this chapter, we draw attention to the historical and contemporary contexts of suboptimal research practices imposed on Indigenous peoples globally. The subsequent interpretations of research findings have not been beneficial and often perpetuate dispossession of land, language and culture that innately reinforce negative stereotypes and explanations that focus on their perceived deficits. Many Indigenous peoples no longer accept such approaches to research (Congress of Aboriginal and Torres Strait Islander Nurses and Midwives [CATSINaM] 2017, Hudson et al 2010, Watego et al 2021). They are wary of research and researchers—Indigenous and non-Indigenous alike—and choose to engage only in research that aligns with their goals, reflects their Indigenous realities and ultimately benefits their communities.

So who are Indigenous peoples? The United Nations (2013) defines Indigenous peoples as those people who first lived in areas or had nomadic lifestyles, and can be identified by distinct cultural practices and structures for social order and control. They have common histories of racialised domination by non-Indigenous settlers that has led to their cultural, social, political and economic disenfranchisement.

Indigenous peoples are identifiable by their links to countries and tribal areas before being colonised and their long-held cultural beliefs and practices along with their own social, economic and political systems.

Today, Indigenous peoples are marginalised within their own countries. However, they resolve to maintain and restore their ancestral and traditional environments and systems as distinct peoples and communities. First peoples, First Nations, Aboriginal, ethnic groups, mobs, iwi (tribe), hapū (subtribe) or Travellers are some of the different terms Indigenous peoples prefer and reflect modern understandings of being 'Indigenous' (United Nations [UN] 2008, World Health Organization 2007).

The Indigenous peoples of Australia, New Zealand, Europe and the United Kingdom (UK) are (respectively): the **Aboriginal and Torres Strait Islander peoples**; **Māori peoples**; and **Gypsy, Roma and Traveller peoples**. They are not homogenous groups, as implied by these broad titles. Instead, they often identify by their nation or country in Australia, their iwi (tribe) and hapū (subtribe) in New Zealand or their ethnic identity as Gypsy, Roma and Traveller in the UK. The UN definition of Indigenous peoples includes those peoples who have nomadic lifestyles (like Sami people of northern Europe). We also include Gypsy, Roma and Traveller peoples living across Europe and the UK as Indigenous because they too have experienced processes that have led to enforced changes to their cultural ways of life, and have marked inequities in health service access, morbidity and premature mortality (Heaslip et al 2019, McFadden et al 2018). While not formally recognised, some groups of Gypsy, Roma and Traveller peoples, like Irish and Scottish Travellers, refer to themselves as Indigenous. Nevertheless, they all share similar histories of **colonisation** resulting in historic injustices that brought about depopulation, socioeconomic and political disenfranchisement and marginalisation that rendered them powerless minority groups within their own countries (Heaslip, Wilson & Jackson 2019). Through processes of colonisation, contemporary Indigenous peoples have lost their land, languages and cultural practices. Notably, they suffer ongoing contemporary injustices and inequities compared to other population groups living in their countries (Mbuzi, Fulbrook & Jessup 2017).

Within the context of research, those advocating Western scientific paradigms invalidate and trivialise Indigenous peoples' well-developed knowledge systems and ways of knowing (Chilisa 2012, McFadden et al 2018, Smith 2012). This chapter explains privileging Indigenous health realities as a way to better understand and address the health disparities they experience. Following this will be an overview of the **social, historical and political contexts** of Indigenous peoples, stressing the relevance of these contexts when reading and interpreting research. We will then discuss and position Indigenous worldviews, ethics, values and protocols as different from the dominant worldviews that generally inform health research. The chapter ends with a discussion about the use of research evidence relating to Indigenous peoples in a **culturally safe** manner to inform nursing and midwifery practice (Wilson 2017).

PRIVILEGING INDIGENOUS REALITIES

Processes of colonisation and enforced cultural change took place in countries such as Australia, New Zealand, the United States (US), Canada and Africa, and across Europe and the UK, where Indigenous peoples' nomadic lifestyles were forcibly constrained. Universally, Indigenous peoples are concerned about inequities in their poor health status and health outcomes because of colonisation and associated loss of the traditional cultural practices that kept them well and safe, the loss of their connection to traditional land and their loss of language (UN 2013). Historically, Indigenous peoples have suffered because researchers have undertaken research in disrespectful ways, silenced Indigenous voices, and reframed and renamed their experiences and cultural values and practices (Chilisa 2012, Garcia et al 2013, Smith 2012, Wilson, Mikahere-Hall & Sherwood 2021). Often, researchers reported their findings in ways that victim blame, reinforce negative stereotypes and provide deficit explanations to explain inequities. Privileging Indigenous realities is about resisting how Indigenous peoples are framed, named and labelled (Penehira et al 2014). The continuation of such approaches is a form of research harm, which perpetuates ongoing colonialism and knowledge that does not reflect Indigenous views of health and wellbeing or their realities. It is from this basis that there is a need to instead privilege Indigenous voices and viewpoints to better understand their health and wellbeing realities (Brannelly & Boulton 2017, Tipa 2020).

Indigenous researchers have been focused on reclaiming Indigenous ways of knowing and functioning, particularly as it pertains to their health and wellbeing (Varcoe et al 2017, Wilson 2017). Recognising Indigenous worldviews as distinct ontological (nature of reality) and epistemological (knowledge and knowing) traditions informed by cultural values (axiology) is essential when using Indigenous health research (Martin 2008, Moreton-Robinson 2013). Western research methodologies remain limited as they generally ignore the importance of Indigenous histories and their influence on contemporary Indigenous peoples—for instance, the unacceptable inequities in health status and health outcomes (Cormack et al 2018).

According to Chilisa (2012, p. 14), oppression in the research context is '... a process of conducting research in such a way that the worldviews of those who have suffered a long history of oppression and marginalisation are given space to communicate from their frames of reference'. Health research knowledge about Indigenous peoples is mostly defined by evidence generated from dominant cultural viewpoints that oppress and pathologise them (Watego et al 2021, Wilson 2017). Therefore, it is imperative that when reviewing health literature and research you ask: through whose eyes and worldview has this research been analysed or interpreted? For instance, non-Indigenous researchers generally construct Māori and their use of health services as non-compliance (Penney, Barnes & McCreanor 2011). This is at odds with Māori accounts of their experiences with health and social services (e.g. Garcia et al 2013, Goodman et al 2017, Mbuzi et al 2017, Wilson et al 2019). Therefore, it is essential to also access Indigenous-focused research where possible (Wilson, Mikahere-Hall & Sherwood 2021).

In appreciating Indigenous worldviews and ways of knowing, nurses and midwives must value the different ways that Indigenous peoples understand health and wellbeing. As we have discussed, the dominant biomedical model, driven by Western science, has influenced what constitutes 'valid' knowledge and evidence, including the methods of producing knowledge via research within the health arena. This research, by focusing mainly on an individual's physical health or illness, influences not only how health services are structured and delivered, but informs nursing and midwifery practice.

Furthermore, research that is driven by a deficit approach ignores the cultural obligations associated with reciprocity, and cultural, social and economic factors and realities that are determinants of health affecting Indigenous peoples' health and lives (Ehrlich et al 2016, McDonald & Lawson 2017). Instead, it generally reports Indigenous 'deficit' accounts and victim-blaming. This ignores the role those systems, structures and health professionals' behaviours and attitudes have in perpetuating Indigenous health inequities (Heaslip et al 2019) and that makes health services difficult for Indigenous peoples to use (see, for example, Makowharemahihi et al 2014, Tipa 2020). When considering published research, it is important to consider Indigenous worldviews; their cultural values, beliefs and practices; and their realities. Miller (2014) stresses the importance of listening carefully with both our ears and our heart, as well as observing and reflecting on what we 'hear' and 'see'.

Rights, Social Justice and Equity

Privileging Indigenous realities is underpinned by ethical, social justice principles including equity and human rights. In addition to basic human rights, the UN *Declaration on the Rights of Indigenous Peoples* affirms Indigenous peoples' 'equal right to the enjoyment of the highest attainable standard of physical and mental health' (UN 2008, Article 24:2). This declaration was endorsed by Australia, New Zealand, the US and Canada. Moreover, the *Geneva Declaration on the Health and Survival of Indigenous Peoples* calls for 'access to quality and culturally appropriate healthcare ... without discrimination' (United Nations Economic and Social Council 2002). In New Zealand, Māori also have rights under the Te Tiriti o Waitangi (Māori language version of the Treaty of Waitangi). This is a historical agreement setting out Māori rights to governance, self-determination and autonomy, equity and spiritual wellbeing that health researchers and service providers are obliged to honour (Wilson & Haretuku 2015). The importance of these rights is highlighted by the need for research that better reflects Indigenous peoples' health experiences. It is important to note that

Gypsy, Roma and Traveller peoples have no such rights in the UK. Indeed, it was only in the 2021 census that Roma was added as a distinct Ethnic Minority group.

In addition to a rights approach, a social justice perspective also involves privileging the voices of Indigenous peoples. It is important to understand that inequities and disparities exist in communities when social structures and systems are in place that unfairly disadvantage minority and marginalised groups, such as Indigenous peoples (Braveman 2014, Braveman & Gottlieb 2014, Browne et al 2016). Therefore, disparities in Indigenous peoples' social and health status are considered unjust and unfair, and are largely a result of social structures and systems. Far from choosing a 'lifestyle', related to increased risks of morbidity and mortality, disadvantaged groups have difficulties in accessing the necessary determinants of health. This is because of structural barriers and **discrimination**, and, for instance, mismatches in understandings and expectations of Indigenous peoples, researchers and healthcare providers (Bell et al 2015). Thus, privileging Indigenous peoples' voices enables them to inform researchers about the systems and processes that oppress and inhibit them and allows them to elaborate on alternative approaches that may optimise their wellbeing and invest in their futures.

Intersectionality offers a way of considering the range of intersecting and compounding forms of oppression that Indigenous peoples encounter. It refers to the interrelated categorisation of people according to their race, class, gender, different abilities and socioeconomic status (for example) applied to individuals and groups of people. Categorisations such as these are intersecting and have compounding effects while being interdependent. They are each systems of discrimination and disadvantage for some groups or privilege for others (Crenshaw 1991). Some researchers are using intersectionality in their research to better understand and present the complexities of individual and collective identities that can simultaneously occur and marginalise people for their characteristics such as being Indigenous, female, queer, blind, deaf or poor.

Equal approaches based on the notions of 'sameness' are not effective. Indigenous peoples are often underserved populations and are viewed as problematic. However, intersectionality is an approach that shows how multiple compounding forms of oppression, including discrimination and **racism**, intensifies the disadvantage of Indigenous peoples. In some circumstances inequalities are: 1. expected and 2. acceptable (for instance, the inequalities in breast cancer between men and women). Equitable approaches, on the other hand, require greater levels of attention and intervention to reduce the morbidity and mortality Indigenous peoples suffer. This invariably requires doing things differently (Braveman 2014). While this is a brief overview of these concepts, it lays the foundation for culturally safe use of research.

STUDENT CHALLENGE

Equity

Using social justice and intersectionality approaches, what individual cultural and social determinants of health might Ahmed wish to explore in his assessment of an 87-year-old Indigenous man?

SOCIAL, HISTORICAL AND POLITICAL CONTEXTS

The colonisation of Australia and New Zealand by people from other countries, predominantly the UK, was an essential part of European and British territorial imperialism. Imperialism, informed by Western knowledge and traditions, involved the applications of laws of the imperial nation-state to justify the invasion and colonisation of other countries to exploit land and resources to benefit the respective empire. Subjugation, control and sometimes negotiating agreements like treaties were common outcomes for Indigenous peoples subject to the imperial forces (Moreton-Robinson 2015). Similar forms of control have also constrained the nomadic lifestyles and cultural practices of Gypsy, Roma and Traveller peoples (Heaslip & Smith 2016, Heaslip, Hean & Parker 2016a, 2016b). Colonisation facilitated an agenda for Indigenous peoples to be the 'same' (assimilation) as settlers and colonisers. Simultaneously, it created Indigenous peoples as 'others' (marginalisation) and disempowered them culturally, economically, politically and cognitively (Chilisa 2012, Smith 2012). In Australia and New Zealand, this was aided by invasion, forcible land acquisition and the destruction of Indigenous political, social, economic and cultural systems that had ensured Indigenous peoples thrived and prospered (Smith 2012). Today, the forces of imperialism and colonisation can be seen in the interpersonal and institutional racism and discrimination Indigenous peoples experience. This is evident in their different access to determinants of health and health services, and the differences in the quality and safety of healthcare they receive that can lead to poorer health outcomes (see Cormack, Stanley & Harris 2018 and Thurber et al 2021 for examples).

It is important to appreciate that Western worldviews formed the basis for the ways Indigenous peoples were constructed and represented, viewing Indigenous peoples as inferior, which negatively stigmatised and stereotyped them. For example, one such construct is the racialisation of Indigenous peoples, which is the belief that darker skin complexion equates to inferiority. This was influenced by social Darwinism which classified Indigenous peoples as a different and inferior human 'species' (Wilkerson 2020). These negative views gave rise to terms such as 'noble savages' to describe Māori, for instance, whereby they were seen as primitive 'savages' but were also seen as 'noble' when compared to peoples of darker races. Those belonging to the dominant cultural group (driven by their Western perspectives and beliefs of being superior to those whose land they stole or took by devious methods) assumed settlers, missionaries and themselves brought Western ideas of civilisation to Indigenous peoples they believed were uncivilised and savages.

Indigenous peoples were usurped from their homes, ways of life and freedom. Colonisation significantly impacted Indigenous peoples globally, resulting in separation from their traditional lands, aided by Western laws and policies that stripped them of their sovereignty, autonomy and status. Smith (2012, p. 21) stated it left a '... legacy of suffering and destruction'. Colonisers, using these Western paradigms, determined what constituted knowledge, who could be a knower and how knowledge would be produced. However, it systematically demeaned and devalued Indigenous knowledge and ways of knowing (i.e. 'research'), and associated racial agendas protected settlers and cast Indigenous peoples in negative ways. For instance, Indigenous peoples needed to be quarantined because they were 'riddled with disease' (Anderson 2002). Such actions and beliefs, often published, highlighted significant differences between the superior and clean Europeans and the primitive, disease-ridden and declining Indigenous peoples (Anderson 2002).

Smith (1999, p. 80) simply concluded, 'they came, they saw, they named, they claimed'. Considerable research on Indigenous peoples has reinforced dominant colonising ways of viewing them. Research was synonymous with being scientific and had profound consequences for Indigenous peoples and their ways of knowing. The positioning of Indigenous peoples as 'other' guaranteed their objectification and marginalisation. Not only did this silence them, but it also denied and invalidated their worldviews and knowledges. It became normal to measure, judge and interpret Indigenous peoples against Western scientific worldviews and standards (Bishop 2008, Chilisa 2012, Denzin, Lincoln & Smith 2008, Smith 2012).

As highlighted earlier, Western ways of knowing silenced Indigenous peoples globally and subjugated their knowledges (Battiste & Henderson 2000, Ermine et al 2004, Smith 2012). According to Ladson-Billings (2000), dominant cultural hegemony promotes and validates one way of viewing the world. Consequently, the negative constructions of Indigenous peoples persisted and informed research and policy that targeted these communities, even when evidence confirmed such constructions were false (Denzin, Lincoln & Smith 2008).

STUDENT CHALLENGE

What Counts as Evidence?

When planning research with young women living with intellectual disabilities and type 1 diabetes, Jamie should take note of the existing evidence and the lack of research undertaken with Indigenous women. Nurses and midwives should consider engagement with Indigenous communities and families to understand the knowledge and strengths they possess.

In the absence of research with young Indigenous women, what other forms of evidence might Jamie need to consider for working with these young women? How would you identify their strengths and support systems, and the intersecting forms of oppression they encounter?

Using Western scientific research tools and approaches, researchers have generally investigated contemporary Indigenous health issues with the perception of Indigenous peoples as problematic dominating the literature. Since the 1970s, Indigenous peoples globally are concerned about the socioeconomic and health disparities they experience and have been increasingly reclaiming and developing their own approaches to research. This includes asserting their right to investigate health and social issues affecting their communities, using tools informed by their own epistemological worldviews (see, for example, Simmonds 2011). Such approaches enable Indigenous peoples to undertake critical, strengths-based and outcome-focused research, rather than problem-oriented research.

WORLDVIEWS

A worldview is a system of knowledge that develops from birth and is shaped by the cultural, social and physical environment you grow up in. It is shaped by your culture, the experiences you have and the belief systems you encounter (Nesdole et al 2014). Worldviews are frameworks for understanding and investigating the world we live in. They support the way we act and relate in the world, are knowledge systems informed by cultural values and beliefs and provide models and contexts for processing, understanding and explaining information and knowledge (Nesdole et al 2014). They can be considered the foundations for the way we perceive and live in the world (Wilson 2017).

Worldviews are generally monocultural conceptual frameworks for the way you see and think about the world (Kovach 2009), informed by the multiple and different cultural groups to which people belong. They guide and determine an entire mode of living,

particularly about how we interpret and order our realities in the world (Wilson, Heaslip & Jackson 2018). The 'truths' produced by worldviews are biased by a particular cultural standpoint (Denzin & Lincoln 2000). What this means is that there are multiple ways of seeing and understanding the world we live in. We must appreciate our own individual worldviews are no more right or better than other people's worldviews, and that there is no right or wrong worldview, just different ways of viewing the world (Wilson 2017, Wilson, Heaslip & Jackson 2018).

Indigenous Worldviews

A paradigm involves a methodological process informed by a philosophical framework about what constitutes knowledge and ways of knowing, and that identifies relevant ethics and values (Chilisa 2012). Indigenous paradigms are informed by Indigenous peoples' knowledge system, ways of being, values and methods of generating knowledge (see Table 10.1). It is important to note that while there is great diversity among the world's Indigenous peoples, there are a number of shared perspectives. Key features of Indigenous worldviews are that they are generally:

- holistic in nature
- ecologically and spiritually based
- based on people's relationships with others and their environments
- collective-oriented (contrasting with dominant individual orientations)
- integrative of the past, present and future (contrasting with dominant Western beliefs that view time in a linear way)
- resistant to colonial imposition.

TABLE 10.1		
Indigenous Research Paradigm		
Axiology	Values	Respectful and ethical practices, grounded in Indigenous cultural beliefs and practices. Indigenous peoples determine the transfer of information and knowledge. Elders play an important role as holders of knowledge and determine who will and can have access to it.
Ontology	Ways of being	Social and relational construction of Indigenous ways of being.
Epistemology	Ways of knowing	Knowledge systems are relational.
Methodology	Ways of doing research	Oral transmission, storytelling, yarning, songs, ceremonies, symbols.

Indigenous peoples have special and enduring connections with their traditional lands. These places are the basis of their survival and spiritual wellbeing, are places of nurturing and define their identity (Wilson, Heaslip & Jackson 2018). Indigenous worldviews are dynamic and responsive to societal changes, ensuring continuous re-informing of ways of knowing and living in the world. Therefore, the many social and technological changes occurring in our world influence many contemporary Indigenous peoples' traditional worldviews.

A particular feature of Indigenous peoples is their collective way of living and the importance of relationships with others (this includes all living and non-living entities and spirits) (Hart 2010, Martin 2008). This promotes collective responsibilities and intrinsic obligations to others and differs notably from dominant cultural groups that endorse self and individual success over the collective group. Chilisa and Tsheko (2014) explain this:

Knowing is something that is socially constructed by people who have relationships and connections with each other, the living and the non-living, and the environment. Knowers are seen as beings with connections with other beings, the spirits of the ancestors and the world around them that informs what they know and how they can know it ... the challenge is on how to bring this cultural knowledge into the research process.

(p. 223)

Therefore, research must reflect Indigenous peoples' views of health and wellbeing. This is holistic and inclusive of the emotional, social, physical and spiritual dimensions of individuals, and their relationships with their families and others within their communities. For example, based on our knowledge of Indigenous worldviews, when researchers (like Ahmed and Jamie) are planning their research, they need to consider how they maintain flexibility and plan for participants' choice of individual or group interviews (Gifford et al 2013). For instance, when Ahmed is planning his research to include older Indigenous peoples who may only speak their Indigenous language, he will need to be flexible in working with them to obtain relevant and meaningful information

that is useful to those working with older Indigenous peoples. As relationships are fundamental to research practice, Ahmed will need to constantly work on overcoming language and cultural barriers in the development and maintenance of relationships with research participants.

INDIGENOUS KNOWLEDGE AND WAYS OF KNOWING

Indigenous ways of knowing are secular and relational. Creation stories and tribal lands are the foundations of knowledge that inform spiritual and cultural praxis (Archibald, Lee-Morgan & De Santolo 2019). Indigenous knowledge systems are regulated through tribal authorities with defined roles and responsibilities, and systems and processes for research (Australian Institute of Aboriginal and Torres Strait Islander Studies [AIATSIS] 2012, Health Research Council of New Zealand 2010, National Health and Medical Research Council [NHMRC] 2018a, 2018b, Smallacombe, Davis & Quiggin 2007). Thus, embedded within traditional Indigenous knowledge are the ways in which people understand and function in the world about them, and what they value. This is relevant for understanding why many Indigenous peoples struggle when using health services—their views, values and practices of health differ markedly, something generally ignored by health professionals. Ideally, Indigenous paradigms are best to research Indigenous peoples. Oral traditions transmit knowledge via storytelling, song, music and designs on visual art forms, for example. The following briefly introduces you to Aboriginal, Torres Strait Islander, Māori and Gypsy, Roma and Traveller peoples' creation stories, as traditional and contemporary ways of knowing.

Aboriginal Dreaming

Customary law has always been in place in Australia since time immemorial, laid down by the creating spirits of the Dreaming. Indigenous Australians maintain that their creation and beginnings were founded by the Dreaming, an era of creation—marking the time that Aboriginal occupation commenced in Australia (Stanner 1979). This way of knowing is universal to all Indigenous Australian groups (Pawu-kurlpurlurnu, Holmes & Box et al 2008, Razani et al 2007). Aboriginal peoples were created through the life force of their

Dreaming ancestors, along with their respective lands, flora and fauna. Each Aboriginal person, no matter where they are from, has metaphysical and geographical relationships with all the living and non-living beings of their respective Dreaming creators (Hume 2002). This is an essential standpoint of Aboriginal Australians' worldview, and is distinctly different from a Western way of knowing them and their history (Grieves 2009, Sherwood 2010).

Torres Strait (Zenadth Kes) Belonging and Standpoint

Central to Zenadth Kes ways of knowing, being and doing is belonging to ged/lag (home), one's land and sea country, family, tribe and Island community (Harvey 2020, Drummond et al 2021). Like Aboriginal people, Torres Strait Islanders' relationship with ancestor and creation spirits remains significant. However, a contrasting feature with Aboriginal peoples is that since colonisation many Torres Strait Islanders also value their relationship with the Christian God. British colonial assaults on their land, bodies and souls continue, although the people of Zenadth Kes prove resilient, navigating the ongoing colonisation and maintaining their agency. They do this by adopting their ways of knowing, being and doing to better respond to immediate and future challenges. This is reflective of Zenadth Kes standpoint and agency within the cultural interface of ongoing colonisation and dispossession (Drummond 2020, Drummond et al 2021, Nakata 2007).

Māori Whakapapa (Genealogy)

Whakapapa provides a way of understanding the Māori world. It links the origin of humankind from Te Kore (a void, state of potential), to Te Pō (the realm of darkness) holding Ranginui (the sky father) and Papatūānuku (the Earth mother), to Te Ao Marama (the world of light) where Ranginui's and Papatūānuku's children were born. The womb (Te Pō) and birthing (Te Ao Marama) symbolically explain aspects of the origins of humankind. Whakapapa explains the genealogy and the connectedness of humans along with other living things, and importantly prescribes the integral relationships humans have to each other, the environment and other living things. In this way, it links past, present and future humans and atua (gods), tūpuna (ancestors), Papatūānuku (tribal area) and the whenua (land), and living things (Mead 2016, Royal 2003). Whakapapa uniquely brings together knowledge of the present with the past and the future. As Graham (2005) explains, it is also concerned with generating new Indigenous knowledge grounded in a Māori world. Embedded within whakapapa is practical knowledge that aids survival and influences the behaviours, obligations and responsibilities that, as Indigenous peoples, they have to one another and the environment and all things within it (Mead 2016, Mikaere 2017).

Gypsy, Roma and Traveller Peoples' Storytelling

Gypsy, Roma and Traveller peoples have a strong oral tradition. As with other Indigenous peoples, stories are a way of communicating family histories, knowledge and values. These stories are told within family groups around campfires, thereby strengthening family structures, and are important in establishing the cultural identity and connections for nomadic peoples. Stories become important ways of undertaking research with Gypsy, Roma and Traveller peoples because of their strong oral traditions (Condon et al 2019).

STUDENT CHALLENGE

Differentiating Indigenous and Western Knowledge Systems

Identify the features of Indigenous knowledge systems using the following headings: epistemology (knowledge and knowing), ontology (realities), axiology (cultural values) and methodology (ways of transmitting knowledge). Then compare these to Western biomedical knowledge systems that inform nursing and midwifery knowledge systems. How may these differences influence Ahmed, Martha and Jamie when they begin to analyse published research?

ETHICAL INDIGENOUS RESEARCH

Researcher contact with Indigenous peoples and communities has often left Indigenous peoples and communities feeling exploited. This is especially the case when research was carried out in ways that lacked relevance, was culturally offensive or failed to benefit the community or contribute to positive change. This exploitation has been identified across various Indigenous communities, including Aboriginal and Torres Strait Islander communities (Bond, Foley & Askew 2016), Gypsy, Roma and Traveller peoples (Greenfields & Home 2006), First Nation, Inuit and Métis communities (Flicker & Worthington 2012) and Māori communities (Furness et al 2016). When considering the scientific and social value of research, non-Indigenous researchers need to be cautious that they do not impose their perspectives on identifying research that Indigenous communities need, especially if it perpetuates a problematising of issues that further stigmatises and marginalises Indigenous peoples. Such approaches can be considered a form of ongoing colonisation.

Indigenous Data Sovereignty (IDS) provides Indigenous principles and a framework that ensures Indigenous peoples control research on or about them. IDS is about Indigenous governance and self-determination about data practices that are inclusive of data collection, use, storage and interpretation. In this way, IDS provides guidance to avoid research that negatively frames Indigenous peoples by disparities, deprivation, disadvantage, dysfunction and difference, all providing deficit-based understandings of their realities (Kukutai & Cormack 2019, Walter & Suina 2019).

Westernised worldviews focus on and privilege individuals, whereas Indigenous communities' philosophies are on the collective group. Flicker and Worthington (2012) highlight that Indigenous worldviews privilege holistic and collaborative relationships, spirituality and reciprocity, which contrasts with Westernised views of rationality and individualism. Such approaches enable researchers to focus on individuals, problems and deficits in ways that ignore the bigger more holistic picture. For example, decolonisation requires consideration of pre- and post-colonisation histories of Indigenous communities and needs to critically appraise the ongoing effects of colonisation and structural discrimination and barriers (Wilson, Mikahere-Hall & Sherwood 2021).

Because of the different understandings of ethical research, researchers undertaking research with Indigenous peoples need to conform to both Western research ethics and Indigenous principles and ethics that are informed by their values, beliefs and ways of living. This is fundamental to ensure research is undertaken in respectful and ethical ways, and that the research findings are grounded in Indigenous worldviews and

realities. Table 10.2 outlines some of the issues and risks that can occur when a broader approach to ethics is not undertaken. In Australia and New Zealand, this has led to the development of ethical guidelines that outline expectations for anyone undertaking research with Indigenous peoples (AIATSIS 2012, Health Research Council of New Zealand 2010, Hudson et al 2010, NHMRC 2018a, 2018b). In the UK and Europe, the *International Ethical Guidelines for Health-related Research Involving Humans* (Council for International Organizations of Medical Sciences [CIOMS] 2016) are useful to guide planning and undertaking research with Gypsy, Roma and Traveller peoples.

In practice, researchers need to clearly explain the research processes and how Indigenous peoples have been involved, to ensure an Indigenous worldview is privileged and captured in the research. The benefits and burdens of any research for Indigenous peoples needs to be explicit at a community level. For instance, you should expect to see a description of the community engagement (collaborative relationships and involvement) of Indigenous peoples during the research process. While the process of dissemination is a vital part of research, researchers often publish academic papers or submit research reports that communities are unable to access and use. When considering how to disseminate research findings, researchers need to also use culturally appropriate and acceptable mechanisms—for example, Gypsy, Roma and Travellers have a cultural tradition of storytelling and oral histories (similar to other Indigenous peoples), so translating the research findings using video monologues and recorded stories may be more meaningful and useful.

Ensuring ethical Indigenous research ultimately requires partnership with the community at each stage of the research process. As an example of this, Jamie could contact local Indigenous communities and enquire as to whether their planned research aligns with their research needs and, importantly, whether any special cultural considerations need to be incorporated into their research plan and process. This enables identifying and negotiating the research agenda, developing the appropriate research design with Indigenous communities, and being collaborators in undertaking the research and disseminating its results. Furthermore, Riddell and colleagues (2017) identify seven key areas of consideration for researchers working with

TABLE 10.2
Examples of Research Issues and the Risks for Indigenous Peoples

Ethical Issue	Risk	Rationale
Non-Indigenous researchers imposing their views about what research is needed.	Disempowers Indigenous communities and perpetuates problematising issues they face. It also risks reinforcing stigma and marginalisation.	Indigenous peoples have the right to self-determination, which includes research agendas. Research should reflect Indigenous aspirations and be beneficial.
Researchers not collaborating or establishing relationships with Indigenous communities, or doing so late in the development of a piece of research.	Research outcomes lack relevance and benefits for Indigenous communities, and there is a risk of placing avoidable burden on sometimes over-researched communities.	Indigenous community engagement is necessary to ensure the research design and process is culturally appropriate and acceptable.
Researchers claim ownership over the data and research outcomes.	Misappropriation of traditional knowledge and cultural artefacts.	Indigenous communities must retain ownership of their traditional knowledge and cultural expression.
Researchers using written information and consent forms aimed at individual participants.	Indigenous peoples are either unable to read written texts or comprehend the language researchers use (especially jargon), and therefore risk consenting to processes that are not informed.	Indigenous peoples' cultural traditions are oral and based on collective responsibilities and obligations to members of their whānau or community, and to the group as a whole. Furthermore, some Indigenous peoples, of all ages, have been educationally disadvantaged and this impacts on their literacy. Consenting processes should be inclusive of individuals and groups, and also provide for oral forms of consent to be provided (e.g. captured on audio-recording).
Researchers not including Indigenous peoples on their research team or advisory groups.	Using Western-based analyses and interpretation that produces research that is not reflective of Indigenous realities.	Indigenous inclusion in research promotes and reflects Indigenous realities observed and interpreted.

Indigenous communities, which you should expect to see in any reported research.

1. Inclusion of traditional values, protocols and norms
2. Critical understanding of the history of research with Indigenous populations
3. Agreeing on the nature of collaboration during the research project
4. The nature of co-creation or collaborative research relationships
5. Co-creating research processes
6. Analysing and interpreting research findings that accurately reflect Indigenous realities
7. Establishing the dissemination process of the research

Ethical Indigenous research involves researchers being respectful, inclusive and ensuring Indigenous voices are heard. Importantly, any ethical research should leave Indigenous peoples feeling culturally safe (Wilson 2017).

STUDENT CHALLENGE
Indigenous Ethics—Similar or Different?

In what ways are Indigenous ethics similar to or different from mainstream or dominant cultural research ethics informed by Western worldviews?

CULTURALLY SAFE USE OF RESEARCH

Fundamental to any research with Indigenous peoples is that they feel culturally safe and that the research is responsive to their needs. This is what Wilson and Neville (2009, p. 73) refer to as '... creating a space for dialogue and negotiation ...'. Both Australia and New Zealand require nurses and midwives to be **culturally safe** and **culturally competent** (CATSINaM 2017, Midwifery Council of New Zealand 2011, Nursing and Midwifery Board of Australia 2018, Nursing Council of New Zealand 2011). However, in the UK, the Nursing and Midwifery Council only asks that nurses consider cultural sensitives in their communication (Nursing and Midwifery Council 2018).

Cultural safety is a way of being, a commitment to accepting that others may have different perceptions and values. This acceptance of difference is in addition to having the necessary knowledge, skills and capabilities to work with Indigenous peoples (Wilson & Hickey 2015). As such, nurses and midwives need a critical understanding of their own worldviews and sociocultural positioning to ensure they act respectfully and responsively, especially to integrate Indigenous peoples' cultural needs into their research plans (Wilson 2008, 2017). This means engaging critically with and questioning the research literature. Caution is required as to how research is framed and then interpreted to avoid perpetuation of stigma, marginalisation and problematisation of Indigenous health issues that lay blame for poorer health status on individuals. Heaslip, Hean and Parker (2016b), Kotz and colleagues (2016) and Wilson and Barton (2012) all argue that Indigenous peoples often provide contrasting perspectives to those of researchers and health professionals about their poorer health status that link more to difficulties engaging with and using health services.

As nurses and midwives, we need to consider how we use research to inform our practice and advocate for health services that meet the needs of Indigenous peoples. Essential in such consideration is the requirement to reflect on and address any individual and institutional values, beliefs and approaches that consciously and unconsciously perpetuate colonial imaginations of Indigenous peoples that support the diminishing, demeaning or disempowering of them (Cox et al 2020). At this point in your career, you may not be able to influence the way research is planned, undertaken and interpreted, but you can begin by being more critical about the way you question the research that informs your practice. Part of cultural safety is how nurses and midwives use research findings for evidence-based practice. In Box 10.1, there is a set of questions (adapted from Smith 2012) that can

---

BOX 10.1

GUIDING QUESTIONS TO REVIEW RESEARCH WITH INDIGENOUS PEOPLES

- Did the research team include Indigenous researchers and/or an Indigenous cultural advisory group?
- Who defined the research problem? Was the relevant Indigenous community(ies) involved in developing the research questions and aims?
- For whom is the study beneficial and relevant? Who says so?
- What knowledge will the Indigenous community(ies) gain from this research?
- What knowledge did the researcher gain from this research?
- What are the positive outcomes from this research?
- What were the potential negative outcomes from this research? How were potential negative outcomes removed?
- In what ways were the research findings communicated? Do the findings reinforce deficit explanations or negative stereotypes associated with Indigenous health or do they highlight a more strengths-based approach?
- To whom was the researcher(s) accountable?
- What processes were in place to ensure cultural support for the research, researched and researcher(s)?

Source: Adapted from Smith LT: Decolonizing methodologies: research and Indigenous peoples, ed 2, London, 2012, Zed Books.

---

be used to review and question the appropriateness of the research being reviewed about Indigenous peoples.

STUDENT CHALLENGE

Understanding Health Information

Indigenous peoples are often referred to as lacking health literacy (the ability to access and fully understand health information to enable appropriate decision-making). This is despite having never received information about their health conditions and their management or having been given information in jargon-laced language that is difficult to understand.

How do researchers portray health literacy for Indigenous peoples? How do they focus or not focus the lens on health professionals in undertaking this research? How can the concept of health literacy be problematic for Indigenous peoples? What advice would you give to Ahmed and Jamie about interpreting and understanding research evidence about Indigenous peoples?

CONCLUSION

Indigenous peoples globally have suffered enforced cultural changes that have resulted in the colonisation of not only their land but also their language, cultural beliefs and values. Such changes have impacted their ways of living everyday life, achieved in part by the invalidation of Indigenous knowledges and their ways of generating knowledge. The subjugation they experience has been enabled by the ongoing domination of what counts as knowledge—thus, research has used a dominant Western cultural lens on which to design and undertake research with Indigenous peoples. This has produced research findings that are often at odds with Indigenous realities and that position them in ways that further marginalises Indigenous peoples in the community. The interpretation of these research findings reinforces negative stereotypes, offers deficit explanations and further stigmatises them. We urge nurses and midwives to become knowledgeable about why Indigenous peoples sit at the margins of our societies, and to critically read and interrogate research. From the perspectives of Indigenous peoples themselves, beneficial research is research that seeks to understand Indigenous realities.

ADDITIONAL RESOURCES

The following documents are useful for getting a fuller and more specific understanding of the considerations in undertaking research with Indigenous peoples.

Cram F: Kaupapa Māori health research. In Liamputtong P (ed), Handbook of research methods in health social sciences. Singapore, 2017, Springer Singapore, pp. 1–19.

Wepa D, Wilson D: Struggling to be involved: an interprofessional approach to examine Māori whānau engagement with healthcare services, Journal of Nursing Research and Practice 3(3):1–5, 2019.

Wilson D, Barton P: Indigenous hospital experiences: a New Zealand case study, Journal of Clinical Nursing 21(15–16):2316–2326, 2012.

Wilson D, Moloney E, Parr JM, et al, Creating an Indigenous Māori-centred model of relational health: a literature review of Māori models of health, Journal of Clinical Nursing 30 (23–24):3539–3555, 2021.

Australia: National Health and Medical Research Council (NHMRC)

NHMRC: Values and ethics: guidelines for ethical conduct in Aboriginal and Torres Strait Islander health research, Canberra, 2003, Commonwealth of Australia. Online. Available: https://nhmrc. gov.au/about-us/publications/values-and-ethics-guidelines-ethical-conduct-aboriginal-and-torres-strait-islander-health-research (accessed 28 November 2021).

Examples of Research Using Indigenous Methodologies

Cram F, Kennedy V: Researching with Whānau collectives, MAI Review (3): 2010. Online. Available: http://www.review.mai.ac.nz/ mrindex/MR/article/download/382/382-2874-1-PB.pdf (accessed 28 November 2021).

Durie M: Understanding health and illness: research at the interface between science and Indigenous knowledge, International Journal of Epidemiology 33(5):1138–1143, 2004.

Graham J: Nā Rangi tāua, nā Tuānuku e takoto nei: research methodology framed by whakapapa. MAI Review (1), Article 3:1–9, 2009. Online. Available: http://www.review.mai.ac.nz/ mrindex/MR/article/download/199/199-1200-1-PB.pdf (accessed 28 November 2021).

Heaslip V, Wilson D, Jackson D, 2019a. Are Gypsy Roma Traveller communities Indigenous and would identification as such better address their public health needs? Public Health Nov;176: 43–49, 2019.

Kurtz DLM: Indigenous methodologies: traversing Indigenous and Western worldviews in research, AlterNative: An International Journal of Indigenous Peoples 9(3):217–229, 2013.

Sherwood J, Kendall S: Reframing spaces by building relationships: community collaborative participatory action research with Aboriginal mothers in prison, Contemporary Nurse 46(1):84–95, 2013.

REFERENCES

Anderson W: The cultivation of whiteness: science, health and racial destiny in Australia, Melbourne, 2002, Melbourne University Press.

Archibald J-A, Lee-Morgan JBJ & De Santolo J (2019). Decolonizing research: Indigenous storywork as methodology. Zed Books.

Australian Institute of Aboriginal and Torres Strait Islander Studies (AIATSIS). 2012, AIATSIS. https://aiatsis.gov.au/sites/default/files/2020-09/gerais.pdf

Battiste M, Henderson JY: Protecting Indigenous knowledge and heritage: a global challenge, Saskatoon, 2000, Purich Publishing.

Bell D, Lindeman MA, Reid JB: The (mis)matching of resources and assessed need in remote Aboriginal community aged care, Australasian Journal on Ageing 34(3):171–176, 2015.

Bishop R: Freeing ourselves from neo-colonial domination in research: a Māori approach to creating knowledge. In Denzin NK, Lincoln YS, editors: The SAGE handbook of qualitative research, ed 3, Thousand Oaks, 2008, SAGE, pp. 109–138.

Bond C, Foley W, Askew D: 'It puts a human face on the researched'—a qualitative evaluation of an Indigenous health research governance model, Australian and New Zealand Journal of Public Health 40(S1):S89–S95, 2016.

Brannelly T, Boulton A: The ethics of care and transformational research practices in Aotearoa New Zealand, Qualitative Research 17(3):340–350, 2017.

Braveman P, Gottlieb L. The social determinants of health: it's time to consider the causes of the causes, Public Health Reports 129(Suppl 2):19–31, 2014.

Braveman P: What are health disparities and health equity? We need to be clear, Public Health Reports 129(Suppl 2):5–8, 2014.

Browne AJ, Varcoe C, Lavoie J, et al: Enhancing health care equity with Indigenous populations: evidence-based strategies from an ethnographic study, BMC Health Services Research 16:544, 2016.

Chilisa B: Indigenous research methodologies, Thousand Oaks, 2012, SAGE.

Chilisa B, Tsheko GN: Mixed methods in Indigenous research: building relationships for sustainable intervention outcomes, Journal of Mixed Methods Research 8(3):222–233, 2014.

Condon L, Bedford H, Ireland H, Kerr S, Mytton J, Richardson Z, Jackson C: Engaging Gypsy, Roma, and Traveller communities in research: maximizing opportunities and overcoming challenges, Qualitative Health Research 29(9):1324–1333, 2019.

Congress of Aboriginal and Torres Strait Islander Nurses and Midwives (CATSINaM): Position statement: embedding cultural safety across Australian nursing and midwifery, 2017. https://catsinam.org.au/2021/01/catsinam-cultural-safety publications/.

Cormack D, Stanley J, Harris R: Multiple forms of discrimination and relationships with health and wellbeing: findings from national cross-sectional surveys in Aotearoa/New Zealand, International Journal for Equity in Health 17(26):1–15, 2018.

Council for International Organizations of Medical Sciences (CIOMS): International ethical guidelines for health-related research involving humans, 2016. https://cioms.ch/wp-content/uploads/2017/01/WEB-CIOMS-EthicalGuidelines.pdf.

Cox LG, Taua C, Drummond A, et al: Enabling cultural safety. In Crisp J, Douglas C, Rebeiro G, Waters D (eds): Potter and Perry's Fundamentals of nursing. 6th ed. Chatswood: Elsevier; 2020, pp. 49–83.

Crenshaw K: Mapping the margins: intersectionality, identity politics, and violence against women of color, Stanford Law Review 43(6):1241–1299, 1991.

Denzin NK, Lincoln YS, Smith LT: Handbook of critical and Indigenous methodologies, Thousand Oaks, 2008, SAGE.

Denzin NK, Lincoln YS: The practices and politics of interpretation, Thousand Oaks, 2000, SAGE.

Drummond A: Embodied Indigenous knowledges protecting and privileging Indigenous peoples' ways of knowing, being and doing in undergraduate nursing education, The Australian Journal of Indigenous Education 49:127–134, 2020.

Drummond A, Mills Y, Mills S, et al: Torres Strait Islander health and wellbeing. In Best O, Fredericks B, editors. Yatdjuligin, Aboriginal and Torres Strait Islander Nursing & Midwifery Care. 3rd ed. Cambridge: Cambridge University Press; 2021, pp. 81–103.

Ehrlich C, Kendall E, Parekh S, et al: The impact of culturally responsive self-management interventions on health outcomes for minority populations: a systematic review, Chronic Illness 12(1):41–57, 2016.

Ermine W, Sinclair R, Jeffery B, et al: The ethics of research involving Indigenous peoples, Saskatoon, 2004, Indigenous People's Research Centre.

Flicker S, Worthington CA: Public health research involving Aboriginal peoples: research ethics board stakeholders' reflections on ethics principles and research processes, Canadian Journal of Public Health 103(1):19–22, 2012.

Furness J, Nikora LW, Hodgetts D, et al: Beyond ethics to morality: choices and relationships in bicultural research settings, Journal of Community & Applied Social Psychology 26(1):75–88, 2016.

Garcia R, Melgar P, Sorde TW, et al: From refusal to getting involved in Romani research. In Mertens DM, Cram F, Chilisa B (eds), Indigenous pathways into social research: voices of a new generation, Walnut Creek, 2013, Left Coast Press, pp. 367–380.

Gifford H, Wilson D, Boulton A, et al: Māori nurses and smoking: what do we know?, New Zealand Medical Journal 126(1384): 53–63, 2013.

Goodman A, Fleming K, Markwick N, et al: 'They treated me like crap and I know it was because I was Native': the healthcare experiences of Aboriginal peoples living in Vancouver's inner city, Social Science & Medicine Apr;178:87–94, 2017.

Graham J: He āpiti hono, he tātai hono: that which is joined remains an unbroken line: using whakapapa (genealogy) as the basis for an Indigenous research framework, The Australian Journal of Indigenous Education 34:86–95, 2005.

Greenfields M, Home R: Assessing Gypsies' and Travellers' needs: partnership working and 'The Cambridge Project', Romani Studies 16(2):102–131, 2006.

Grieves V: Aboriginal spirituality: Aboriginal philosophy, the basis of Aboriginal social and emotional wellbeing, Darwin, 2009, Cooperative Research Centre for Aboriginal Health.

Hart MA: Indigenous worldviews, knowledge, and research: the development of an Indigenous research paradigm, Journal of Indigenous Voices in Social Work 1(1):1–16, 2010.

Harvey M: Caring for Saibai Island stories: conducting research and creating a performative story in an ethical and culturally appropriate way. [Dissertation thesis on the Internet] Monash University, 2020, p. 113. https://bridges.monash.edu/articles/thesis/Caring_for_Saibai_Island_Stories_conducting_research_and_creating_a_performative_story_in_an_ethical_and_culturally_appropriate_way/12095580/1.

Health Research Council of New Zealand: Guidelines for researchers on health research involving Māori, 2010. https://www.hrc.govt.nz/resources/guidelines-researchers-health-research-involving-maori.

Heaslip V, Hean S, Parker J: Lived experience of vulnerability from a Gypsy Roma Traveller perspective, Journal of Clinical Nursing 25(13–14):1987–1998, 2016a.

Heaslip V, Hean S, Parker J: The etemic model of Gypsy Roma Traveller community vulnerability: is it time to rethink our understanding of vulnerability? Journal of Clinical Nursing 27 (17–18):3426–3435, 2016b. doi:10.1111/jocn.13499.

Heaslip V, Smith S: Working with people from diverse cultures: cultural competence, a knowledge domain, or way of being?, International Journal of Therapy & Rehabilitation 23(11):553–554, 2016.

Heaslip V, Vanceulebroeck V, Kalkan I, et al: Student nurse perceptions of Gypsy Roma Travellers: a European qualitative study. Nurse Education Today Nov;(82):1–7, 2019.

Heaslip V, Wilson D, Jackson D: Gypsy Roma Travellers: an indigenous population? Public Health Nov;176:43–49, 2019a. https://doi.org/10.1016/j.puhe.2019.02.020.

Hudson M, Milne M, Reynolds P, et al: Te Ara Tika Guidelines for Māori research ethics: a framework for researchers and ethics committee members, Auckland, 2010, Health Research Council of New Zealand. https://www.hrc.govt.nz/resources/te-ara-tika-guidelines-maori-research-ethics-0.

Hume L: Ancestral power: the Dreaming, consciousness and Aboriginal Australians, Melbourne, 2002, Melbourne University Press.

Kotz J, Munns A, Marriott R, et al: Perinatal depression and screening among Aboriginal Australians in the Kimberley, Contemporary Nurse 52(1):42–58, 2016.

Kovach M: Indigenous methodologies: characteristics, conversations, and contexts, Toronto, 2009, University of Toronto Press.

Kukutai T, Cormack D: Mana motuhake ā-raraunga: datification and social science research in Aotearoa, Kotuitui: New Zealand Journal of Social Sciences 14(2):201–208, 2019

Ladson-Billings G: Racialized discourses and ethnic epistemologies, ed 2, Thousand Oaks, 2000, SAGE.

Makowharemahihi C, Lawton BA, Cram F, et al: Initiation of maternity care for young Māori women under 20 years of age, New Zealand Medical Journal 127(1393):52–61, 2014.

Martin KL: Please knock before you enter, Aboriginal regulation of outsiders and the implications for researchers. Teneriffe (Qld), 2008, Post Pressed.

Mbuzi V, Fulbrook P, Jessup M: Indigenous peoples' experiences and perceptions of hospitalisation for acute care: a metasynthesis of qualitative studies, International Journal of Nursing Studies Jun;71:39–49, 2017.

McDonald MI, Lawson KD: Doing it hard in the bush: aligning what gets measured with what matters, Australian Journal of Rural Health 25(4):246–251, 2017.

McFadden A, Siebelt L, Gavine A, et al: Gypsy, Roma and Traveller access to and engagement with health services: a systematic review, European Journal of Public Health 28(1):74–81, 2018.

Mead HM: Tikanga Māori: living by Māori values, Wellington, 2016, Huia.

Midwifery Council of New Zealand: Statement on cultural competence for midwives, 2011. https://www.midwiferycouncil.health.nz/common/Uploaded%20files/Registration/Statement%20on%20Cultural%20Competence.pdf.

Mikaere A: The balanced destroyed, Otaki, 2017, Te Wānanga o Raukawa.

Miller K: Respectful listening and reflective communication from the heart and with the spirit, Qualitative Social Work 13(6):828–841, 2014.

Moreton-Robinson A: The white possessive: Property, power and Indigenous sovereignty. Minneapolis, 2015, University of Minnesota Press. pp. 19–20.

Moreton-Robinson A: Towards an Australian Indigenous Women's standpoint theory, Australian Feminist Studies 28(78): 331–347, 2013.

Nakata M: Disciplining the savages, savaging the disciplines. Canberra, 2007, Aboriginal Studies Press, p. 247.

National Health & Medical Research Council (NHMRC): Australian Code for responsible conduct of research, Canberra, 2018a, Commonwealth of Australia. https://nhmrc.gov.au/about-us/publications/australian-code-responsible-conduct-research-2018.

National Health & Medical Research Council (NHMRC): Keeping research on track II: a companion document to ethical conduct in research with Aboriginal and Torres Strait Islander peoples and communities: guidelines for researchers and stakeholders. Canberra, 2018b, Commonwealth of Australia. https://www.nhmrc.gov.au/about-us/resources/keeping-research-track-ii.

Nesdole R, Voigts D, Lepnurm R, et al: Reconceptualizing determinants of health: barriers to improving the health status of First Nations peoples, Canadian Journal of Public Health 105(3):e209–e213, 2014.

Nursing and Midwifery Board of Australia: NMBA and CATSINaM joint statement on culturally safe care, Melbourne, 2018, Nursing and Midwifery Board of Australia. https://www.nursingmidwiferyboard.gov.au/codes-guidelines-statements/position-statements/joint-statement-on-culturally-safe-care.aspx.

Nursing and Midwifery Council: The Code. 2018. https://www. nmc.org.uk/globalassets/sitedocuments/nmc-publications/nmc-code.pdf.

Nursing Council of New Zealand: Guidelines for cultural safety, the Treaty of Waitangi, and Māori health in nursing education and practice. 2011. https://www.nursingcouncil.org.nz/Public/ Nursing/Standards_and_guidelines/NCNZ/nursing-section/ Standards_and_guidelines_for_nurses.aspx.

Pawu-kurlpurlurnu WJ, Holmes M, Box LA: Ngurra-kurlu: a way of working with Warlpiri people. Alice Springs, 2008, Desert Knowledge CRC.

Penehira M, Green A, Smith LT, et al: Māori and Indigenous views on R and R, MAI Journal 3(2):96–110, 2014.

Penney L, Barnes HMB, McCreanor T: The blame game: constructions of Māori medical compliance, AlterNative: An International Journal of Indigenous Peoples 7(2):73–86, 2011.

Razani J, Burciaga J, Madore M, et al: Effects of acculturation on tests of attention and information processing in an ethnically diverse group, Archives of Clinical Neuropsychology 22(3):333–341, 2007.

Riddell JK, Salamanca A, Pepler DJ, et al: Laying the groundwork: a practical guide for ethical research with Indigenous communities, Internal Indigenous Policy Journal 8(2):1–20, 2017.

Royal TAC: The woven universe: selected writings of Rev. Otaki, 2003, Māori Marsden. Te Wānanga o Raukawa.

Sherwood J: Do no harm: decolonising Aboriginal health research, Sydney, 2010, School of Social Work. University of New South Wales.

Simmonds N: Mana wahine: decolonising politics, Women's Studies Journal 25(2):11–25, 2011.

Smallacombe S, Davis M, Quiggin R: Desert knowledge: scoping project on Aboriginal traditional knowledge, Northern Territory, 2007, Desert Knowledge CRC.

Smith LT: Decolonizing methodologies: research and Indigenous peoples, Dunedin, 1999, University of Otago Press.

Smith LT: Decolonizing methodologies: research and Indigenous peoples, ed 2, London, 2012, Zed Books.

Stanner WEH: White man got no Dreaming: essays 1938–1973, Canberra, 1979, Australian National University Press.

Thurber KA, Walker J, Batterham PJ, et al: Developing and validating measures of self-reported everyday and healthcare discrimination for Aboriginal and Torres Strait Islander adults, International Journal for Equity in Health 20(14).1–10, 2021. http://doi.org/10.1186/s12939-020-01351-9.

Tipa Z: Mahi ngātahi: Culturally responsive ways of working with whānau accessing Well Child/Tamariki Ora services. [Doctoral thesis] Auckland University of Technology, 2020. https://openrepository.aut.ac.nz/handle/10292/14007.

United Nations: Declaration on the rights of Indigenous peoples. 2008. https://www.un.org/development/desa/Indigenouspeoples/declaration-on-the-rights-of-Indigenous-peoples.html.

United Nations: Indigenous peoples and the United Nations human rights system: fact sheet No. 9/Rev. 2, New York and Geneva, 2013, United Nations.

United Nations Economic and Social Council: Geneva Declaration on the health and survival of Indigenous peoples, New York, 2002, United Nations. https://dialoguebetweennations.com/N2N/PFII/English/HealthAnnex1.htm.

Varcoe C, Browne AJ, Ford-Gilboe M, et al: Reclaiming our spirits: development and pilot testing of a health promotion intervention for Indigenous women who have experienced intimate partner violence, Research in Nursing & Health 40:237–254, 2017.

Walter M, Suina M: Indigenous data, Indigenous methodologies and Indigenous data sovereignty, International Journal of Social Research Methodology 22(3):233–243, 2019.

Watego C, Whop LJ, Singh D, et al: Black to the future: Making a case for Indigenist Health Humanities, International Journal of Environmental Research and Public Health 18(16):1–10, 2021. http://doi.org/10.3390/ijerph18168704.

Wilkerson I: Caste! The origins of our discontent, New York, 2020, Random House.

Wilson D, Barton P: Indigenous hospital experiences: a New Zealand case study, Journal of Clinical Nursing 21(15–16):2316–2326, 2012.

Wilson D: Culturally safe research with vulnerable populations (Māori). In Liamputtong P (ed), Handbook of research methods in health social sciences, Singapore, 2017, Springer Singapore, pp. 1–19.

Wilson D, Haretuku R: Te Tiriti o Waitangi/Treaty of Waitangi 1840: its influence on health practice. In Wepa D (ed), Cultural safety in Aotearoa New Zealand, Melbourne, 2015, Cambridge University Press, pp. 79–99.

Wilson D, Heaslip V, Jackson D: Improving equity and cultural responsiveness with marginalised communities, Journal of Clinical Nursing 27(19–20):3810–3819, 2018.

Wilson D, Hickey H: Māori health: Māori- and whānau-centred practice. In Wepa D (ed), Cultural safety in Aotearoa New Zealand, Melbourne, 2015, Cambridge University Press, pp. 235–251.

Wilson D, Mikahere-Hall A, Sherwood J, et al: E Tū Wāhine, E Tū Whānau: Wāhine Māori keeping safe in unsafe relationships, 2019, AUT Taupua Waiora Māori Research Centre. https://open-repository.aut.ac.nz/handle/10292/13068.

Wilson D, Mikahere-Hall A, Sherwood J: Using Indigenous kaupapa Māori research methodology with constructivist grounded theory: generating a theoretical explanation of Indigenous women's realities, International Journal of Social Research Methodology 25(3):1–16, 2021. http://doi.org/10.1080/13645579.2021.1897756.

Wilson D, Neville S: Culturally safe research with vulnerable populations, Contemporary Nurse 33(1):69–79, 2009.

Wilson S: Research is ceremony: Indigenous research methods, Nova Scotia, 2008, Fernwood.

Wilson D: The significance of a culturally appropriate health service for Indigenous Māori women, Contemporary Nurse 28 (1–2):173–188, 2008.

World Health Organization: Health of Indigenous peoples, Geneva, 2007, World Health Organization. https://www.who.int/mediacentre/factsheets/fs326/en/.

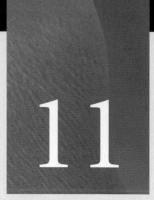

11

DIVERSITY AND INCLUSION IN RESEARCH

CALVIN MOORLEY ■ RUTH NORTHWAY ■ RUTH OSHIKANLU

LEARNING OBJECTIVES

After reading this chapter and following critical reflection, readers should be able to:

- discuss the meanings of equity, diversity and inclusion
- understand the impact of exclusion from the research process
- identify ways of increasing inclusion in research
- apply a social justice lens to research participants, researchers and research.

KEY TERMS

co-production

diversity

equity

inclusion

inclusive research

justice

reflexivity

stereotypes

vulnerability

ABSTRACT

If ignored, lack of equity, diversity and inclusion (EDI) can lead to bias in research and to research which is unjust since it marginalises and excludes the experiences and views of key groups. This chapter takes the reader on a journey that identifies EDI issues that every student should be cognisant of when reading, appraising, planning or undertaking research. It focuses on the key domains of diversity, equity and inclusion, and provides examples and discussions of how these can be incorporated into any research project. The chapter focuses on exclusion from research and drivers for inclusive practice, including intersectionality and how to develop a trusting relationship in research. Furthermore, readers are introduced to applying a social justice lens to research.

STUDENT QUOTE

I think too often equity, diversity and inclusion (EDI) focuses on the research sample OR those conducting the research, when equal attention on both sides simultaneously is what's important. Proper EDI should permeate the whole research process for more valid, reliable and unbiased results. (Mental Health student nurse, UK)

INTRODUCTION

As stated in earlier chapters of this book, research is pivotal to informing the care that nurses and midwives provide to patients/clients and the wider community. It can help to make decisions on treatment for best possible outcomes, provide rationale for treatment protocols and guide future research. This chapter explores four main areas that impact good and ethical research practices: 1. diversity, equity and inclusion; 2. exclusion from research; 3. drivers for inclusive research; and 4. promoting inclusion. The chapter starts with a case study, which sets the scene for imagining what a diverse community may look like. The chapter uses challenge activities to help the reader to critically explore diversity and inclusivity in research.

CASE STUDY 11.1

Saint Peter's Street is situated on the edge of the City of London. It is a lively street with a corner pub opposite the Seacole Estate (a welfare housing development) where the residents socialise. There is a small greengrocer's shop on the estate and a general practice. There is a large park 5 minutes' walk away, a church and a mosque all within walking distance. The Seacole Estate is made up of six buildings, including a 20-floor tower block, apartments and terrace houses. On the same street are private houses and apartment blocks. There is a shared community space used for social activities, including a community garden project. The community is a mixture of people from different backgrounds. The residents look out for each other through the neighbourhood watch group, collect each other's mail and assist each other through citizenship.

MEANINGS OF EQUITY, DIVERSITY AND INCLUSION (EDI)

In this section, we will explore and discuss the meaning of equity, diversity and inclusion (EDI). We examine how diversity in research is recognised, respected and celebrated. The section ends with a discussion on intersectionality as a critical guide to inclusive research practice.

STUDENT QUOTE

For me, EDI in research represents the thoughts, views and experiences of a diverse population.

STUDENT CHALLENGE

Considering Diversity

1. Based on the case study scenario of Saint Peter's Street, can you think of the diverse groups that may exist on the street?
2. Now that you have identified these groups, can you think of any health inequities that may exist in the community?

Diversity

Diversity is usually accompanied by the terms 'equity' and 'inclusion', and you will learn more about these as you continue to read this chapter. For research contexts, if you are embracing diversity as a researcher, this means you should be inclusive and equitable in your practice.

Diversity is a term that has been mainstreamed into research as a standard practice for researchers and they should be mindful not to trivialise this concept. **Diversity** can be defined as ensuring we recognise, respect, value and celebrate the differences between individuals. In research, diversity is ensuring we capitalise on the differences that each person brings to the work we do. This includes researchers, participants and geographic locations. Diversity is a complex yet simple concept. The characteristics of individuals and populations contribute to diversity and include personal and social aspects (Fuentes, Zelaya & Madsen 2021). Some examples are race, gender, age, sexual orientation, disability, religious beliefs and practices, languages, socioeconomic status and includes people from various groups such as migrant, disabled, ethnic minority, asylum seeker, refugee, Indigenous peoples and single parents. Importantly, when you read research, you may see some of these characteristics as variables or used to describe the participants. When reading research, you should always try and identify the extent of diversity within the participants.

When exclusion of diverse groups takes place, discrimination occurs. This can also happen in research, meaning that research findings only have limited use. International events have led to a greater awareness of diversity in research. For example, the killing of Black American George Floyd in 2020 has led to discussions and actions of how Black people are treated and discriminated against in society. It raises the awareness that people from minority groups may also face discrimination as research participants and researchers. They may also be misrepresented in research findings. Exclusion can take many forms and can include the following:

- (mis)treatment of gay men and women in some countries
- non-recognition of transgender people
- ghettoisation of people based on gender identity or sexuality
- use of religion to deny human rights to people who identify as gender diverse
- struggle for gender equality and recognition of women

- discriminatory treatment of people living with mental illness, physical and intellectual disabilities.

The effects of some of this exclusion is evidence in the health disparities that emerged during the COVID-19 pandemic.

Equity

Equity focuses on overcoming the challenges and obstacles that detract from ensuring **justice** and fairness. As a researcher, a key skill is to be able to recognise the unique attributes that members of your research team and participants bring to the study. More importantly, you need to possess the knowledge and/or identify the resources that will be needed to ensure fairness in all stages of the research process. This involves the researcher changing their gaze towards structural and social determinants and processes that leads to inequities in health research, and not be limited to the traditional and dominant frames (e.g. biomedical and behavioural models) in which health is perceived, defined and operationalised. It also requires that we rethink what might be viewed as 'traditional' approaches to how we do research.

Inclusion

Promoting and planning for **inclusion** needs to be undertaken from the very beginning of the research process. We live in a world of systematic exclusion, which provides a challenge for inclusive research. Inclusion is not as simple as it sounds; it is not merely including individuals and groups with different characteristics. When undertaking, reviewing or reading research, you will need to develop your thinking and practice to ensure inclusion covers creating and or changing the organisational and environmental culture that would allow your research team members and participants (from diverse backgrounds) to inhabit and thrive. **Inclusive research** practices should give all involved a sense of belonging and the ability to function as required. Inclusive research practice should align with your research protocol and those involved should feel a sense of belonging and identify the relevance of the research (Mitchell et al 2020). Including people in research is a decision and process that involves reflection on the systems of privilege that exist. For the researcher, it implies a capacity, ability and willingness to examine how they can mitigate power imbalances that are deeply rooted in the histories of inequity based on enslavement, colonisation, class, race, gender and wealth. Sometimes we can include researchers from other disciplines who may be instrumental in helping to answer complex research questions. It is worth remembering that interdisciplinary collaborations can help build on the inclusive and diverse research practices that each discipline applies to answering a research question. Nursing and midwifery researchers must recognise how discipline heterogeneity in research teams can impact achieving diversity in research.

WHY DIVERSITY AND INCLUSION IN RESEARCH?

The people we research (sample/participants) and those who constitute our research teams (researchers) are the people who make up our society. They belong to social groups that are diverse, with their own unique and identifying characteristics, which are personal, cultural and religious beliefs and customs. These customs and practices are important to individuals and impact their health and wellbeing, in terms of how they view and access health, social care and healthcare systems, and how they are viewed by healthcare providers. People with learning and physical disabilities, sexual and gender minority groups, different ethnicities and those from lower socioeconomic status can be marginalised within both society and research. Importantly, diversity is multilayered and multifaceted. For example, an individual can belong to a lower socioeconomic group, identify as Black and non-binary and have a physical disability. Therefore, health and social care researchers need to take an intersectional approach. The individual should be viewed as a unique whole, where different characteristics and identifying factors contribute to them as a person. This leads to inclusive person-centred research.

Most regulatory bodies, associations and councils, through their code or principles of practice, have mandated nurses and midwives as advocates and agents of change. Nurses and midwives are seen to be professionals who can mobilise interdisciplinary healthcare teams to improve the health and outcomes for those who are unable to speak or act for themselves. Therefore, diversity and inclusion, through a social justice

approach, in nursing and midwifery research can help give a voice to the voiceless, and empower individuals, families and communities from a capacity and strengths perspective.

In this chapter, we approach diversity and inclusion as tenets for research and explore them through a social justice lens. Social justice in nursing and midwifery is about balancing the benefits and burdens experienced by citizens aiming for a just society (American Association of Colleges of Nursing 2017). It is to do with using social criticism and social change towards an end goal for 'more equitable distribution of social and economic benefits and burdens, greater personal, social, and political dignity; and a deeper moral vision for society' (American Nurses Association 2015, p. 5). In essence, social justice in nursing and midwifery research should 'advocate for understanding causes of inequities and taking responsible action to eliminate inequities' (Canadian Nurses Association 2010, p. 10).

EXCLUSION FROM RESEARCH

Some groups of people are at particular risk of being excluded from health and social care research despite having specific and additional needs. For example, a review of 300 randomly selected clinical trials identified that only 2% included people with intellectual disabilities (Feldman et al 2014). Another systematic review found that almost 27% of the trials reviewed had an upper age limit stated as an exclusion criterion, thus excluding older people from participation (Thake & Lowry 2017). No explanations for these exclusions were given by the authors of the papers reviewed.

The reasons for such exclusion are many and varied. Some are conscious (such as setting an upper age limit for participation) while others occur due to factors such as prejudice, a lack of awareness or a lack of accessibility. Even where conscious actions lead to exclusion, these can be founded on misunderstandings. For example, certain groups (such as those with intellectual disabilities and those living with mental health issues) are often viewed as being 'vulnerable' in the context of research. Such a belief is not unfounded given history reveals examples of such groups of people being exploited, coerced and harmed in the context of research (for more on this see Chapter 6). One response to such perceptions of **vulnerability** is then to exclude all those who are considered to belong to that group from participation in future research. However, considering entire groups of people as 'vulnerable' ignores the diversity of individuals to whom the group label is applied. It also fails to question what it is that they may be vulnerable to and whether this can be removed or any potential harm reduced.

A commonly cited reason for exclusion from studies is a lack of capacity to consent to participation. It is essential that valid and informed consent is obtained wherever possible and that individuals are not coerced into participating in research against their will. However, it is sometimes the case that researchers assume that (for example) all those who are considered to have an intellectual disability or dementia will lack the capacity to provide consent or that it would be too difficult to obtain informed consent. Such a position ignores the fact that the terms 'intellectual disability' and 'dementia' are applied to groups of people with very diverse strengths and needs. Many in either of these groups will be able to provide valid informed consent, and adaptations could easily be made to the way study information is provided to support and extend this capacity. Of course, the way study information is provided does not just impact people with intellectual disabilities or dementia. Others may be excluded by a failure to provide information in different languages, formats (e.g. braille) or culturally acceptable ways.

Perceptions of capacity can, however, also extend beyond capacity to consent and some groups of people are at risk of being excluded from participation in research due to prejudiced views regarding the value of their knowledge and their potential to meaningfully contribute. People with intellectual disabilities have been stereotyped as being unable to contribute to research and so are not invited to participate. They do not then get the opportunity to participate and therefore have no experience of research, meaning that they may find participation difficult. Such **stereotypes** may also be internalised, as members of these groups do not see themselves represented in research, feel that research is therefore not for them, do not participate and thus lose the opportunity to gain experience and to challenge misperceptions (Barden 2021). Stereotypes can continue to perpetuate exclusion, creating a continuing cycle of exclusion.

Other reasons for exclusion can include a failure on the part of researchers to consider diversity at the stage of study design. Increasingly online data collection methods are being used which may enhance the participation of some groups but exclude those who lack digital access or skills. Similarly, a focus group may provide an opportunity to bring together people with diverse views, but its timing may preclude participation by those who work, its location could exclude those without transport, and the level of commitment may mean that those with caring responsibilities are unable to take part. Exclusion can also occur at the stage of study recruitment if researchers fail to recognise the need to reach out to different groups in different ways: people may be excluded simply because they do not know that there is an opportunity to participate. The effects of exclusion from research can also be far-reaching and are perhaps best considered in terms of exploring the factors that make clear the case for a more inclusive approach at all stages of the research process.

STUDENT QUOTE

For me, EDI in research means equitable representation, but acknowledging limitations until it/we reach the representative target audience better. It also means more evidence-based practice, especially to enable closing the health inequalities gap.

STUDENT CHALLENGE

Barriers to Participation in Research

Take some time to reflect on the Seacole Estate case study presented at the beginning of the chapter. Think about the diversity of residents that are likely to reside on the Seacole Estate. What factors may impact their inclusion in research? What barriers to participation might they experience?

INTERSECTIONALITY IN RESEARCH

EDI are not unilateral dimensions of research. Rather, they are a thread woven throughout the research process from design to final write-up, dissemination and translation and implementation of findings.

Researchers should be able to recognise that individuals possess multiple characteristics that are pivotal to shaping who they are and their experience in society and that together these impact how they access healthcare as well as how healthcare is offered and delivered to them. Taking an intersectional approach to your research can make your study more robust, inclusive, diverse and ethically sound.

Intersectionality is a concept that allows us to consider how a variety of socially constructed dimensions come together or intersect while contributing to shaping an individual's life (see Chapter 10 for more on intersectionality). An individual's life comprises their experiences, actions and meanings. Taking an intersectional approach to our research allows recognition of multiple dimensions such as race, ethnicity, gender, sexual orientation, religion, disability, class, socioeconomic status, geographical location and physical characteristics such as weight, height, physical disability and/or distinguishing marks. These dimensions can contribute to oppression or advantage concerning healthcare. Cole (2009) describes intersectionality as an approach in research that aims to help understand the lived experience through the lens of multiple intersecting dimensions. Intersectionality can also be extended and applied to how researchers view the phenomena under investigation; for example, using a multiple lens or multidimensional approach such as individual, community and organisational approaches. Intersectionality can help to better understand the role that oppression and inequality plays in the role that oppression and inequity play in the health of individuals, groups and communities. Intersectional research can present challenges in data collection and analysis; however, its conclusions are much more inclusive and contextual.

Intersectional methodology allows research participants to self-identify as intersectional. Although the research may be focused on a topic such as health access, an intersectional approach will also allow consideration of factors such as gender, ethnicity and disability status. This approach can promote more-inclusive and more-reflexive practice. It can also allow researchers to model inclusion, privilege voices that are silent or remain unheard and allow for all consideration of the intersection of all identities leading to a more inclusive rather than a unidimensional approach.

It can lead to changing researchers' mindsets to become linguistically and culturally skilled, where researchers recognise the heterogeneity of the intersecting identities. Intersectionality can create and build links to social networks that address barriers to inclusive research. Intersectionality in research can lead to the creation of decolonised knowledge, as data analysis takes contextual and critical approaches that can help to empower disadvantaged groups. By taking an intersectional approach, researchers can co-produce the research and its findings, leading to greater accountability and symbiotic learning.

CASE STUDY 11.2

When undertaking a literature review as part of their research project, Jamie has initially found only limited evidence relating specifically to type 1 diabetes among people with learning disabilities. Jamie has, therefore, looked more broadly at the wider evidence regarding management of type 1 diabetes to consider how this might inform the care of the young woman who is the focus of the case study. However, when reviewing this literature, Jamie notices that in several studies people with learning disabilities have been excluded from participation. Jamie reflects on why this might be the case and how the research might have been undertaken differently to facilitate their participation.

DRIVERS FOR A MORE INCLUSIVE APPROACH

Reflecting on this case study can help you to understand how research can become more inclusive. Research is concerned with the creation of knowledge. If we deny the capacity of individuals to contribute knowledge then we are wronging them at a very fundamental level of their humanity (Jones et al 2021). There is a compelling ethical reason for making research as inclusive as possible since to do otherwise is to contribute to injustice and results in findings that are of limited use. Participants in nursing and midwifery research often are not representative of the populations for which interventions are needed, preventing research findings from being robust and transferable. Certain groups are deemed 'hard to reach' and are excluded from the research.

NIHR-INCLUDE is a project funded by the National Institute for Health Research (NIHR) in the United Kingdom (UK) that seeks to promote the inclusion of underserved groups in research (https://www.nihr.ac.uk/documents/improving-inclusion-of-under-served-groups-in-clinical-research-guidance-from-include-project/25435) and identifies several groups at risk of being underserved or excluded from research. These include those excluded due to demographic, socioeconomic, health or disease-specific factors. They also identify the consequences of failing to adopt an inclusive approach. This may include the fact that research findings may not be generalisable to those groups and that a failure to test an intervention with a particular group may mean it is not feasible in practice due to logistical, cultural, psychological and biological factors. They suggest that if an intervention has not been tested on a specific patient group, then clinicians may be reluctant to prescribe its use for that population, potentially meaning that they are denied access to beneficial treatments.

Many of the groups identified as being at risk of exclusion from research are also those who experience health disparities. For example, Milner and Frawley (2019) describe the shifting mindsets of people with disabilities from research focusing 'on' them to research 'with' as research with disabled people is often absent from mainstream healthcare research. Similarly, Pugh and colleagues (2021) argue that despite efforts to reverse the situation, Black and minority ethnic populations in the United States continue to experience a lack of representation in research.

This issue has been brought into sharp focus in the context of the COVID-19 pandemic. During the pandemic, many of the groups at increased risk of infection and its effects have been those commonly excluded from research, such as those from Black and minority ethnic communities, disabled people and those living in care homes (Witham et al 2020). Witham and colleagues (2020) argue that inclusive COVID-19 research is a necessity and calls for the inclusion of groups often excluded at all stages of the research process. They also suggest that healthcare researchers need to have prepared platforms and study designs, networks and identify key questions before the next pandemic to help ensure inclusive research. Treweek and colleagues (2021) developed the INCLUDE Ethnicity Framework to guide researchers on ethnicity. Crowell and colleagues (2021) suggest the development of training programs to sensitise healthcare providers on transgender research, capacity-building programs for socio-behavioural researchers and administrative support programs to build capacities of community-based organisations representing transgender people.

PROMOTING INCLUSION

In this section, inclusion in research and the way to promote it will be discussed. Areas that are covered include developing a trusting relationship, recognising and addressing power imbalances and how to take an inclusive approach to the research process.

Developing a trusting relationship

Trust is the basis for any successful research and is considered essential in the researcher/participant relationship. It is important because it allows open and transparent communication between both parties, thus eliminating the biases and misconceptions that can lead to a relationship breakdown resulting in poor research outcomes. Two cases that populate mistrust among oppressed populations are the Tuskegee syphilis study (Brandt 1978) and the use of Henrietta Lacks (Editorial 2020) cell line. You can read about these using the links provided in the Additional resources at the end of the chapter.

Trust is a key ingredient for a successful research relationship, both within teams and with participants. Trust is the intrapersonal relationship between the researcher and the participant. It is where each expects the other to act respectfully, which should be guided by ethical principles such as beneficence, nonmaleficence, justice, candour and veracity (Doody & Noonan 2016). Fernandez and colleagues (2021) explain that trust and relationship-building are messy and may differ according to researchers' own identity and standpoint. They highlight that research processes are a series of deliberate judgments with consequences that affect the wellbeing of communities with whom we engage. If done well, strategies such as using a patient and public involvement model can help the development of inclusive and trusting relationships.

Based on the student challenges earlier in this chapter (Barriers to participation in research and Recognising hard-to-reach groups) let's explore how you can develop a trusting research relationship with the residents of Seacole Estate. You may want to start with how your research is conceived and designed. Researchers may find themselves acting in isolation and make decisions on what is needed for a group (such as the Seacole residents) based on the information they have acquired from desktop research. Or, if they undertake primary research, they focus on participants who are viewed as 'easy to reach' or who readily engage. We propose that to build a trusting relationship, researchers should include participants from the outset of the research design.

Researchers and participants working in partnership to decide on the topic, the project, its design and the desired outcomes is an essential building block in the trusting relationship. A good starting point will be to use any previously established relationships with the Seacole residents (e.g. with community groups and key individuals within them), as often groups and communities may otherwise be closed to researchers.

The existence of power differentials can contribute to complexity when undertaking research. Researchers must recognise that they may hold more power than research participants and should take a proactive approach towards addressing these. Even where they seek to work in ways that share such power, they may still be perceived by others as being more powerful. Some of the power differentials between researchers and participants can be influenced by policies and procedures, budget constraints, organisational position, researcher privileges and the fact that individuals have varying levels of 'agency' or individual power and authority. These can also be shaped by the fact that community members may not have previous experience of engaging in research and it is important to stress that what they will bring to the research is their expertise and experience concerning their situation and priorities.

Humility is required to ensure that research is designed with participants in mind. A gold-standard practice is to include patient and public involvement in the design and development of your research. Jackson and Moorley (2022) explain that the phrase 'nothing about us without us' captures the idea that services and policymakers involve the engagement and participation of members of communities and groups whose voice is not always represented. This is also applicable to those undertaking research, as this approach can provide specialist feedback from disability advocates, special interest groups (e.g. environmental health), LGBTQIA+ groups and those that are minoritised or at risk of being marginalised in society.

Researchers must ensure their projects are undertaken in a culturally safe way, recognising and respecting the spiritual and cultural identities of participants, and ensuring that their needs and voice take a dominant role. This may require undertaking a process of decolonisation, learning and acknowledging the role that colonisation and history may have impacted some participants and their lives. Studies examining workplace cultures, cultural safety or interprofessional research should include knowledge about the history of the community and individuals being researched, the researchers and the system in which the researchers work. Researchers should also examine the impact it has had on those being researched; this may help researchers act with cultural sensitivity and use cultural competence (for more on cultural competence see Chapter 10).

Participants should be treated equitably regardless of their cultural differences, and every effort should be made to ensure that the researcher's actions do not demean, diminish or disempower others. Increasing PPI can lead to **co-production**, which is a collaborative model that shares the power researchers hold with stakeholders, policymakers and anyone who falls into the PPI category. Together they co-produce the research, from developing the agenda, to designing the study, to carrying it out and then interpreting, disseminating and implementing the findings. The co-production model is applicable across the health and social care sector and researchers should apply reflexivity to achieve the best possible outcome.

Reflexivity differs from being reflective. All researchers reflect and make judgments about their data and draw conclusions. Reflexivity goes further and examines the individual making the judgments. It is a measure of how much a researcher admits influence over a study (von Unger 2021). Researchers cannot reduce biases about which they are unaware. Therefore, they must examine their assumptions, practices and beliefs throughout the research process. The objective is to identify personal beliefs that may introduce bias into any research. By implementing reflexive practice, the researcher can better inspect the integrity of the decisions made, transparency and authenticity, thereby adding rigour to the study. When working with and carrying out research with diverse participants, researchers should employ a reflexive approach while maintaining cultural safety.

STUDENT CHALLENGE

Research in Communities 2

Many of the residents living on Seacole Estate are Black and Asian. Health data shows that women from these backgrounds have poorer pregnancy outcomes, with increased morbidity. Several women from the estate have died in the perinatal period over the last 2 years. You have been asked to undertake some research to explore the reasons behind this phenomenon. How would you approach this project?

Black women are four times more likely than white women to die in pregnancy or childbirth. Women from Asian ethnic backgrounds face a twofold risk, and women living in the most deprived areas of the UK are almost three times more likely to die during childbirth than those in the most affluent areas. Stillbirth rates for Black and Black British babies were over twice those for white babies, while neonatal death rates were 45% higher. For babies of Asian and Asian British ethnicity, stillbirth and neonatal death rates were both around 60% higher than for babies of white ethnicity (Knight et al 2021).

Mothers and Babies: Reducing Risk through Audits and Confidential Enquiries across the UK (MBRRACE-UK) is a national audit program commissioned by all UK governments to collect information on all late fetal losses, stillbirths, neonatal deaths and maternal deaths across the UK. You can find a link to learn more about the MBRRACE-UK report in the Additional resources at the end of this chapter.

With these statistics in mind, the researcher should use cultural humility along with a reflexive approach. This involves the process of checking power imbalances, employing humility to develop and maintain mutually respectful and dynamic partnerships with communities. Regular critical self-reflection is also required to enable researchers to become self-aware and consider how their beliefs, values and actions influence interaction with participants (Foronda 2020).

Researchers should be mindful of cultural and community mores, especially if they hold a different ethnic background or different social and biological characteristics to the participants. The primary goal is to form a trusting relationship with participants while striving to understand their lived experiences. Once rapport has been established, continuous critical self-reflection will enable a better understanding of what benefits the participants may receive from the research project for it to be co-produced. For example, the female residents of Seacole Estate would want improved perinatal outcomes for themselves and their babies. Some of them may not have English as their first language and may require interpreters to facilitate communication. Others may have poor literacy skills and require support to understand the project to be fully included in it. Yet others may have had traumatic experiences during pregnancy and childbirth or heard of such experiences from family members which may further traumatise them. Researchers may require additional training such as trauma-informed care to recognise and respond to the signs, symptoms and risks of trauma to better support the health needs of participants who have experienced trauma. Recognising these aspects of research may require extra funding and additional time to enlist the support of counsellors and therapists during the research project. Many researchers maintain a reflective journal throughout the project to help aid a process of ongoing critical self-reflection.

RECOGNISING, RESPECTING AND CELEBRATING DIVERSITY, EQUITY AND INCLUSION IN RESEARCH

There is a wealth of research on/with diverse groups in health and social care and in other areas such as education. Studies in gender and disease—for example stroke and African women (Aradine et al 2021, Molokhia et al 2021); men's experience of traumatic brain injury (D'Souza 2019); South Asian people and diabetes (Davidson et al 2021); lesbian and transgender parenting (Malmquist & Nieminen 2021); children with intellectual disability and restrictive practices (Singh & Mckie 2021)—all provide insights into diversity in the context of health, illness and disability. Although these examples, and others, show the breadth of diverse research, often diversity in research goes unrecognised, and is not respected or celebrated.

Research is often viewed as an adjunct role to nursing or midwifery practice. It must be recognised that nursing and midwifery research make a vital contribution to the evidence base that improves care, treatment and the lives of healthcare recipients. Researchers need to be mindful that conducting and undertaking diverse and inclusive research is not just about promoting their careers. Most research regarding health and social care, education and workforce is concerned with improving the lives of patients, their families and their communities.

On an international level, the knowledge and evidence derived from research activities contribute to achieving aims of organisations such as the International Council of Nurses and the World Health Organization. Therefore, it is important to recognise the worth and contribution of research nurses and midwives and those who work in health and social care. Some health and social care workers apply a social justice lens to their research and have looked at areas such as poverty and socioeconomic status concerning health (e.g. Fliesher, Neumann & Curtis [2021] looking at poverty and school nurse poverty education). Research on poverty also helps to equip students to work with those impacted (Voth Schrag 2021).

All this research, no matter where it occurs or is undertaken, should have recognisable aspects of diversity. As outlined earlier in this chapter, anyone reading or reviewing your research should be able to recognise how an inclusive and diverse lens was applied and how the findings would be translated into practice to improve the health outcomes for the community. A lack of diversity and inclusion in any study can mean the work can have limited applicability.

Respecting diversity is a core value for researchers. When diversity in research is respected, it means that it is recognised and that researchers have considered the existing inequalities, the perspectives of diverse groups and how to work within systems of inequity. Researchers are expected to respect and acknowledge that all findings are not homogenous and to report findings in a manner that illuminates the diversity of the research participants representing the population they constitute. Below are some areas that demonstrate respecting diversity in research:

- respecting the role of language barriers and linguistics in applied research
- demonstrating respect through understanding and applying cultural competence
- respecting the position of research participants
- respecting that different genders are treated and experience the world differently
- recognising that adjustments may be required to the research process to enable the participation of key groups
- respecting that what may be important to one group may matter little to another group
- respecting that structural inequalities contribute to the experiences of individuals and communities
- respecting that other disciplines can bring diverse perspectives to any research

■ recognising and respecting gatekeepers in various communities and the importance of their role (this may include religious, cultural and community leaders).

STUDENT CHALLENGE

Reflections on Learning

After reading this chapter, can you list how you can recognise, respect and celebrate diversity in research?

BEYOND THE EDI STATEMENT— DEVELOPING DIVERSE, EQUITABLE AND INCLUSIVE RESEARCH PRAXIS

Some funders request an EDI statement and others do not require one. It is good practice to always provide an EDI statement as it can help to guide your research to areas of PPI and co-production. Once the grant has been awarded, the researcher or research team would need to move beyond the EDI statement and think critically about how they become diverse, equitable and inclusive researchers. Here are a few tips on actualising EDI research praxis.

■ How diverse is your team? Have you included researchers from a similar background to the phenomenon being investigated? For example, if you are doing a project on mental health among Black, Latino or Indigenous people, are any members of your research team from these groups? You may want to advertise for a research assistant in non-traditional places to ensure that you reach a population that has not had the opportunity to engage in research because they are advertised in spaces they don't access. Research participants must be able to identify with researchers as this may lead to greater participation and engagement with the study and provide better quality data. A diverse team will help to consider how participants are included and how questions are asked or experiments set up for diverse groups.

■ Consider setting up a steering group to support the research and ensure there is representation that fits a diverse background. You can co-design the research with members that may have experienced the healthcare system and phenomenon you are investigating. You will need to look at the time of meetings and seminars as they may impact those with childcare and other caring commitments. You also need to consider the location and format of meetings since these can exclude potential participants due to a lack of transport, physical barriers and information that is not presented in an accessible format. Your own position, how you view the phenomenon you are investigating and how you situate yourself can be a drawback of the study. Therefore, a steering group can help bring diverse perspectives and steer the research into the direction that is required.

■ Consider reaching out to any people who may usually be excluded from undertaking research, such as single parents who cannot make late-evening meetings, those with care commitments or disabled people, who may be excluded as others are reluctant to change their ways of work (e.g. repeating information and/or using clearer language).

■ Consider the term 'hard-to-reach groups'; are they hard to reach or do you need to rethink the frame that you are viewing them through?

■ You will want to make your research equitable and will need to think about how you have mitigated privilege and power bias that leads to less-diverse and less-inclusive practice. As a researcher, your identity is not fixed and you should be able to adapt and situate your perspective. This calls for a reflexive approach that acknowledges the personal, subjective, structural and intellectual position of the research.

By using a EDI approach in your research, you would begin to influence and change the research environment and culture in your organisation and redress the power balance and areas of privilege that lead to bias and systematic exclusion. Some communities are described as hard to reach, and this may be for many reasons such as social class, cultural differences, language barriers and geographical location. Communities and groups that are often labelled as hard to reach include ethnic minorities, LGBTQIA+ people, those with intellectual and/or physical disabilities, older people and people with mental health issues. Researchers should reconsider using the term 'hard to reach' and begin to conceptualise new and innovative ways to reach the groups and communities with whom they encounter difficulty. Using a PPI strategy can be instrumental in reaching and working with such groups and communities.

CONCLUSION

Research has the potential to improve patient and population health. Diversity and inclusion are essential to conducting good research. EDI are not unidimensional, must be integrated into the research from the study's conception and remain a key consideration throughout the research process. There are different ways to promote and undertake inclusive research as well as drivers to achieve diverse, equitable and inclusive research praxis. Reflection and reflexivity are equally important tools of governance to ensure you eliminate any bias regarding EDI, particularly around the areas of race, gender identity, sexual orientation, religion, age, disability, socioeconomic status, geographical location and culture. This chapter has explored the importance of diversity and inclusion in the context of research and considered the implications of failing to consider these issues in the planning and implementation of research. Some practical strategies to assist with promoting diversity and exclusion have been explored and it has been argued that these need to be adopted from the outset of a research project. By actively promoting diversity and inclusion, we can ensure more representative research and address existing inequities.

ADDITIONAL RESOURCES

Further reading

Mir G: Cultural competence in health and social care. In: The Ethnicity Training Network, 2009–10, Leeds, 2011, University of Leeds.

Helpful websites

INVOLVE: https://www.nihr.ac.uk/documents/ improving-inclusion-of-under-served-groups- in-clinical-research-guidance-from-include- project/25435

Henrietta Lacks cell line: https://www.hopkins medicine.org/henriettalacks/

MBRRACE-UK Mothers and Babies: Reducing Risk through Audit and Confidential Enquiries across the UK: https://www.npeu.ox.ac.uk/ mbrrace-uk

The Social Inclusive Cities Network: promoting global equity: https://www.youtube.com/ watch?v=BBtF7TcH1TY&t=5s

Tuskegee syphilis study: https://www.cdc.gov/ tuskegee/timeline.htm

REFERENCES

American Association of Colleges of Nursing: Diversity, inclusion, & equity in academic nursing 12(01), 2017.

American Nurses Association (ANA): Code of ethics for nurses with interpretative statements. Silver Spring, 2015, ANA.

Aradine EM, Ryan KA, Cronin CA, et al: Black-white differences in ischemic stroke risk factor burden in young adults, Stroke Mar;53(3):e66–e69, 2021.

Barden O: Getting inside histories of learning disabilities, Educational Action Research 29(4):1–17, 2021.

Brandt AM: Racism and research: the case of the Tuskegee syphilis study, Hastings Centre Report 8(6):21–29, 1978.

Canadian Nurses Association: Social justice: a means to an end an end itself, Ottawa, Canada, 2010, Canadian Nurses Association.

Cole ER: Intersectionality and research in psychology, American Psychologist 64:170–180, 2009.

Crowell TA, Fast PE, Bekker LG, Sanders EJ: Response to: 'Inclusion as illusion: erasing transgender women in research with MSM', Journal of the International AIDS Society 24(1):e25662, 2021.

D'Souza A: The gendered experiences of men with traumatic brain injury (TBI): a qualitative study [Doctoral dissertation, University of Toronto, Canada], 2019.

Davidson EM, Krasuska M, Jenum AK, et al: Developing a realist informed framework for cultural adaptation of lifestyle interventions for the prevention of type 2 diabetes in South Asian populations in Europe, Diabetic Medicine Nov;38(11):e14584, 2021.

Doody O, Noonan M: Nursing research ethics, guidance and application in practice, British Journal of Nursing 25(14):803–807, 2016.

Editorial: Henrietta Lacks: science must right a historical wrong, Nature Sept;585(7823):7, 2020. http://doi.org/10.1038/d41586- 020-02494-z.

Feldman MA, Bosett J, Collet C, Burnham-Riosa P: Where are persons with intellectual disabilities in medical research? A survey of published clinical trials, Journal of Intellectual Disability Research 58(9):800–809, 2014.

Fernandez M, Mowatt RA, Shinew KJ, et al: Going the extra mile: building trust and collaborative relationships with study participants, Leisure Sciences 43(3–4):418–435, 2021.

Fliesher S, Neumann L, Curtis MP: School nurse poverty education: why it is important to your practice, NASN School Nurse Nov;36(6):323–327, 2021.

Foronda C: A theory of cultural humility, Journal of Transcultural Nursing 31(1):7–12, 2020.

Fuentes MA, Zelaya DG, Madsen JW: Rethinking the course syllabus: Considerations for promoting equity, diversity, and inclusion, Teaching of Psychology 48(1):69–79, 2021.

Jackson D, Moorley C: 'Nothing about us without us': embedding participation in peer review processes, Journal of Advanced Nursing May;78(5):e75–e76, 2022.

Jones SC, Gordon CS, Akram M, et al: Inclusion, exclusion and isolation of autistic people: community attitudes and autistic people's experiences, Journal of Autism and Developmental Disorders 52(3):1131–1142, 2021.

Knight M, Bunch K, Tuffnell D, et al (eds) on behalf of MBRRACE-UK: Saving lives, improving mothers' care—lessons learned to inform maternity care from the UK and Ireland Confidential Enquiries into Maternal Deaths and Morbidity 2017–19, Oxford, 2021, National Perinatal Epidemiology Unit, University of Oxford.

Malmquist A, Nieminen K: Negotiating who gives birth and the influence of fear of childbirth: Lesbians, bisexual women and transgender people in parenting relationships, Women and Birth 34(3):e271–e278, 2021.

Milner P, Frawley P: From 'on' to 'with' to 'by': people with a learning disability creating a space for the third wave of inclusive research, Qualitative Research 19(4):382–398, 2019.

Mitchell M, Baker D, Moorosi N, et al: Diversity and inclusion metrics in subset selection. Proceedings of the AAAI/ACM Conference on AI, Ethics, and Society Feb:117–123, 2020.

Molokhia M, Yousif S, Durbaba S, et al: Social determinants of diabetes, hypertension, stroke, and coronary heart disease in Black Caribbean and Black African women aged 40 years or older in south London: findings from 70,582 primary care records from 2000–18, The Lancet, 398, S96, 2021.

Knight M, Bunch K, Tuffnell D, et al (eds) on behalf of MBRRACE-UK: Saving lives, improving mothers' care—lessons learned to inform maternity care from the UK and Ireland Confidential Enquiries into Maternal Deaths and Morbidity 2017–19, Oxford, 2021, National Perinatal Epidemiology Unit, University of Oxford.

Pugh E, Robinson A, De Vito AN, et al: Representation of US Black Americans in neuropsychology research: how well do our reporting practices show that Black lives matter? The Clinical Neuropsychologist 1–13: 2021.

Singh S, McKie J: A survey of the use of seclusion and physical restraint at school and at home for children under the care of the NHS Lanarkshire CAMHS–learning disability team, BJPsych Open 7(S1):S222, 2021.

Thake M, Lowry A: A systematic review of trends in the selective exclusion of older participant from randomised clinical trials, Archives of Gerontology and Geriatrics 72:99–102, 2017.

Treweek S, Banister K, Bower P, et al: Developing the INCLUDE Ethnicity Framework—a tool to help trialists design trials that better reflect the communities they serve, Trials 22(1):1–12, 2021.

Voth Schrag RJ, Mitschke D, Orwig T, Kunkel L: Outcomes of an inter-professional education event for social work and allied health professional students working with families in poverty: implications for social work education, Journal of Teaching in Social Work 41(2):135–150, 2021.

von Unger H: Ethical reflexivity as research practice, Historical Social Research/Historische Sozialforschung 46(2):186–204, 2021.

Witham MD, Anderson E, Carroll CB, et al: Ensuring that COVID-19 research is inclusive; guidance from the NIHR INCLUDE project, BMJ Open 10:e043634, 2020.

Witham MD, Gordon AL, Henderson EJ, Harwood RH: Pandemic research for older people: doing it better next time, Age and Ageing 50(2):276–278, 2021.

12

KNOWLEDGE TRANSLATION OF RESEARCH FINDINGS: CHALLENGES AND STRATEGIES

JULIAN GRANT ■ TINEKE WATER ■ ROB ION

CHAPTER OUTLINE

LEARNING OBJECTIVES

*After reading this chapter and following critical reflection, readers
should be able to:*

- understand the concept of knowledge translation
- know how to translate evidence in to practice
- know how to use evidence to inform clinical guidelines
- understand the role nurses and midwives play in
knowledge translation
- know the steps to take to explore how culture change
can happen.

KEY TERMS

clinical guidelines

evidence-based practice

evidence-informed
practice

evidence-informed
decision-making

impact

integrated knowledge
translation

know-do gap

knowledge translation

README

research literacy

research translation

ABSTRACT

Knowledge translation (KT) is the process by which research findings are made relevant and accessible for use in clinical practice, education or policy. At the conception of any research activity, nursing and midwifery researchers have an ethical responsibility to consider how this will be achieved. This must be done in ways that are experienced by end users as useful and respectful.

As users of translated findings, nurses and midwives also have responsibilities to develop their research literacy skills. These skills include the ability to critically appraise, translate and apply research evidence, considering the needs of diverse populations in different contexts and practice settings.

This chapter will help to build your understanding of KT. The key message is that KT is a core research skill that bridges the gap between a research project and the world of practice. You will learn how a commitment to KT can be built into research designs and how this enhances the likelihood that findings will be used to address real-world problems. Finally, we present a range of strategies to develop individual research literacy and consider organisational readiness for KT.

INTRODUCTION

The reason we undertake research is to increase our understanding of the world and make impactful changes to practice, healthcare and education. In healthcare, this is usually to improve some aspect of end-user experience. We might, for example, be interested in finding out how best to improve the uptake of a service by a marginalised group, or to understand how to improve support for student nurses during practice placement. We might want to assess if a new intervention to reduce self-harm in young people is more effective than existing approaches, or to establish how frequently student midwives encounter poor clinical practice and what, if anything, they do about this. Finding answers to these questions is not, however, the endpoint. If research is to be of value, we need to take steps to ensure that findings can quickly and easily move from the desktop of the researcher to the community, hospital, boardroom or classroom. We know that this is often not an easy process. Indeed, a lapse of 17 years is reported as the average time between

research being undertaken and its implementation in clinical practice (Morris, Wooding & Grant 2011).

WHAT IS KNOWLEDGE TRANSLATION?

There are many different terms that you may come across concerning **knowledge translation** (KT) (also known as **research translation**). These include research utilisation, research dissemination, research diffusion, knowledge uptake or knowledge to action (Curtis et al 2017). KT is a useful umbrella term that encompasses these. The World Health Organization (2012a) defines KT as: 'the synthesis, exchange, and application of knowledge by relevant stakeholders to accelerate the benefits of global and local innovation in strengthening health systems and improving people's health'. It is the process through which research knowledge is created, circulated and adopted into practice (Curtis et al 2017). The process is one that requires active commitment on the part of researchers, practitioners and sometimes policymakers to work together (Duhamel 2017). In many cases, this will also require an early and ongoing commitment to collaboration with end users.

The end user of a KT activity is not simply a passive recipient of new knowledge at the end of a project. KT is also more than direct messaging. It is an ongoing complex process of exchange between different actors such as nurses midwives, researchers, recipients of care, individuals and communities (Kitson et al 2018). It can start from an issue being raised by any individual or group, then progress to designing a study together, working through the project together and analysing findings from a range of cultural, social, economic or political viewpoints. Collectively the group will chart how the findings will be used and all the while knowledge is being shared and translated throughout the entire course of the study. When everyone is involved in the creation of new knowledge, less knowledge is 'lost in translation' between health professionals and patients/communities.

As outlined, KT involves applying the best evidence into practice, which results in better care and patient outcomes. Evidence-based solutions have been discussed earlier in Chapter 4; thus, it is important when applying KT you are aware of the research evidence that needs to be developed and applied to practice.

Integrated knowledge translation (IKT) is argued to increase the chances of research findings being integrated into practice through co-production and collaboration (Graham, Tetroe & MacLean 2014). It is an active collaboration between researchers and research users in all parts of the research process, including the shaping of the research questions, decisions about the data collection methods and tools development, interpretation of the findings and the dissemination and implementation of findings (Graham & Tetroe 2007). Like other participatory approaches, the core values and principles of IKT include 'co-creation, reciprocity, trust, fostering relationships, collaboration, respect, co-learning, active participation, democratisation of knowledge and shared decision-making in the generation and application of knowledge' (Nguyen et al 2021, p. 15).

These values make the use of IKT particularly relevant when working across cultural domains where the nature and value of knowledge may differ between cultural groups. They reflect the responsibilities of researchers expressed in the Australian Institute of Aboriginal and Torres Strait Islander Studies (AIATSIS) and Te Ara Tika research ethics framework (AIATSIS 2020, Hudson et al 2010). Such responsibilities include: recognition and respect; engagement and collaboration; informed consent; cultural capability and learning; First Nation/tangata whenua (people of the land) led research; First Nation/tangata whenua perspectives and participation; First Nation/tangata whenua knowledge and data; benefit and reciprocity; **impact** and risk; First Nation/tangata whenua land and waters; ongoing First Nation/tangata whenua governance, reporting and compliance; and First Nation/tangata whenua customary practices.

STUDENT CHALLENGE

Your Understanding of Knowledge Translation

1. Write a paragraph that describes your understanding of KT and its relevance to your practice as a nursing or midwifery researcher.
2. Describe a case when you translated research evidence into practice to provide or inform appropriate care for a person.
3. Consider the case study about Jamie. Who might they need to talk with when designing the research project to make sure that the research findings can be translated at the end of the study?

STUDENT CHALLENGE

Knowledge Translation Approach

See Box 12.1 for an example of a research exemplar. We suggest you check in to the exemplar throughout your chapter reading to see how it illustrates different points related to KT. Think about why a KT approach was used in the study. Was it appropriate?

WHY IS KNOWLEDGE TRANSLATION IMPORTANT?

There are many reasons why KT is important. First, people should receive and benefit from evidence-informed care that is efficient and effective (Dickinson & Ledger 2018), equitable and sustainable (cost-effective). At the same time, individuals should not be exposed to unnecessary, outdated, wasteful or potentially harmful care (Braithwaite 2018). However, globally, healthcare continues to be undertaken without being based on the latest evidence (Braithwaite 2018, Kristensen, Nymann & Konradsen 2016). This is due to several factors, including that the number of papers published every month on any given topic can be overwhelming and that the skills and lack of time for many health professionals to find, read, synthesise and utilise the latest evidence can be a significant barrier. Finally, for many communities and countries, the barrier of English being the primary language of published work inhibits the uptake of findings.

Although **evidence-based practice** (EBP) or **evidence-informed practice** (EIP) strive to be generalisable, this does not result in equitable outcomes. Currently, some people benefit from the latest knowledge, but not everyone. This is particularly the case in marginalised communities. For example, Gould and colleagues (2017) found that the lack of culturally appropriate cessation smoking programs for the prevention and treatment of tobacco use during pregnancy in Indigenous communities in countries such as Australia and New Zealand contributed to increased adverse health outcomes for women and their babies. Similar findings exist for the United Kingdom where, despite smoking cessation programs, people living in poverty or who identify as LBGT are disproportionately impacted by the effects of tobacco (ASH 2019).

BOX 12.1
RESEARCH EXEMPLAR

Collaboration was core to an IKT pilot study that explored the cultural acceptance of the Pēpi-Pod program as an alternative safe sleep space for First Nations families in metropolitan Adelaide, South Australia (SA) (Grant et al 2021). Following the processes of IKT, the project began with community and industry members identifying a problem in practice, working with researchers to synthesise evidence of possible solutions, collaboratively shaping the research question and making decisions about the methods of data collection. This active collaboration and co-production (Graham, Tetroe & MacLean 2014) continued through data analysis and dissemination of findings.

The team included Aboriginal cultural consultants (ACCs), child and family health nurses, clinicians and leaders from SA Aboriginal Health Services and the Aboriginal Family Birthing Program, the SA Health Public Health Service, Kidsafe SA, the Aboriginal Health Council of South Australia, SIDS and Kids SA, and researchers from Flinders University.

While the project outcomes found that the design could be improved to make the sleeping devices more culturally appropriate, the research found that families identified feelings of comfort and safety when sleeping their babies in the Pēpi-Pods. Confusion around safe sleep education and processes were also identified. This information was shared in real time through the very well-connected project team, resulting in a drive to dive deeper into the problem with a larger KT project. This pilot IKT project captures the core values of 'co-creation, reciprocity, trust, fostering relationships, collaboration, respect, co-learning, active participation, democratisation of knowledge, and shared decision-making in the generation and application of knowledge' (Nguyen et al 2020, p. 15).

These very values meant that the team worked well together and were comfortable and safe to keep working collaboratively to scale the project for a larger national successful bid through the Medical Research Future Fund (MRFF) Rapid Applied Research Translation grant fund. As a model for working across cultural domains, the values and principles of IKT enabled centrality of First Nations' ways of knowing and being. This was essential when scaling the project to increase culturally appropriate participant use of new knowledge alongside working to decolonise mainstream health service delivery. Families and community members (end users) were core to all aspects of the project. For examples see https://sites.flinders.edu.au/ssabsa/ and https://sites.flinders.edu.au/ssabsa/families/

The second reason why KT is important is an ethical one. Participants and healthcare organisations invest resources such as time, access, experience and funding into research. It stands that they should see some benefit, even if the research is not directed at individuals. The World Health Organization (2012b) states that to not share research findings, either positive or negative, is unethical as it may either expose future participants to harm or prevent sharing of benefits to some people or groups. This has relevance not only to where and how research is conducted, but where the findings or subsequent interventions are implemented.

The development of the founding document for the ethical conduct of research, the World Medical Association (WMA) Declaration of Helsinki, offers an example. In the 1990s, concerns were raised that drug companies were undertaking clinical trials in low-income countries. These trials included participants who did not have access to other drugs or interventions which would be classified as standard care. They used this to justify offering some intervention through research rather than no intervention (Angell 1997, Lie et al 2004). In this example, researchers from high-income countries exploited more vulnerable participants in lower-income countries who had less access to healthcare, less economic security and limited protective legislation. Further, the benefits of the drug trials were exported to high-income countries. This led to revisions of the Declaration of Helsinki in 1996 and 2000 (Bošnjak 2001, Carlson, Boyd & Webb 2004). Later revisions included the determination to disseminate all research findings, including negative or inconclusive studies, an imperative to ensure research benefited communities in which the research is undertaken and greater protection of research participants (Carlson, Boyd & Webb 2004).

KT explicitly enables the use of knowledge synthesis to support safe practice. This third reason relates specifically to impactful practice change. Knowledge synthesis is a process of evaluating and summarising all available evidence on a particular topic. **Clinical guidelines** are an example of knowledge synthesis. They constitute essential guidance for practice, based on the latest available high-quality evidence. Clinical practice guidelines for young people with diabetes would be a clear starting point for Jamie (in the case study in earlier chapters) to investigate current clinical practice. The application of clinical guidelines would then need to be contextualised with information about the 14-year-old's learning challenges, mental health concerns and family living context.

Examples of clinical guidelines include:
- Guidelines International Network—https://guidelines.ebmportal.com/
- National Institute for Health and Care Excellence (NICE)—https://www.nice.org.uk/guidance
- Guideline Central—https://www.guidelinecentral.com/summaries/organizations/new-zealand-guidelines-group/.

There is also a range of regional guidelines such as the Royal Children's Hospital Melbourne guidelines for diabetes mellitus at https://www.rch.org.au/clinicalguide/guideline_index/Diabetes_mellitus/.

WHAT ARE NURSING AND MIDWIFERY RESEARCHERS' ROLES IN KNOWLEDGE TRANSLATION?

The traditional research model has been one in which researchers worked alone or in research teams to identify research questions, design and undertake studies and then share findings, usually with other researchers or academics. Generally, there was little or no involvement with those individuals and communities who were the focus of the research. This way of working may be highly effective in some circumstances; for example, during the COVID-19 pandemic there was an urgent need for researchers to develop medical treatments to combat the virus. The traditional researcher-led model ('brilliant scientists develop miracle medicine') worked well in this context, and effective vaccines were developed and delivered in months rather than the usual timeframe of years.

For all its successes, however, there is a recognition that this model is sometimes limited, particularly in contexts that require an understanding of aspects of lived experience, or where research may significantly impact the culture in which findings will be operationalised. The slogan, 'Nothing about us without us', has

come to represent a view that seeks to include those who are the focus of research and/or its end users in the identification of research questions, as well as the design and execution of the study and dissemination of findings (for more about diversity and inclusion in research, see Chapter 11).

This means that researchers must now do more to engage and work in partnership with participants, end users and/or stakeholders to ensure that findings are gathered, shared and communicated in ways that are appropriate and accessible (not lost in translation). KT should, therefore, bridge the **know-do gap** between what we know and what we do in practice by focusing on the needs of end users or stakeholders to break down barriers and enable mutual sharing and learning between the knowledge users and researchers (Nguyen et al 2021). Breaking down the barriers includes: careful consideration of the context of the research before starting the project; consultation with the community on the research approach and potential issues the researchers may not have anticipated; being clear about the purpose of the research throughout; and sharing the findings in a way that acknowledges different audiences.

Let's start with consideration of context, end-user needs and shared identification of purpose. It is often an ethical challenge for researchers to consider *how* participants or groups of people are represented in findings. Many marginalised groups, such as young people or those from cultural minorities, are tired of being overrepresented in negative statistics, which may reflect only one aspect of their life or reflect research approaches that are not culturally sensitive. For example, many women who have experienced intimate partner violence, or human trafficking, do not like the terminology of 'victims'; and young people who are experiencing poverty argue for perspectives in the findings that also focus on their strengths (Berentson-Shaw 2018, Thaggard 2016).

Working in partnership with communities from the outset is an important part of ensuring the relevance and applicability of the findings later. An example of this is the study of Huntington's disease for Māori in New Zealand. Dr. Melanie Cheung (Ngāti Rangitihi, Te Arawa) says building respectful relationships with Tangata Whenua/First Nation people takes time and it took 6 years before the researchers were ready to start the project. The result of the consultation, partnership and listening saw the research underpinned by tikanga Māori that ensured continuity of the physical and spiritual worlds, and combined experimental neuroscience, bioethics, tikanga (ceremony/customary practice) and the mātauranga Māori (Māori traditional knowledge) brain plasticity-based training program to treat Huntington's disease (Kinita 2013). Fundamental to this was the respect for the brain, which belonged to a human being, who also belonged to a family and community. For Cheung and the research team, it was important to acknowledge the passing of the person, the family's grief and the gift to the researchers (Kinita 2013). The impact of this trust, developed through the engagement process, was the gifting of brains and early postmortem results by Māori peoples that was not seen in other studies.

This also points to the importance of the researcher's role in sharing findings with a range of audiences. Eljiz and colleagues (2020) argue that matching communication mediums to relevant audiences and stakeholders increases the impact of healthcare research. They introduce the **README** checklist and STEP tool to refine how researchers and clinicians can work collaboratively to effectively translate research findings. The README checklist stands for REAch and Diffusion of health iMprovement Evidence. It encompasses nine communication methods to translate knowledge: research reports, posters, healthcare industry and academic presentations, peer-reviewed articles, elevator pitches, podcasts, webinars and infographics (Eljiz et al 2020). The Strategic Translation and Engagement Planning or STEP tool is used to determine which forms of communication would be most useful given the level of interaction with stakeholders and the complexity of information to be shared. Decisions can be based on how actively involved in the research or application of the research the stakeholders might be.

CASE STUDY 12.1

Ahmed might consider a range of KT strategies to communicate his findings. These could include a series of posters for the 87-year-old man with COPD and a research report or podcast for care workers. Can you think of any other strategies Ahmed could use to increase KT?

Not all nurses and midwives are producers or communicators of research; however, all have a role in KT by developing their **research literacy**, which refers to 'the ability to read and understand research literature' (Hines et al 2018, p. 1). This understanding supports nurses and midwives to use evidence to inform their practice and decision-making to provide relevant care. This includes nurses and midwives being consumers of research by knowing how to access research and being able to understand and critique research and findings and then make judgments around whether they can trust applying these findings in their clinical practice.

Mallidou and colleagues (2018) identified a core approach that underpins this practice. This includes the ability to ask meaningful research questions and appraise literature or other research findings. This is relevant for all nurses and midwives. Some may take this further to include selecting a relevant study design and collaborating to implement their research to challenge normative perspectives, then responding to barriers and facilitators to implement new knowledge. All nurses and midwives have responsibility for KT by using research findings to inform decision-making, policies, procedures, standards of care and practices in the clinical setting.

STUDENT CHALLENGE

Applying Knowledge Translation to Your Project

You are planning a research project to look at peer-to-peer education with young people who identify as LGBTQIA+.
1. When might you involve the end users and stakeholders?
2. What steps might you take to determine a relevant study design?
3. Who else might you need to consult with? How will you do this?
4. What actions will help maximise the successful implementation of the findings at the end of the research project?

DEVELOPING A CULTURE THAT IS READY FOR KNOWLEDGE TRANSLATION

An organisational culture that values knowledge and research and where decisions are routinely based on evidence is more likely to be receptive to KT. Opening the door for KT and **evidence-informed decision-making** (EIDM) requires us to take up a culture of inquiry, having an open mind to possibilities across disciplines, practice and culture. The following section offers strategies for adopting a culture of inquiry.

Create the Organisational Context

Just as farmers need to prepare their fields before planting crops and then nurture them as they grow, nursing and midwifery leaders need to spend time making their organisations research-ready. This might be done through role modelling, where leaders are active and visible researchers or consumers of research, or by their support and reward of research conducted by others. Support and reward in this context are not just about congratulations on a website or in a newsletter; they may require allocation of resources, including time, money or equipment. Without these, serious research and its translation into practice are unlikely.

Leaders can also do much to create a culture in which reflection and critical questions are encouraged and where suggestions for improvement and positive change are welcomed. This culture should be one in which all stakeholders—including patients, staff and students—feel able to comment on practice at any level and know that their comments will be heard. There are some strategies to help nurses and midwives support KT environments.

QUESTION CLINICAL PRACTICES

We may still be putting butter on burns if someone had not questioned the practice. 'Sacred cows' of practice are often based on tradition rather than evidence (Hanrahan et al 2015) and need questioning. As a new nurse or midwife, you may find this challenging, but it is essential to respectfully question the evidence underpinning practices. You can try the following activities.

- Write a list of questions about practices in your workplace. You can then raise these with your supervisor in supervision meetings.
- Listen to your colleagues to see if they are questioning the same practices.
- Think about the 'sacred cows' that might be hanging on in your practice environment. These

might seem contrary to practices you have seen or learned about during clinical education or they may simply be illogical or time-consuming. Talk these over with other staff; they might be thinking the same things!

- Read peer-reviewed journals and consider how your reading might differ from what you are experiencing in practice.

Listen to Recipients of Care

For example, Aboriginal maternal infant care workers would never have been introduced into maternal, child and family health practice across South Australia if midwives had not listened to First Nations families. Due to historic and ongoing colonisation in mainstream health services, families from First Nations backgrounds are fearful and cautious of accessing services from nurses and midwives who are not First Nations people. In 2003, in response to birthing concerns from senior First Nations women in South Australia, a statewide consultation was held. This led to the introduction of a birthing program in regional towns of Port Augusta where Aboriginal Maternal Infant Care (AMIC) workers practised alongside midwives (Stamp et al 2008). The strategy is now embedded in the statewide Women and Children's Health Network. You can practise listening by:

- paying attention to how recipients of care respond to procedures, checking their body language and engagement
- asking how those with and for whom you care experience their healthcare
- pay attention to aspects of care that people might be resistant to; ask what it is about the care that is not meeting their needs
- develop skills in culturally safe practice to support questioning your clinical practice alongside active listening.

Engage in Professional Development Activities

Finishing your study is not the end of learning. As a professional, lifelong learning is key to maintaining currency with developments in healthcare and clinical practice. This includes both formal and informal learning, which can be self-directed or provided by workplaces or professional organisations. Approaches to engagement may include:

- making time on a regular weekly or fortnightly basis to read relevant literature to stay updated about the latest research and developments in your practice area
- joining or initiating a journal club or professional reading group where you can discuss ideas and approaches with colleagues
- accessing resources in your workplace such as the intranet and online library resources
- identifying key quality peer-reviewed journals that publish research relevant to your area of practice and setting up email alerts for these.

Join Relevant Organisational and Professional Groups/Committees to Influence Change

Professional bodies bring together a critical mass of interested, enthusiastic clinicians, researchers, leaders and educators. It is this critical mass that enables change. It doesn't matter how much you know individually; you cannot change the world on your own. Joining national and/or international professional organisations provides an opportunity for social learning and the development of professional networks. Remember that both KT and EIDM require collaboration, development of relationships and trust. Joining a professional network enables you to develop these skills and work towards collaborative identification of key issues that could benefit from further investigation. The following strategies will support your development.

- Join a relevant professional organisation linked to your area of practice or a national or international nursing group. Most nursing and/or midwifery organisations provide a range of resources for members to access, which may include journals, online resources and workshops and other professional activities discounted to members.
- Identify and join relevant committees or working parties in your workplace where you will be exposed to the development and/or review of practice guidelines or clinical audit activities and outcomes.
- Find out if your organisation has a research or knowledge development/translation unit and identify opportunities to become involved in research activities undertaken by the unit and to learn from the staff in the unit.

- Identify a mentor who can assist you to develop knowledge and skills related to EIDM and support you to become involved in clinically focused projects (Gagliardi et al 2017).

STUDENT CHALLENGE

Developing a Culture of Inquiry

1. Look for evidence that supports common practices in your workplace. If you find conflicting evidence, think about who you could talk this over with. Consider barriers to changing practice and how you might address these.
2. Review your current strategies for lifelong learning. Look for relevant professional nursing organisations and identify how these might benefit your readiness for EIDM and KT.
3. Discuss with your manager or supervisor how you can be involved in activities in your workplace; for example, reviewing clinical practice guidelines or shadowing researchers across the service.

CONCLUSION

There is broad global agreement that nurses and midwives demonstrate their professional practice through their use of the best available research evidence in their clinical decision-making, tailored to the needs of the person or group and context. KT, IKT and EIDM are key processes in achieving desired equitable and quality care outcomes. KT aims to address the evidence–practice gap and ultimately improve quality healthcare and health outcomes.

In this chapter, we used the example of a study where IKT principles were operationalised from the outset, leading to culturally safe research with collaboration and co-construction with end users throughout the entire process. This chapter presented a range of strategies to develop individual research literacy and EIDM behaviours and improve organisational readiness for KT in healthcare systems. The strategies could be adopted by managers and nurse leaders, nurses, midwives and undergraduate students. They strengthen organisational environments, facilitate individual research literacy and, importantly, help bridge the gap between research and practice to improve outcomes. KT is a core skill for all nurses and midwives.

ADDITIONAL RESOURCES

Campbell Collaboration, an international organisation that conducts systematic reviews of education, social welfare, and social science research: http://www.campbellcollaboration.org

Canadian Institutes of Health Research (CIHR), a federal agency responsible for funding health research in Canada for KT research, development and dissemination: http://www.cihr-irsc.gc.ca/e/29529.html

Cochrane, an international organisation that conducts systematic reviews of health and medical research: http://www.cochrane.org

The Cochrane Library: http://www.cochranelibrary.com

Cochrane Public Health: http://ph.cochrane.org

Consolidated Framework for Implementation Research: https://isrn.net/blog/consolidated-framework-implementation-research-cfir

JBI, an international nursing organisation that conducts systematic reviews in health and provides resources to undertake critical appraisals: https://jbi.global/

Knowledge Translation Program (KTP) (University of Toronto, Canada), a multidisciplinary academic program developed to address the gap between research evidence and clinical practice and the need to focus on the processes through which knowledge is effectively translated into changed practices: https://knowledgetranslation.net/kt-tools

Knowledge Utilization Studies Program (University of Alberta, Canada) focuses on nursing, social sciences and research utilisation in nursing: https://www.ualberta.ca/nursing/research/research-units/knowledge-utilization-studies-program/index.html

National Health Service (NHS) Centre for Reviews and Dissemination (University of York, England) conducts systematic reviews of research and disseminates research-based information about the effects of interventions used in health and social care in the United Kingdom: http://www.york.ac.uk/inst/crd/welcome.htm

REFERENCES

Angell M: The ethics of clinical research in the Third World, New England Journal of Medicine 337(12):847–849, 1997.

ASH: Health inequities and smoking, 2019. https://ash.org.uk/wp-content/uploads/2019/09/ASH-Briefing_Health-Inequalities.pdf.

Australian Institute of Aboriginal and Torres Strait Islander Studies (AIATSIS): AIATSIS Code of Ethics for Aboriginal and Torres Strait Islander Research, 2020. https://aiatsis.gov.au/sites/default/files/2020-10/aiatsis-code-ethics.pdf.

Berentson-Shaw J: Telling a new story about 'child poverty' in New Zealand, Auckland, 2018, The Workshop and The Policy Observatory. https://thepolicyobservatory.aut.ac.nz/.

Bošnjak S: The declaration of Helsinki: the cornerstone of research ethics, Archive of Oncology 9(3):179–184, 2001.

Braithwaite J: Changing how we think about healthcare improvement, BMJ (Clinical Research Ed.) 17 May;361:k2014, 2018. https://doi.org/10.1136/bmj.k2014

Carlson RV, Boyd KM, Webb DJ: The revision of the Declaration of Helsinki: past, present and future. British Journal of Clinical Pharmacology 57(6):695–713, 2004. http://doi.org/10.1111/j.1365-2125.2004.02103.x.

Curtis K, Fry M, Shaban RZ, Considine J: Translating research findings to clinical nursing practice, Journal of Clinical Nursing 26 (5–6):862–872, 2017.

Dickinson H, Ledger J: Accelerating research translation in healthcare: the Australian approach. In McDermott A, Kitchener M, Exworthy M, Managing improvement in healthcare, Champaign, Illinois, 2018, Palgrave Macmillan, pp. 201–216.

Duhamel F: Translating knowledge from a family systems approach to clinical practice: Insights from knowledge translation research experiences, Journal of Family Nursing 23(4):461–487, 2017.

Eljiz K, Greenfield D, Hogden A, et al: Improving knowledge translation for increased engagement and impact in healthcare, BMJ Open Quality 9, e000983, 2020. http://doi.org/10.1136/bmjoq-2020-000983.

Gagliardi AR, Kothari A, Graham ID: Research agenda for integrated knowledge translation (IKT) in healthcare: what we know and do not yet know. Journal of Epidemiology and Community Health Feb;71(2):105–106, 2017.

Gould GS, Patten C, Glover M, et al: Smoking in pregnancy among Indigenous women in high-income countries: a narrative review, Nicotine & Tobacco Research 19(5):506–517, 2017.

Graham I, Tetroe J: CIHR research: how to translate health research knowledge into effective healthcare action, Healthcare Quarterly 10(3):20–22, 2007.

Graham I, Tetroe J, MacLean R: Chapter 1: Some basics of integrated knowledge translation research. In Graham ID, Tetroe J, Pearson A (eds), Turning knowledge into action: practical guidance on how to do integrated knowledge translation research, Philadelphia, 2014, Lippincott Williams & Wilkins, p. 196.

Grant J, Sivertsen N, Deverix J, Steeb A: 'It looks like a breadbox': a pilot study investigating implementation of the Pēpi-Pod® program with Aboriginal families in metropolitan South Australia, Primary Health Care Research & Development 22:E29, 2021. http://doi.org/10.1017/S1463423621000293.

Hanrahan K, Wagner M, Matthews G, et al: Sacred cow gone to pasture: a systematic evaluation and integration of evidence-based practice, Worldviews on Evidence-based Nursing Feb;12(1):3–11, 2015. http://doi.org/10.1111/wvn.12072.

Hines S, Ramsbotham J, Coyer F, Lizarondo L: Best practice information sheets: Interventions for improving the research literacy of nurses, JBI EBP Database 20(12):1–4, 2018. http://doi.org/10.1111/nhs.12799.

Hudson M, Milne M, Reynolds P, et al: Te ara tika. Guidelines for Māori research ethics. A framework for researchers and ethics committee members. Pūtaiora Writing Group 9 Feb, 2010. https://www.fmhs.auckland.ac.nz/assets/fmhs/faculty/tkhm/tumuaki/docs/teara.pdf.

Kinita D, Science finds a fit with tradition, Rotorua Daily Post 1 Oct, 2013. https://www.nzherald.co.nz/rotorua-daily-post/news/science-finds-fit-with-tradition/NUFSQKDZ5RRHQWDVPYFTXA4HMA/.

Kitson A, Brook A, Harvey G, et al: Using complexity and network concepts to inform healthcare knowledge translation, International Journal of Health Policy and Management 7(3):231–243, 2018. https://doi.org/10.15171/ijhpm.2017.79.

Kristensen N, Nymann C, Konradsen H: Implementing research results in clinical practice – the experiences of healthcare professionals, BMC Health Services Research 16(48), 2016. http://doi.org/10.1186/s12913-016-1292-y.

Lie RK, Emanuel E, Grady C, Wendler D: The standard of care debate: the Declaration of Helsinki versus the international consensus opinion, Journal of Medical Ethics 30(2):190–193, 2004.

Mallidou AA, Atherton P, Chan L, et al: Core knowledge translation competencies: a scoping review, BMC Health Services Research 18(502), 2018. https://doi.org/10.1186/s12913-018-3314-4.

Morris ZS, Wooding S, Grant J: The answer is 17 years, what is the question: understanding time lags in translational research, Journal of The Royal Society of Medicine 104(12):510–520, 2011. http://doi.org/10.1258/jrsm.2011.110180.

Nguyen T, Graham ID, Mrklas KJ, et al: Birthing on Country for the best start in life: Returning childbirth services back to Yolu mothers, babies and communities in East Arnhem, Northern Territory, 2020 Nhulunbuy Workshop Report, 2021.

Stamp G, Chamption S, Anderson G, et al: Aboriginal maternal and infant care workers: Partners in caring for Aboriginal mothers and babies. Rural and Remote Health 8:3:1–12, 2008.

Thaggard S: The mosaic of a superhero: a Ricoeurian hermeneutic construction of life and identity after intimate partner violence. [Doctoral dissertation] Auckland University of Technology, 2016.

World Health Organization: Knowledge translation framework for ageing and health, 2012a, WHO. https://www.who.int/publications/m/item/knowledge-translation-framework-for-ageing-and-health.

World Health Organization: The WHO strategy on research for health, 2012b, WHO.

World Medical Association. WMA Declaration of Helsinki: ethical principles for medical research involving human subjects Oct, 2013. www.wma.net/en/30publications/10policies/b3/index.html.

13

DEVELOPING A RESEARCH CAREER IN NURSING AND MIDWIFERY

HELEN WALTHALL ■ MICHELE BRIGGS ■ MARILYN CRUICKSHANK

CHAPTER OUTLINE

LEARNING OBJECTIVES

After reading this chapter and following critical reflection, readers should be able to:

- define the terms 'research nurse/midwife' and 'academic nurse/midwife'
- outline the different roles of the research nurse/midwife and academic nurse/midwife
- outline some research career pathways for nurses and midwives.

KEY TERMS

academic nurse/midwife

clinical academic

good clinical practice (GCP)

research nurse/midwife

research capacity

research capability

ABSTRACT

Not all nurses and midwives realise that, like management, education or clinical specialty practice, research can be a fulfilling career pathway. If you are new to research and are unsure what roles and career pathways are open to you, it can be difficult to navigate the system. When thinking about research pathways, various roles are available to nurses and midwives. Internationally, there is not a common career pathway, and some countries are more developed in nursing and midwifery research roles and career opportunities than others. There are, however, two types of roles that you may encounter. They have similar names but are very different roles. A **research nurse/midwife** often works within a team undertaking specific roles such as patient recruitment, clinical assessment and data collection in a project led by an academic researcher, who may or may not be a nurse or midwife. An **academic nurse/midwife** can be employed by a university or clinical organisation and either leads research themselves or collaborates with an investigator team to lead research. Both of these roles offer great opportunities for nurses and midwives to gain skills in research and to participate in and lead research activities. With a degree of knowledge, resilience and determination, you will be able to build your career choices in research and influence nursing or midwifery research in such areas as workforce, education or practice.

INTRODUCTION

The preceding chapters have highlighted the importance of research to nursing and midwifery practice. This chapter will look at how nurses and midwives can build a research career. There is a strong association between a scientific basis for healthcare interventions with quality care, safety and cost-effectiveness (Maben & King 2019). Evidence has shown that organisations that engage in clinical research have better patient outcomes compared to their non-research-active counterparts (Jonker, Fisher & Dagnan 2020). Research activity has also been associated with reduced staff turnover for organisations and staff recommending the organisation as a place to work (Newington, Alexander & Wells 2021, Jonker & Fisher 2018). It is key for practice to develop and provide the best

evidence-based care to patients that all nurses and midwives are aware of the research in the area. Whether you're a student or newly qualified nurse, or a more experienced nurse or midwife, it is important to familiarise yourself with research that is being undertaken in your area of practice so that you can discuss this with patients and give them an opportunity to participate in the research relevant to them. Being research-aware and using the most up-to-date evidence in your practice is also important.

Nurses and midwives have a unique role in working with people/patients to bring about cultural or behavioural change that could have a direct impact on practice (Curtis et al 2017). As professionals, we are well placed to undertake research into many aspects of our practice, whether that is how we educate aspiring nurses and midwives (education), how we enable the delivery of care (workforce) or how we support and care for people (practice). Nurses and midwives are often concerned with the experiences of people and how a difficult journey can be made more tolerable. For example, a midwife may be interested in a new mother's experience of breastfeeding to explore if and how this experience could be enhanced. Or a nurse may research the experience of a patient who is diagnosed with a long-term condition and how this condition has impacted their employment. You will notice both examples are aligned to a qualitative methodology (see Chapter 8 for more details); however, nursing and midwifery can also involve research with a more quantitative focus (see Chapter 7). For example, a midwife may be interested in testing if the education program implemented for first-time mothers who breastfeed has an impact on their wellbeing, by using validated tools to test the mothers' quality of life or anxiety or depression levels; or a nurse could implement a return-to-work intervention for a person with a long-term condition and use validated tools to measure how effective it was.

If you are interested in pursuing a research-focused role, these two examples illustrate how nurses or midwives could lead or work within research that seeks to develop practice and improve the care received by patients. However, nurses or midwives can also work within teams to support the delivery of research which is led by another member of the multidisciplinary team. For example, a midwife could work in a team led by obstetricians supporting a study exploring a new drug treatment for hyperemesis in a group of prenatal women, or a nurse could work in a team which is supporting a study that is delivering a new drug regimen for people diagnosed with heart failure. These examples show the nurse or midwife is working in research, supporting the research being delivered to participants, but not leading the research. These are illustrating two different roles in research which will be explored as the chapter progresses and both offer career opportunities and pathways for nurses and midwives.

STUDENT CHALLENGE

Roles in Research

1. What are your thoughts on what research roles are available in nursing or midwifery?
2. Consider each of the following questions and record your answers.
   a. What roles do you think nurses or midwives do who want to do research?
   b. What do you think the difference in the roles are?
   c. Would you consider any of these roles in your career? Why or why not?

As a student nurse or midwife who may be thinking about which area of practice you would like to explore on qualification, it is important to define the distinct roles nurses and midwives can have in research and the expectations for each of these roles. In the literature, there is no agreement between countries on titles and/or expectations of roles in nursing and midwifery research. Some international titles and definitions are summarised in Table 13.1. In this chapter, we will refer to an academic nurse/midwife and research nurse/midwife so please ensure you are aware of the definition of these roles.

Before we can look at the career opportunities available for nurses and midwives who want to work in these roles, it is important to outline the difference in the roles.

RESEARCH NURSE/MIDWIFE

There is no agreement on a international definition for a research nurse or midwife; however, many countries use the definition outlined by the United States and Canadian association, the International Association of

---

TABLE 13.1
Research Roles

Role Title	Definition of Role	Country of Origin
Clinical academic nurse/midwife	A nurse or midwife who is engaged concurrently in both clinical and academic activities and can provide clinical leadership in the pursuit of excellent evidence-based healthcare; usually has a doctorate	United Kingdom (Baltruks & Callaghan 2018)
Clinical researcher	A clinician who has been given time to do research within a clinical setting as part of their role	Australia (Pain, Fernando & Peterson 2018)
Research nurse/midwife	A nurse or midwife who supports the delivery of research through recruitment, informed consent, data collection and entry	United Kingdom (NIHR 2020, Tinkler & Robinson 2020)
Clinician researcher	A clinician who undertakes research activities, including writing for publication	Australia (Smith et al 2018a)
Embedded researchers	Nurse or midwife researchers who work in both academic and healthcare institutions	Australia (Mickan & Coates 2022)
Academic nurse/midwife	A nurse or midwife who works in an academic institution or in a healthcare organisation	United Kingdom, Australia and New Zealand
Nurse/midwife consultant	A leading expert clinician who leads practice and who has research as an essential component of the role	United Kingdom, Australia and New Zealand

Clinical Research Nurses (IACRN) (Tinkler et al 2018). Hastings and colleagues (2012) define clinical research nursing and/or midwifery as a specialised practice that is focused on maintaining equilibrium between the care of the research participant and the requirements of the research protocol. This area of practice incorporates: human participants' protection; care coordination and continuity; contribution to clinical science; clinical practice; and study management throughout a variety of professional roles, practice settings and clinical specialties (IACRN 2012). This definition is supported in the United Kingdom (UK) through the National Institute of Health Research (NIHR) and Royal College of Nursing (RCN). As Smith and colleagues (2018b) outline, in Australia this role is known as clinical trials nurse/midwife, but ultimately the roles outlined in this chapter are the same.

McCabe and colleagues (2019) describe the role as being based on the following five domains:

1. the protection of human participants
2. coordination and continuity of therapeutic care
3. nursing clinical practice
4. contributing to the research knowledge base
5. the management of trials.

What is the role?

The research nurse/midwife role is to undertake the research as agreed in the research protocol in clinical practice (Fitzpatrick 2019). This research is often led by researchers from other disciplines who employ a research nurse or midwife to undertake the day-to-day running of the study, including protocol development and ethical approval, participant recruitment, informed consent, collection of data, clinical care delivery and protocol management. All these elements enable safe and ethical research to be undertaken, and the findings help to develop practice and improve outcomes for patients.

McCabe and colleagues (2019) found that research nurses were often the only members of the research team with in-depth knowledge of patient care, research process and training in problem-solving. Kunhunny and Salmon (2017) identify two key elements to the role. The first is professional practice, including to identify the responsibility, values, attitudes and beliefs of nursing, exposure to ethical dilemmas and challenges from clinical practice. The second

is drawing on prior nursing experience, team and management support and the clinical research training and education obtained. This role is seen as enabling nurses or midwives to deliver research in practice through supporting patients to make informed decisions, delivering research in an ethical framework which supports safe patient care and by learning and developing new skills in the research process.

CASE STUDY 13.1

Ahmed is an undergraduate student in the second year of his degree. As an assessment task he has to learn about conducting research and its implications for practice. Ahmed has to explore best practices in caring for an 87-year-old man living with chronic heart failure and newly diagnosed COPD, who also has carer responsibilities for his 85-year-old wife who is living with dementia.

Ahmed has been assigned a placement with the lead research nurse within the respiratory research group who is responsible for the delivery of several studies exploring treatment options for patients with COPD. One of these is a new drug regimen to manage COPD in the community. It is the research nurse's responsibility to make sure this study can recruit participants who meet the inclusion and exclusion criteria and who consent to participate once they have been fully informed about what the study entails. Ahmed learned the following on his placement that enabled him to write his assignment:

- working with the clinical team to identify patients who would meet the inclusion and exclusion criteria
- how to communicate with potential participants to see if they were interested in being involved in research
- how important the conversation is to ensure any potential participant is fully informed of the study and what is involved so that the right decision for them can be made around participation
- how important it is for a participant to see what commitment is required for them to participate in the study (e.g. how many trips and for how long to the research unit or any extra activities they need to do that would impact their time)

- how essential it is to collect the right data at the right time to ensure the research is conducted as per the protocol
- how important it is to monitor for any breaches to the protocol or any issues with the safety of the drug being administered
- how the clinical research nurse acts as the participants' advocate at all times while they are engaged in the study.

ACADEMIC NURSE/MIDWIFE

In comparison to the research nurse/midwife role, a **clinical academic** nurse/midwife leads or collaborates in leading research to acquire new knowledge relevant to nursing/midwifery practice, patient outcomes, education or workforce issues (Newington, Alexander & Wells 2022, Carrick-Sen et al 2016). Academic nurses or midwives do this through using rigorous research methodologies and methods which have the potential to uncover evidence that could improve patient care or progress the profession (Theofanidis 2021). They lead a research team for the whole research process of the study from conception to publication/dissemination or are collaborating members of the investigator team.

What is the role?

This role involves leading and/or guiding the research team along the pathway from identifying the problem to finding the solution. The academic nurse/midwife identifies the problem in practice in partnership with the stakeholders (patients, carers or health professionals) and then applies all aspects of the research process to lead the investigation of the problem through to implementing the findings back into practice. The academic nurse/midwife has demonstrated expertise in the research process, including a knowledge base of research methodologies, data collection methods and analysis techniques.

COMPARING THE ROLES

The research nurses/midwives role involves supporting the research projects, whereas the academic nurses/midwives develop ideas into robust research questions and projects. Academic nurses/midwives lead research, ensuring it is undertaken in an ethical framework that supports patient safety and meets all research governance requirements before the study begins. Academic nurses/midwives can either be employed by a university or in healthcare organisations, or they may hold a joint appointment between both a clinical organisation and a university. The research ideas emerge from their specific area of expertise, whether this is practice, workforce or educational research. The academic nurse/midwife is leading the research to improve patient outcomes. Table 13.2 summarises the difference in the two research roles.

TABLE 13.2
The Difference in the Two Research Roles

Research Nurse/Midwife	Academic Nurse/Midwife
Works on studies where the idea is from a lead researcher (principal investigator)	Has the idea and either leads or is a collaborator of a research study (principal investigator)
Ensures the delivery of the study is within the study's protocol	Has written and developed the study's protocol
Collects data determined by the lead researcher (principal investigator)	Is the lead or co-lead researcher (principal investigator) who determines what data needs to be collected
Produces the data for the lead researcher (principal investigator) to analyse	Is the lead or co-lead researcher (principal investigator) who analyses the data
Works in a team to ensure the research is delivered ethically and safely	Leads or contributes to the team to ensure the research is delivered ethically and safely
Works in the relevant area (healthcare provider or university) to deliver the research	May work in either clinical practice or academia to develop the research

Jamie is a final year undergraduate undertaking a core research module. Jamie must undertake a research project to demonstrate an understanding of evidence-based practice applied to a case study. They have been assigned to investigate the care required for a 14-year-old female living with learning disabilities who is newly diagnosed with type 1 diabetes. She is in foster care and has a history of mental health issues including self-harming behaviours.

Jamie has been assigned a supervisor for this research project. Jamie's supervisor is the lead academic nurse in diabetes who has published many papers and undertaken many studies on juvenile-onset of type 1 diabetes mellitus. Time with the supervisor has given Jamie great insight into leading a research project from the inception of the problem to completing the study. Jamie has learned the following aspects:

- how to identify a focused research problem
- how to search the literature to identify the current evidence of the topic area
- how important it is to appraise the literature to determine the quality of the evidence
- how to write a clear research question with focused aims and objectives for the research project
- how to analyse the data to enable the research question to be answered
- how important the write up of the project is to ensure transparency of the results and implications for practice.

Jamie feels that working with the supervisor has provided valuable insights into the research process to enable the completion of the prescribed assignment.

HOW CAN I GET INVOLVED IN RESEARCH?

As we have seen throughout this book, research is fundamental to all nursing and midwifery practice. What is key for a nurse or midwife is to know how to get involved in research once they have completed their pre-registration qualification (at either bachelor degree or masters academic degree level) and are working as a nurse or midwife.

Finding a pathway into a research career can present some challenges for nurses or midwives interested in continuing to advance their clinical practice and generate the knowledge to ensure that patients have the best outcomes possible. Pattison and colleagues (2021) indicated there are challenges in developing an academic nursing or midwifery workforce globally. Most research in this area describes a form of a partnership model, in which academics (employed in the university; Baltruks & Callaghan 2018) work on projects in clinical practice. However, globally there is evidence this partnership model is gaining momentum for academics to be employed in the healthcare organisation, and examples of how to implement academic nurses or midwives in healthcare organisations are emerging at a great pace (e.g. Edelman et al 2021, Olive et al 2022, Oulton et al 2022).

If you think you are interested in developing your research knowledge and skills and want to know more, Box 13.1 gives you some easy tips for engaging in research while working in practice.

STUDENT CHALLENGE

Exploring Research Roles

1. Why are these research roles important in practice?
2. Consider each of the following questions and record your answers.
   a. What do you think is important in choosing a research role?
   b. Have you seen either of these research roles in healthcare organisations or in a university?
   c. What attributes do you think you need to do these roles?

CAREER OPTIONS FOR NURSES AND MIDWIVES IN RESEARCH

There is not one clearly defined pathway for nurses and midwives to enter a research career, nor is there international consistency in the nomenclature of these kinds of research roles (Kunhunny & Salmon 2017, Cleaver 2020). Globally, there is a range of approaches to support these career opportunities and a range of roles that nurses and midwives can explore.

What is common in a research career is an individual's enthusiasm for learning, questioning and finding solutions to problems and issues of concern. Developing a research career usually involves going the extra yards in undertaking small, less complex activities such as quality improvement projects or joining research teams to gain key skills. Being actively involved in professional organisations will provide a network and role models, mentoring opportunities and a setting for presenting studies and listening to others presenting their research. Academic research education at bachelor honours or master level will provide coursework and projects that expose nurses and midwives to research. They will also develop essential skills such as searching the literature, awareness and familiarity with ethical issues and understanding appropriate methods and analysis, as well as having the opportunity to apply this knowledge through small projects under the supervision of a nurse or midwife researcher. In a recent UK national survey carried out by the Council of Deans of Health to assess the current landscape of research education provision in the UK, several areas of good practice were revealed in integrating research into the curricula to prepare nurses for professional life (McCormack, Baltruks & Cooke 2019). Further research training and education at the doctoral level enables capacity development to equip the nurse or midwife with the necessary skills to independently lead research and provides the theoretical components to underpin leading and developing a research project from inception to completion.

Research Nurse/Midwife

Often research nurse/midwives are employed on short-term, fixed contracts for the life of a research project. This can make the career progression challenging for the research nurse/midwife. However, several researchers have explored what the role is and its requirements and thus have outlined the support and development needed for nurses who undertake the role, and employing organisations are now supporting the development and career progression of this role. Both Tinkler and colleagues (2018) and Cleaver (2020) identify the need for a period of time to enable the nurse or midwife to develop from a clinical nurse or midwife into the role of a research nurse/midwife. Both identified that this transition period needs to commence with a clear induction program into the role and what the role entails. They found this was often not supported and left research nurses/midwives feeling anxious and unprepared. Similarly, Kunhunny and Salmon (2017) identified the need to establish a structured induction program as well as a well-defined educational pathway for research nurses/midwives to recruit to this role, retain them and offer clear personal and professional development within the role.

Not all research nurse/midwife jobs require you to have had research experience beyond a bachelor degree when you commence the role. Opportunities for training and education in the research nurse/midwife role include knowledge of the research process and the delivery of a research study. Study-specific training and education will be discussed according to individual needs and informed by the needs of the role, and the individual research nurse/midwife. There are no internationally agreed standards for research governance and ethics, but it is important to know and understand when working in a research nurse/midwife role what the processes are in your organisation and country. Usually, local training supports each individual nurse or midwife in ensuring an understanding of ethical research practice, as this is mandatory for the role and tends to include the internationally recognised certificate of **good clinical practice (GCP)** training. Everyone involved in research must be trained or appropriately experienced to perform the specific tasks they are being asked to undertake. GCP training is a requirement in the UK and is set out in the Policy Framework for Health and Social Care Research (NHS Health Research Authority 2020) for researchers conducting clinical trials of investigational medicinal products (CTIMPs)—a quantitative experimental research study (as discussed in Chapter 7)

Key national research strategies for research nurses/midwives aim to develop pathways for career opportunities. One of the strategic goals of both the National Institute for Health Research in the UK (https://www.nihr.ac.uk/documents/developing-our-clinical-research-nursing-strategy/11500) and the New Zealand Health Research Strategy 2017–2027 (Ministry of Business, Innovation and Employment and Ministry of Health (2017) is to improve the awareness, understanding, contribution and impact of the research nurse, including development and support within this role. It is important to engage in nursing organisations (such as the Royal College of Nursing in the UK, the Australian Nursing and Midwifery Federation or the New Zealand Nurses Organisation, Sigma Global Nursing Excellence) to ensure awareness of all opportunities available. Often these roles can be in small teams and additional activities and support can assist in reducing feelings of isolation and imposter syndrome.

Academic Nurse/Midwife

An academic nurse or midwife can be employed in several roles, including advanced nurse practitioner, consultant practitioner, clinical professor or academic researcher/professor in a university. The key to the role of an academic nurse/midwife is the research knowledge and skills required to be part of the leadership team or to lead a research project independently. This accumulation of knowledge is usually through an academic pathway that has started at bachelor honours and/or a master research degree pathway and culminated in progressing to a doctorate, either through a professional doctorate in nursing or midwifery research or a doctorate in philosophy (PhD). To find out more about what this entails and how you can progress on this path, talk to your local institution or professional organisation about the best options available for your own professional development.

Developing as an academic researcher requires formal research training in specific research methodologies, methods and analysis before focusing on a chosen design which usually involves a single study with a single methodology for the doctoral thesis. The end product of the doctoral training program is to complete a research project that adds to the knowledge base of the nursing and/or midwifery professions and equips the graduate with the skills to develop, manage a research project and independently undertake a research project in practice as they progress in the postdoctoral route.

Many approaches have been proposed in the international arena to develop the nursing and midwifery academic research career pathway. These approaches have proposed partnership models between universities and healthcare organisations. The academic researcher pathway is an established pathway for medical and dentistry disciplines and thus nursing and midwifery strategic leaders are trying to apply this good practice to the nursing and midwifery professions. Carrick-Sen and colleagues (2019) outline that although this pathway has been in existence for over 25 years within the UK, the pace of implementation is slow and other countries are developing this pathway in the clinical setting and are making clear progress. Internationally, there are pathways in the United States, Australia, China and the Nordic regions. Reflecting on the pace within the UK, only 0.1% of nursing, midwifery and allied health professionals have recognised academic research posts compared to 5% of medical consultants (Baltruks & Callaghan 2018).

With an international shortage of nurses and mid-wives, the clinical academic role could promote and support nurses and midwives to remain in practice developing patient care and with a career pathway that supports them remaining in practice. In the UK, local universities and healthcare organisations develop local frameworks to support staff on an academic pathway to recruit and retain nurses and midwives. One such adapted pathway is illustrated in Fig. 13.1. This has been adapted for local use from the Health Education England (HEE)/NIHR Integrated Clinical and Practitioner Academic (ICA) Programme by Michele Briggs in Manchester (with permission from Professor Michele Briggs). The five stages of the clinical academic pathway

from the HEE/NIHR model are acknowledged. It is feasible to adapt the model from a range of perspectives relevant to different environments.

The pathway implies, but does not define, when the start of the pathway is; is it after registration or during pre-registration training? Many academics and policymakers believe for nursing and midwifery to develop the clinical academic role in line with stronger research-based disciplines such as medicine and dentistry, research needs to be introduced in the pre-registration curriculum to a far greater degree than it is at present, to engage students with research. This can be on placement, by shadowing researchers and research nurses/midwives, and through your academic

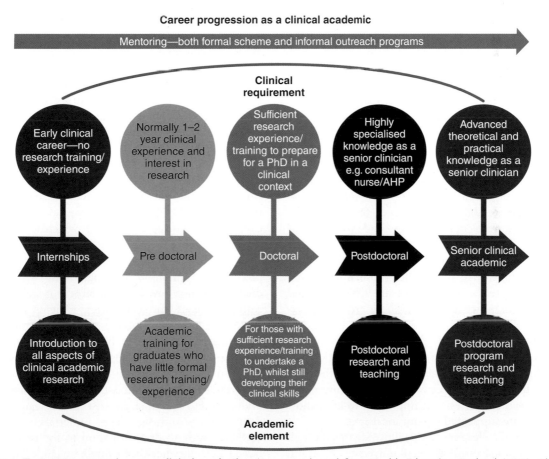

Fig. 13.1 ■ **Career progression as a clinical academic.** (Source: Adapted from Health Education England (HEE): Clinical academic careers framework: a framework for optimising clinical academic careers across healthcare professions, revised edition February 2018. https://www.hee.nhs.uk/sites/default/files/documents/2018-02%20CAC%20Framework.pdf.) AHP = allied health professional

studies. Indeed, there needs to be a realisation that being research-active is a core component of any nursing or midwifery career.

Pattison and colleagues (2021) developed a model for clinical academic involvement where there are four groups in the nursing and/or midwifery workforce: *toe dippers*, *waders*, *trackers* and *spearheaders*. These four groups encompass the wide breadth and levels of clinical academic involvement, from those who 'dip their toes' in clinical academia through to clinical professors who are leading programs of research. This relationship between clinical and research practice is particularly key for new clinical academics. The **toe dippers** may be motivated to pursue a career in academia when they can get the research support to take forward their ideas from clinical practice into a piece of research. An example of a toe dipper may be taking part in a research internship (see, for example, the NIHR Applied Research Collaboration Greater Manchester at https://arc-gm.nihr.ac.uk/). These individuals may then become **waders** who understand and perceive the value of clinical academia, and who will be connected to a research group/supervisor and develop funding bids for training at the doctoral level. The **trackers** are those who have completed doctoral studies, and who continue through to postdoctoral work which informs their area of clinical practice. Doctorally prepared nurses or midwives can raise clinical practice standards; however, there is often a deficit of career opportunities and postdoctoral positions. This impacts delivering the evidence for improving patient outcomes and service delivery. It is therefore imperative that postdoctoral nursing and midwifery career opportunities are developed and embedded in practice. Finally, there are the **spearheaders** who, underpinned by a joint institutional commitment, act as role models and clinical and research experts in their area, as well as foster clinical academic careers for others. How this pathway is funded differs both between hospitals and universities and between countries. It is important to know how programs are supported in your local area.

Weber and colleagues (2022) illustrate this through showcasing a successful model of university and health organisation partnership which developed and refined a family management intervention for parents of preterm infants. The partnership was achieved by the integration of clinical staff (in this case, nurses) with the research team members. The outcome of the study illustrated a positive outcome for the mothers and the clinical academic partnerships promoted excellence in nursing practice, research and education. A similar example is showcased by Mickan and Coates (2022) who explored the embedded researcher model in Australia and found 36% of embedded researchers were from nursing and midwifery. The majority of these reported having a research nurse or midwife within their teams, but also had a role to play in building research capacity and influencing the culture of their organisations. Further reading on the opportunities of a research career is recommended. There are several reviews that have explored developing the clinical academic workforce (Edelman et al 2021, Henshall et al 2021) and the approaches needed to establish and sustain a clinical academic partnership (Baptiste, Whalen & Goodwin 2022).

The COVID-19 pandemic placed research and the value of research in the global limelight. Research nurses/midwives and academic nurses/midwives have been at the forefront of supporting patients and healthcare systems as the world was confronted by the pandemic. The vaccine studies would not have been delivered and the vaccine not brought into the public arena if it were not for research nurses and midwives working around the clock to deliver the many vaccine trials (Hilton 2020). The recovery trial (RECOVERY Collaborative Group et al 2021), which transformed clinical care as the pandemic took hold within the acute setting and saved many patients needing mechanical ventilation and many who would have died, would not have been possible if it were not for research nurses and consenting patients at a very frightening and vulnerable period of their lives and collecting essential data on the progression of the virus and the impact on the drug interventions. Academic nurses/midwives have also played a role in leading COVID-19 research about issues impacting nurses and midwives. For example, in Australia, a team of academic nurses/midwives have undertaken a mixed methods study to draw attention to the issues being faced by primary healthcare nurses in clinical practice. This work highlighted the loss of jobs, negative psychological impacts and impact on care (Ashley et al 2021, Halcomb et al 2020, Halcomb et al 2022).

CONCLUSION

The importance of research to the continued development of nursing and midwifery practice is undeniable. Various roles and entry points are available. These roles can be supported from within a university or a healthcare organisation, or a combination of both, but regardless of where the support comes from, the focus of these roles is on how research informs practice, education or workforce elements of professional nursing and midwifery practice.

ADDITIONAL RESOURCES

Online

Clinical Academic Training & Careers Hub (CATCH): http:www.catch.ac.uk

Council of Deans of Health: Report: Becoming research confident—research placements in pre-registration nursing, midwifery and allied health programmes in the UK. Report: Becoming research confident—research placements in pre-registration nursing, midwifery and allied health programmes in the UK, 7 June 2021. https://www.councilofdeans.org.uk/2021/06/report-becoming-research-confident-research-placements-in-pre-registration-nursing-midwifery-and-allied-health-programmes-in-the-uk/

National Institute for Health and Care Research: https://www.nihr.ac.uk/

National Health and Medical Research Council: https://www.nhmrc.gov.au/

Health Research Council of New Zealand: https://www.hrc.govt.nz/

FURTHER READING

Bramley L, Manning JC, Cooper J: Engaging and developing front-line clinical nurses to drive care excellence: evaluating the chief nurse excellence in care junior fellowship initiative, Journal of Research in Nursing 23(8):678–689, 2018.

Cowley A, Diver C, Edgley A & Cooper J: Capitalising on the transformational opportunities of early clinical academic career training for nurses, midwives and allied health professionals, BMC Medical Education 20:418, 2020. https://doi.org/10.1186/s12909-020-02348-2

Richardson A, Avery M, Westwood G: A cross funder survey of enablers and barriers to progressing a research-related academic career in the nonmedical health professions, 2019, University of Southampton.

Topping A: Review: research excellence across clinical healthcare: a novel research capacity building programme for nurses and midwives in a large Irish region, Journal of Research in Nursing 23(8):707–710, 2018.

REFERENCES

Ashley C, James S, Williams A, et al: The psychological wellbeing of primary health care nurses' during COVID-19: a qualitative study, Journal of Advanced Nursing 77(9):3820–3828, 2021. http://doi.org/10.1111/jan.14937.

Baltruks D, Callaghan P: Nursing, midwifery and allied health clinical academic research careers in the UK, 2018. https://councilofdeans.org.uk/wp-content/uploads/2018/08/Nursing-midwifery-and-allied-health-clinical-academic-research-careers-in-the-UK.pdf/

Baptiste D, Whalen M, Goodwin M: Approaches for establishing and sustaining clinical academic partnerships: a discursive review, Journal of Clinical Nursing 31:329–334, 2022.

Carrick-Sen D, Richardson A, Moore A, Dolan S: Transforming healthcare through clinical academic roles in nursing, midwifery and allied health professions: a practical resource for healthcare provider organisations. AUKUH Clinical Academic Roles Development Group, 2016. https://www.medschools.ac.uk/media/2325/aukuh-transforming-healthcare.pdf.

Carrick-Sen D, Moore A, Davidson P, et al: International perspectives of nurses, midwives and allied health professionals clinical academic roles: are we at tipping point? International Journal of Practice-based Learning in Health & Social Care 7(2):1–15, 2019.

Cleaver C: Experiences of nurses transitioning to the role of research nurse, Nursing Times 116(2):55–58, 2020.

Curtis K, Fry M, Shaban R, Considine J: Translating research findings to clinical nursing practice, Journal of Clinical Nursing 26:862–872, 2017.

Edelman A, Gauld R, Ovseiko P, Murray R: Developing the multiprofessional clinical academic workforce in Australia and New Zealand: a scoping review, Evidence Base 2021(1), 2021.

Fitzpatrick S: Day in the life of a clinical research nurse, Cancer Nursing Practice 18(6):18–20, 2019.

Halcomb E, Fernandez R, Ashley C, et al: The impact of COVID-19 on primary health care delivery in Australia, Journal of Advanced Nursing 78(5):1327–1336, 2022. https://doi.org/10.1111/jan.15046

Halcomb E, McInnes S, Williams A, et al: The experiences of primary health care nurses during the COVID-19 pandemic in Australia, Journal of Nursing Scholarship 52(5):553–563, 2020. http://doi.org/10.1111/jnu.12589.

Henshall C, Kozlowska O, Walthall H, et al: Interventions and strategies aimed at clinical academic pathway development for nurses in the United Kingdom: a systematised review of the literature, Journal of Clinical Nursing Jun;30(11–12):1502–1518, 2021.

Hilton Z: Perspectives: Leadership as a Research Nurse during the pandemic, Journal of Research in Nursing 25(8):749–752, 2020.

Hastings CE, Fisher CA, McCabe MA, et al: Clinical research nursing: a critical resource in the national research enterprise, Nursing Outlook 60:149–156, 2012.

Jonker L, Fisher SJ, Dagnan D: Patients admitted to more research-active hospitals have more confidence in staff and are better informed about their condition and medication: results from a retrospective cross-sectional study, Journal of Evaluation in Clinical Practice 26(1):203–208, 2020. https://doi.org/10.1111/jep.13118.

Jonker L, Fisher SJ: The correlation between National Health Service trusts' clinical trial activity and both mortality rates and care quality commission ratings: a retrospective cross-sectional study, Public Health 157:1–6, 2018.

Kunhunny S, Salmon D: The evolving professional identity of the clinical research nurse: a qualitative exploration, Journal of Clinical Nursing 26(23–24):5121–5132, 2017. http://doi.org/10.1111/jocn.14055.

Maben J, King A: Engaging NHS staff in research, BMJ 17;365:14040, 2019.

McCabe M, Behrens L, Browning S et al: The clinical research nurse: exploring self-perceptions about the value of the role, American Journal of Nursing 119(8):24–32, 2019.

McCormack B, Baltruks D, Cooke R: Becoming research confident: Research in pre-registration curricula for nursing, midwifery and allied health programmes in the UK, London, 2019, Council of Deans of Health. https://councilofdeans.org.uk/wp-content/uploads/2019/05/CODH.RIPR_.report_v3-002.pdf.

Mickan S, Coates D: Embedded researchers in Australia: Survey of profile and experience across medical, nursing and midwifery and allied health disciplines, Journal of Clinical Nursing 31:417–426, 2022.

Ministry of Business, Innovation and Employment and Ministry of Health: New Zealand health research strategy 2017–2027: summary of submissions and consultation. Wellington, 2017, Ministry of Health.

Newington L, Alexander CM, Wells M: What is a clinical academic? Qualitative interviews with healthcare managers, research-active nurses and other research-active healthcare professionals outside medicine. Journal of Clinical Nursing 31:378–389, 2022.

Newington L, Alexander CM, Wells M: Impacts of clinical academic activity: qualitative interviews with healthcare managers and research-active nurses, midwives, allied health professionals and pharmacists, BMJ Open 11:e050679, 2021.

NHS Health Research Authority: UK policy framework for health and social care research, London, 2020, NHS.

Olive P, Maxton F, Bell C, et al: Clinical academic research internships: What works for nurses and the wider nursing, midwifery and allied health professional workforce, Journal of Clinical Nursing 31:318–328, 2022.

Oulton K, Wray J, Kelly P, et al: Culture, cognisance, capacity and capability: the interrelationship of individual and organisational factors in developing a research hospital, Journal of Clinical Nursing 31:362–377, 2022.

Pain T, Fernando M, Peterson M: Building allied health research capacity at a regional Australian hospital: a follow-up study, Internet Journal of Allied Health Sciences and Practice 16:1–10, 2018.

Pattison N, Deaton C, McCabe C, et al: Florence Nightingale's legacy for clinical academics: a framework analysis of a clinical professorial network and a model for clinical academia, Journal of Clinical Nursing 31(3–4):353–361, 2021. http://doi.org/10.1111/jocn.15756.

RECOVERY Collaborative Group, Horby P, Lim WS, et al: Dexamethasone in hospitalized patients with COVID-19, New England Journal of Medicine 25 Feb;384(8):693–704, 2021. http://doi.org/10.1056/NEJMoa2021436.

Smith S, Gullick J, Ballard J, Perry L: A proposed clinical research support career pathway for noninvestigators, International Journal of Nursing Practice 24(3):e12641, 2018b.

Smith S, Gullick J, Ballard J, Perry L: Clinician researcher career pathway for registered nurses and midwives: a proposal, International Journal of Nursing Practice 24(3):e12640, 2018a.

Theofanidis D: Research nurse and clinical academic nurse: differences and similarities, Health and Research Journal 7(4):151–154, 2021.

Tinkler L, Robinson L: Clinical research nursing and factors influencing success: a qualitative study describing the interplay between individual and organisational leadership influences and their impact on the delivery of clinical research in healthcare, Journal of Research in Nursing 25(4):361–377, 2020.

Tinkler L, Smith V, Tiannakou, Robinson L: Professional identity and the Clinical Research Nurse: a qualitative study exploring issues having an impact on participant recruitment in research, Journal of Advanced Nursing 74:318–328, 2018.

Weber A, Voos K, Bakas T, et al: A clinical-academic partnership to develop a family management intervention for parents of preterm infants, Journal of Clinical Nursing 31:390–405, 2022.

14

BRINGING IT ALL TOGETHER: APPLYING THE RESEARCH PROCESS

JENNY SIM ■ RUTH HARRIS ■ CLAIRE MINTON

CHAPTER OUTLINE

LEARNING OBJECTIVES

*After reading this chapter and following critical reflection, readers
should be able to:*

■ develop a research question from an identified problem

■ appreciate the steps involved in planning a study,
   including accessing support people, developing a
   research proposal and navigating ethics approvals

■ describe the importance of designing a study to answer
   the specific research question

■ discuss the data collection and analysis methods for
   different types of research designs

■ recognise the importance of disseminating research
   findings

■ explain the importance of translating research findings
   into practice.

KEY TERMS

literature review

mentor

mixed methods research

research dissemination

research proposal

research question

knowledge translation

qualitative research

quantitative research

189

ABSTRACT

This chapter brings together the knowledge on research gained from reading this text and aims to help you navigate the research process. We start with identifying a research problem or an area of interest and the steps taken to understand what is already known on the issue. We provide guidance on how to access support from more-experienced researchers and encourage you to identify a research mentor. For people interested in undertaking research, we provide guidance on how to write a research proposal, plan a research project and then consider how research needs to be both disseminated and translated into practice settings. We understand that research can be daunting, but we hope to inspire you and encourage you to participate in a research project, and maybe even become a future nurse or midwife researcher.

Don't wait for the light to appear at the end of the tunnel—stride down there and light the bloody thing yourself.

(Henderson 1993)

INTRODUCTION

In this chapter, we bring together all the pieces of the research puzzle that you have been exploring as you have learned about nursing and midwifery research. We refer to important information in other chapters that set the foundations for your knowledge and guide you through the steps of the research process. We use exemplars from published research to demonstrate how you can identify a problem, undertake a **literature review**, develop a **research question** and design a study to answer the research question. We provide tips for success (Box 14.1) and recommend identifying a research **mentor** to support you in your research journey. We aim to help 'pull it all together' and inspire you to consider undertaking your own research in the future.

SO, YOU'VE GOT A PROBLEM

All good research begins with a problem that you want to explore. Your problem can relate to your

---

BOX 14.1
TIPS FOR SUCCESS WHEN COMPLETING A RESEARCH PROJECT

- Identify a problem that interests you
- Review the literature on the topic
- Narrow down your topic so it is manageable
- Discuss your research idea with healthcare professionals in the relevant setting
- Find a research mentor
- Develop a clear research question
- Make sure your research design is appropriate to answer your question
- Write a comprehensive research proposal
- Undertake training in research ethics and integrity
- Prepare and submit your ethics application with the support of a mentor or more-experienced researcher
- Develop a realistic timeline and do not underestimate how long it may take to complete the research process
- Keep a research diary to capture your thoughts and decision-making throughout the study
- Apply for funding to help cover the costs of your research

---

experiences in clinical practice settings or it may relate to a workforce problem or an education concern. You may experience this problem personally, or you may become aware of it by talking with others or reading a research paper. Regardless of how the problem was identified, you now have the skills to explore it using the research process.

Clarifying Your Ideas

The first step involves clarifying your ideas. Depending on the problem, this may include talking to colleagues, more-experienced nurses/midwives or members of the multidisciplinary team. It may also include looking for guidelines and policy documents about the problem. This is likely to lead you to review the literature to explore existing research on the topic. To ensure you examine the problem comprehensively, we encourage you to ask an answerable question. Your question is the key to everything in research. It might be very specific, quite broad or exploratory, depending on how much knowledge is already out there about the area you are interested in.

Searching the Literature

To gather a comprehensive answer to a research question, you will need to search the literature for research that helps to either answer the question or clarify the gaps in knowledge related to the problem. The reason for undertaking the literature search will determine how comprehensive the search process will need to be. Let's look at our case studies. Both Ahmed and Jamie will need to search the literature to look for research papers to help them complete their assignments. Ahmed may choose to look for studies that examine the lived experiences of carers who have chronic health conditions. Jamie may choose to explore guidelines to support evidence-based interventions for type 1 diabetes among women with learning disabilities. The strategies you learned in Chapter 2 on finding research evidence will help you to search the academic literature rapidly and find studies that can help you answer your research questions.

If you intend to conduct a research project, then you need to do a more comprehensive search of the literature to determine what is already known on your topic and where the gaps in knowledge exist. Revise the steps in Chapter 3 on conducting a literature review. We also recommend that you consult a health librarian to help you get started. You may have access to a librarian in your workplace or at a local university.

We will explore an example to illustrate these steps (See Box 14.2).

BOX 14.2
AN EXAMPLE OF A SYSTEMATIC REVIEW OF THE LITERATURE ON PRESSURE INJURY PREVALENCE

SYSTEMATIC REVIEW OF PRESSURE INJURY PREVALENCE IN AUSTRALIAN AND NEW ZEALAND HOSPITALS

Rodgers K, Sim J & Clifton, R

Abstract

Background: Pressure injuries have a major impact on patients and healthcare organisations. The complications of pressure injuries increase morbidity and mortality rates and are costly to individuals and healthcare systems. The total prevalence rate of pressure injuries within acute-care hospitals in Australia and New Zealand is unknown and despite a focus on prevention, pressure injuries still occur within these hospital settings.

Aim: To report the prevalence of pressure injuries within acute-care settings in Australian and New Zealand hospitals and to identify the stage and location of pressure injuries and analyse the methods used to conduct pressure injury point prevalence studies.

Methods: A systematic review of studies published in CINAHL, MEDLINE and Cochrane databases and a two-part grey literature search, including a customised Google search and a targeted website search, was undertaken up to July 2019. The systematic review was prospectively registered with PROSPERO (CRD42018105566).

Findings: The overall prevalence of pressure injuries in acute-care hospitals in Australia and New Zealand is 12.9% (95% CI, 9.5%–16.8%) and the hospital-acquired pressure injury prevalence is 7.9% (95% CI, 5.7%–10.3%). Stage I and stage II are the most common pressure injuries. The most frequent locations for pressure injuries are the sacrum/buttock/coccyx area (41%) and the heels (31%). The reporting of details about methodology varies considerably between studies.

Discussion: Pressure injuries remain a significant problem within acute-care hospital settings. Total prevalence rates are decreasing over time with the numbers of stage I and II pressure injuries decreasing faster than other pressure injuries.

Conclusion: The findings from this study can be used to set performance benchmarks within acute-care hospitals in Australia and New Zealand. Pressure injuries are preventable and pressure injury prevalence studies can be used to monitor the effectiveness of nursing care processes to improve patient outcomes.

Keywords: Australia, New Zealand, prevalence, pressure injury, pressure ulcer, HAPI, hospital-acquired, adverse event, acute care

Source: Rodgers K, Sim J, Clifton R: Systematic review of pressure injury prevalence in Australian and New Zealand hospitals, Collegian 28(3), 310–323, 2021. http://doi.org/10.1016/j.colegn.2020.08.012.

Undertaking a Literature Review (an Exemplar)

The first author of this chapter was asked by a final-year Bachelor of Nursing student how common pressure injuries (also called pressure ulcers) were in Australian hospitals. This led to the student commencing a Bachelor of Nursing (Honours) project that sought to answer the question: 'What is the prevalence of pressure injuries among patients who are admitted to acute-care hospitals in Australia and New Zealand?' (Rodgers, Sim & Clifton 2021). PICO(T) was used to structure the question and then the search strategy was developed (see Table 14.1). This literature review was conducted as a systematic review and meta-analysis because the research question sought to estimate pressure injury prevalence among patients admitted to acute-care hospitals in Australia and New Zealand and there was sufficient literature to answer this question. There are many different types of literature reviews, and the type of review chosen will depend on the research question. You can refer back to Chapter 3 to revise the different types of literature reviews.

In this example, critical appraisal and data extraction were completed using the JBI checklist and data extraction tool for studies using prevalence data (Munn et al 2014). Data was then presented in a summary table and data on prevalence was combined using meta-analysis to answer the research question(s).

You will find more details about all these steps in Chapter 3.

PLANNING A RESEARCH PROJECT

Once you have done a literature review, you will be able to identify any gaps in current knowledge. This will help you identify any questions that you might want to answer in a future research project. Even though you have identified a knowledge gap, the thought of doing a research project might be daunting. It is often at this stage that you need the support of an experienced researcher, who can guide you on how to frame a research question and support you to develop a research design that answers the research question. Reading the literature on your topic area and about the methodology and methods you are likely to use will also help you to plan your project. Reading examples of other research projects can help you understand how best to describe your research design and the procedures you will be using. It is sometimes helpful to also consider the methodologies that have been used in similar studies in your research area of interest, to see their appropriateness to answer your research question.

Accessing Support and Finding a Mentor

When you start participating in research, you generally do so on a small scale with an experienced researcher

TABLE 14.1		
Developing a Question and Search Strategy for a Literature Review Using PICO(T)		
Focused Research Question: What is the Prevalence of Pressure Injuries Among Patients who are Admitted to Acute-Care Hospitals in Australia and New Zealand?		
Population	The population was people admitted to hospital.	'Acute care' OR hospital* OR inpatient*
Intervention/issue	The 'issue' was pressure injuries (also called pressure ulcers, bed sores, decubitus ulcers etc.)	'pressure injur*' OR 'pressure ulcer' OR 'bed sore' OR 'decubitus ulcer'
Comparison	We wanted to quantify the number of people who develop a pressure injury, so there is no true comparator in this research.	N/A
Outcome	We are trying to estimate how many people have a pressure injury as a proportion of the total number of people in hospital, and will therefore use prevalence of pressure injuries as the outcome of interest.	'prevalence'
Type of study	Cross-sectional observational studies that examined pressure injury prevalence as a percentage of patients in hospital.	('prevalence')

to guide you. Identifying a person who can support you to develop your research skills will be invaluable. You may even be invited to join their research team and start out by getting involved in existing research projects. Undertaking research as part of a team enables you to learn from others by doing and collaborating (especially in multidisciplinary teams), and helps you see the research questions from different perspectives. Another advantage of working in a team is that you can undertake the research in a few different settings, which can lead to a larger and more diverse study that can have an impact on a wider range of settings.

You may want to consider approaching someone to become a research mentor. Possible mentors may be experienced researchers who work in your organisation or nursing/midwifery academics from a nearby university. Talk to your nursing/midwifery leaders about your interests and ask them to help you identify a suitable mentor. Make sure to read any publications they have authored and ask others who have worked with them what the experience was like, so you can identify if the two of you might work well together. Professional organisations such as Sigma Nursing and the International Confederation of Midwives provide resources to support education and networking among members. National organisations, such as the Royal College of Nursing in the United Kingdom (UK) and the Australian College of Nursing, also provide mentoring programs that can support connections.

STUDENT CHALLENGE

Identifying a Research Mentor

How would you go about identifying a research mentor? Think about people you could approach in your workplace or at your local university. If you are interested in research, then make an appointment to meet them and have a conversation.

Developing a Research Proposal

Whether you are undertaking a small or larger research project, you generally need to start with a **research proposal**. The research proposal describes the blueprint or plan for the study and must persuade the reader that the research:

- is important to nursing/midwifery practice
- has been informed by previous research

- has a clear research question
- is scientifically rigorous
- is feasible and you have the skills and knowledge to complete it
- is worthy of any funding that may be requested
- has a realistic and achievable timeline.

It is important to have a well-developed plan before writing up the research proposal. You should consider collecting all the information that you will require and begin to develop the research proposal well before you apply for ethical approval for your research. Key stakeholders in the settings where you are considering conducting the research should have input into the planned research. This engagement helps to develop support for the project and can increase the feasibility of the research project due to the input of stakeholders.

Most ethics committees or organisations in which you work will have a template for a research proposal. Ask for a copy of this template and work with a mentor or experienced researcher to develop the proposal.

Timeline and Budget

Your proposal is likely to include a timeline and a budget. The purpose of the timeline is to show that the research is both realistic and feasible. The timeline will help you and others know how much time you must allocate to the research given your other roles and responsibilities, and whether the time anticipated for carrying out the study is realistic. The timeline needs to reflect these aspects and should indicate:

- when each component will commence and finish
- how long each of the components of the research will take you to carry out
- the duration of the project
- if tasks will be occurring consecutively or concurrently.

Some of the research components that may need to be accounted for in a timeline are ethical approval, staff training for research protocols, recruitment, data collection, intervention, data entry, data analysis, report writing and **research dissemination**.

The budget outlines the costs of undertaking the research project. It is important to carefully consider the resources you need and what they will cost. The budget is likely to include costs for personnel (such as research assistants, statisticians and people to enter data or transcribe audio files), equipment (such as computers, digital recorders or diagnostic equipment such as calorimeters or activity trackers), maintenance costs for existing equipment (such as in a laboratory or clinical setting) and travel expenses.

You may be lucky enough to get money from a funding source, such as your university if you are a student or health service where you work, to assist with any research costs. While gaining access to large amounts of funds is unlikely until you are a more-experienced researcher, this may occur if you are part of a research team. It is important to keep track of all funding you are awarded in your curriculum vitae as it helps to convince people later on that they should fund your research.

The next section will explore some of the important concepts related to conducting a research project.

STUDENT CHALLENGE

Developing a Research Proposal

Do you have a research problem you would like to explore? You can start by using a research proposal template. Most universities have examples of the research proposal that they would expect for a research degree, and these can be adapted based on your circumstances.

A guide to developing a research proposal is also available at this link: https://www.ucl.ac.uk/ioe-writing-centre/plan-your-assignment/write-a-research-proposal.

DESIGNING YOUR STUDY

Developing Your Research Question

Formulating a research question is one of the most important aspects of your study. It will determine the scope and direction of your study and the research design and methods you will use. Research questions are not always written well. Good research questions are clear and focused, enabling the study to lead to a reliable and useful answer. When a research question is poorly formulated, it is likely to lead to difficulties in designing a study to answer it and an uncertain answer which may cause confusion. Bad questions include those that are:

- too simple, and perhaps can be answered by a simple yes or no answer
- focused on more than one topic or issue
- unanswerable

- too broad
- not new and don't extend knowledge beyond what has already been answered.

We can illustrate how to create a research question by thinking about our case studies. Ahmed could ask: 'Does regular support by the nursing team enable older adults with multiple comorbidities to continue to undertake their caring responsibilities?' Do you think is a good or bad question? Think about why.

Jamie could ask: 'Can a young person living with a learning disability who has newly diagnosed type 1 diabetes self-manage their care and treatment?' or 'Do more young people living with a learning disability require foster care?' What do you think about these questions? Refer to Chapter 4 and try to improve the research questions for Jamie.

Different questions will require different research designs, and the design you choose is influenced by the type of knowledge you are trying to generate. We will now provide a summary of quantitative, qualitative and mixed methods research (please refer back to Chapters 7, 8 and 9 for more detailed explanations).

Quantitative Research Designs

Quantitative research was explored in detail in Chapter 7. Quantitative research uses systematic and objective processes to gather and analyse data that has been measured by some type of instrument. Quantitative research projects seek to describe, examine relationships and compare groups. Data collection tends to be structured and the methods tightly defined and controlled to reduce bias and ensure the sample is representative of the population being studied. The data collection may be via survey, existing administrative datasets, medical records, physical measurements, validated instruments and tests. The variables (factors, conditions or traits) must be measured using reliable and valid measurement tools; for this reason, a description of how the variables are defined and measured is necessary. Statistical data analysis is carried out on quantitative data.

An example of a quantitative study is the Impact of COVID-19 on Nurses (ICON) longitudinal survey that was developed in response to the COVID-19 pandemic. The research team were aware of the high levels of stress and burnout experienced by nursing staff before the COVID-19 pandemic and sought to identify the personal and workplace factors associated with well-being among nurses (Couper et al 2022). The outcome of greatest importance in quantitative research is called the primary outcome measure, and it is this outcome that informs how many participants are required (Malone et al 2016). In the ICON survey, the primary outcome measure was the prevalence of posttraumatic stress disorder, which was measured using the validated Impact of Events Scale—Revised (IES-R) (Creamer et al 2003) at each time point. Additional outcome measures included: depression, anxiety, stress, job satisfaction, burnout and the participant's intention to leave both their current role and healthcare employment.

Qualitative Research Designs

Qualitative research was explored in Chapter 8. Qualitative designs are generally used when little information is available or when an in-depth understanding of a process or experience is required. The strength of qualitative designs is that they can generate theory or deep understanding. Qualitative designs are not useful for testing hypotheses, nor are the results of this research necessarily applicable to a larger population, as they tend to use small numbers of participants to gain greater depth in each context. Qualitative designs tend to use less-structured forms of data collection such as interviews, focus groups or observations. Analysis of the data can be carried out by various methods, which are influenced by the type of qualitative research being conducted. For example, a qualitative descriptive study may use thematic analysis and grounded theory uses constant comparative analysis.

Building on the ICON longitudinal survey, the research team were aware that a quantitative study would not be able to provide detailed insights into the experiences of nursing staff during the COVID-19 pandemic. Therefore, a separate study, called the ICON longitudinal interview study, was developed to better understand and explore the full impact of COVID-19 on UK nurses with a specific focus on nurses' psychological, psychosocial and emotional health needs along the trajectory of the pandemic (Maben et al 2022).

Mixed Methods Research

Mixed methods research involves the collection and integration of both quantitative and qualitative data within one study to gain a better understanding of the topic under investigation. One of the benefits of mixed methods research is that it enables a researcher to draw on the strengths of both quantitative and qualitative methods to develop a multifaceted perspective on the research topic. Chapter 9 provides an in-depth description of mixed methods research.

An example of a mixed methods study is a large research project undertaken in the UK to evaluate intentional rounding. A mixed method design was used to investigate the impact and effectiveness of intentional rounding in hospital wards in relation to the organisation, delivery and experience of care from the perspective of patients, their family members and staff (Harris et al 2017, Harris et al 2019, Sims et al 2020). This approach allowed researchers to gain a more complete picture of how intentional rounding was working, from a range of perspectives, which would not have been possible with a purely quantitative or qualitative study.

Ethical Considerations in Conducting Research

Before commencing data collection, you must gain ethical approval from the most appropriate ethics committee. Chapter 6 provided a comprehensive overview of the requirements and processes involved in gaining ethical approval for your study. We would encourage you to go back and review this chapter as well as Chapters 10 and 11, which explore important issues on vulnerable populations and equality, inclusion and diversity. There is no doubt that research conducted in nursing and midwifery presents multiple ethical considerations, and an ethical design is a moral requirement (Pietilä et al 2020). For example, if Jamie were to undertake research with young people under 18 years of age with a learning disability, there would be significant ethical issues to consider and address (McNeilly, Macdonald & Kelly 2020). Principles of integrity, respect for persons, beneficence and justice need to be considered throughout the research process.

STUDENT CHALLENGE

Ethical Considerations in Conducting Research

Think about the case study related to Jamie, Martha or Ahmed. If a researcher was to conduct a research project related to one of these scenarios, what are some of the ethical considerations?

Disseminating Your Research

After you have collected and analysed your data, it is important to disseminate the findings from your study. This should include sharing the outcomes with all key stakeholders and depending on the research design used may also include sharing the findings with participants. We encourage you to work with your mentor or an experienced researcher to write a publication from the study and share your findings at local, national and international conferences, as well as on social media. Writing for publication and presenting your research at conferences can be daunting, but this is an important step in the research process so that the knowledge generated by your research is shared.

TRANSLATION OF YOUR RESEARCH INTO PRACTICE

An important part of the research process is **knowledge translation**. Knowledge translation is a multistage process of implementing practice change to align with new evidence. This process has been described in Chapter 12. Numerous organisational and individual factors impact the uptake of new research findings into practice. Many of these barriers relate to human behaviours; therefore, successful implementation of research findings into practice involves changing behaviour and building relationships in the practice setting. For this reason, it is important when planning your project to consider how you will translate your findings into the practice setting.

CONSOLIDATING YOUR RESEARCH SKILLS

As you have seen throughout this book, research is important to all roles in nursing and midwifery and research is 'everybody's business'. Using high-quality research to guide practice is of the utmost importance and a fundamental responsibility of nurses and midwives. Some people reading this text will be keen to develop the research component of their role further and there are many opportunities to further these ambitions. Some of these opportunities include.

- Undertake an honours/master degree. Enrolling in an honours or master degree may enable you to complete coursework focused on research methods or a thesis on a research topic. This will enhance your research skills.
- Undertake a doctorate of philosophy (PhD). You may choose to complete a PhD that involves undertaking a research project to contribute new knowledge to the field of nursing or midwifery. A PhD is considered a comprehensive research training program. Look out for funded scholarships, fellowships and internships, which can provide excellent support to develop an academic or clinical academic career (Long 2019). See Chapter 13 for more discussion on academic careers.
- Apply for a research assistant or research fellow role. There is a range of research roles in research centres and higher education institutes, such as universities, that support the development of research skills and knowledge. These posts are usually to work on a specific project or program of funded research but provide a great opportunity to gain experience and insight into research.
- Take up a clinical research role. Clinical research nurses and midwives have a vital role in delivering clinical research. Clinical research nurse and midwife roles can include supporting a patient through their treatment as part of a clinical trial, preparing trial protocols and other trial-related documentation and collecting data. More information on clinical research roles is available in Chapter 13.

There are many useful resources providing more information about developing a career that includes research work, such as the following from the UK:

- Royal College of Nursing: https://www.rcn.org.uk/Professional-Development/research-and-innovation/Research-training-and-careers
- National Institute for Health Research (NIHR): https://www.nihr.ac.uk/health-and-care-professionals/career-development/.

STUDENT CHALLENGE

Next Steps in Consolidating Your Research Skills

Make some notes on what next steps you can take to develop your research skills. You might want to explore simple actions like reading more research papers or developing your search skills.

For those interested in being a part of a research project, what steps can you take to make this a reality?

CONCLUSION

Research in nursing and midwifery can seem quite daunting. We have all experienced that feeling of apprehension and not knowing where to start! In this final chapter, we have sought to 'bring together' what you have learned in this text and show how you can apply the research process. We hope you will feel confident in examining the literature on a topic, and that if there is a gap in the literature, you feel prepared to consider undertaking a research project. We encourage you to identify a research mentor or an experienced researcher to guide you if you seek to develop a research project. When you are working on your project, it will be important for you to meet with your mentor regularly and seek help and advice from a range of people with the expertise you need. You don't need to do this on your own—in fact you shouldn't! Research is a team activity. It underpins our practice in nursing and midwifery and, regardless of what setting you work in, understanding and using research is pivotal to providing high-quality, safe and effective care to patients and consumers.

ADDITIONAL RESOURCES

When you read research articles, look for evidence of the research process—there should be a clear decision trail laid as to how the study was planned and conducted. We encourage you to read the methods and results sections of papers to help familiarise you with the research process.

There are excellent resources on many websites to assist you in understanding the research process; for example:

JBI—Critical Appraisal Tools: https://jbi.global/critical-appraisal-tools
Cochrane: https://www.cochrane.org/
Campbell Collaboration: https://www.campbellcollaboration.org/
NIHR Evidence: https://evidence.nihr.ac.uk/
EQUATOR Network: https://www.equator-network.org/
Clinical Information Access Project (CIAP), Introduction to Evidence-Based Practice and CIAP: https://www.ciap.health.nsw.gov.au/training/ebp-learning-modules/module1/index.html

HETI (Health Education and Training Institute NSW): Research Module: https://www.heti.nsw.gov.au/education-and-training/courses-and-programs/research-introduction-for-beginners
EBSCO Health/CINAHL: 7 Steps to the Perfect PICO Search: https://www.ebsco.com/sites/g/files/nabnos191/files/acquiadam-assets/7-Steps-to-the-Perfect-PICO-Search-White-Paper_0.pdf
Vitae: Realising the potential of researchers: https://www.vitae.ac.uk/

See if you can find other useful resources on the web more generally or in electronic databases. Nearly all university libraries will have resources to support your understanding of the research process.

REFERENCES

Couper K, Murrells T, Sanders J, et al: The impact of COVID-19 on the wellbeing of the UK nursing and midwifery workforce during the first pandemic wave: a longitudinal survey study, International Journal of Nursing Studies Mar;127:104155, 2022. https://doi.org/10.1016/j.ijnurstu.2021.104155.

Creamer M, Bell R, Failla S: Psychometric properties of the impact of event scale—revised. Behaviour Research and Therapy 41(12):1489–1496, 2003.

Harris R, Sims S, Leamy M, et al: Intentional rounding in hospital wards to improve regular interaction and engagement between nurses and patients: a realist evaluation, Health Services and Delivery Research 7(35):1–168, 2019. https://doi.org/10.3310/hsdr07350.

Harris R, Sims S, Levenson R, et al: What aspects of intentional rounding work in hospital wards, for whom and in what circumstances? A realist evaluation protocol, BMJ Open 7(1):e014776, 2017. https://doi.org/10.1136/bmjopen-2016-014776.

Henderson S: From strength to strength: an autobiography, Melbourne, 1993, Sun Books.

Long T: Why undertake a clinical academic internship? A novice researcher's reflection. Nurse Researcher 7 Jun;30(2), 2019. http://doi.org/10.7748/nr.2019.e1664.

Maben J, Conolly A, Abrams R, et al: 'You can't walk through water without getting wet': UK nurses' distress and psychological health needs during the Covid-19 pandemic: a longitudinal interview study, International Journal of Nursing Studies Jul;131:104242; 2022. https://doi.org/10.1016/j.ijnurstu.2022.104242.

Malone HE, Nicholl H, Coyne I: Fundamentals of estimating sample size, Nurse Researcher 23(5):21–25, 2016. http://doi.org/10.7748/nr.23.5.21.s5.

McNeilly P, Macdonald G, Kelly B: Ethical considerations when conducting research with children and young people with disabilities in health and social care, Nurse Researcher 7 Jun;30(2), 2020. http://doi.org/10.7748/nr.2020.e1645.

Mum Z, Moola S, Lisy K, Riitano D: Joanna Briggs Institute Reviewers Manual: 2014 edition/supplement, Adelaide, 2014, Joanna Briggs Institute. https://nursing.lsuhsc.edu/JBI/docs/ReviewersManuals/Prevalence-and-Incidence-Data.pdf.

Pietilä A-M, Nurmi S-M, Halkoaho A, Kyngäs H (eds): Qualitative research: ethical considerations. In Kyngäs H, Mikkonen K, Kääriäinen M, The application of content analysis in nursing science research, 2020, Springer International Publishing, pp. 49–69. https://doi.org/10.1007/978-3-030-30199-6_6.

Rodgers K, Sim J, Clifton R: Systematic review of pressure injury prevalence in Australian and New Zealand hospitals, Collegian 28(3):310–323, 2021. http://doi.org/10.1016/j.colegn.2020.08.012.

Sims S, Leamy M, Levenson R, et al: The delivery of compassionate nursing care in a tick-box culture: Qualitative perspectives from a realist evaluation of intentional rounding, International Journal of Nursing Studies Jul;107:103580, 2020. https://doi.org/10.1016/j.ijnurstu.2020.103580.

GLOSSARY

Aboriginal and Torres Strait Islander peoples The first peoples or Indigenous peoples of Australia.

Alternative hypothesis States that there is a relationship between the two variables being studied (one variable has an effect on the other). This is an alternate to the null hypothesis.

Appraisal tool A structured guide to undertaking a critical appraisal.

Autonomy The right to self-determination. This assumes that the individual or a group of people have the wisdom to make the best choice for themselves.

Beneficence The concept of doing good. This assumes the performance of actions leading to outcomes that would be regarded as worthwhile.

Bias In scientific research, this occurs when conscious, unconscious or unintentional influences impact a study's outcomes.

Blinding The process of keeping study participants and sometimes those involved in the conduct of a trial unaware of which treatment or intervention is being administered.

Call number Number–letter combination used to identify each individual item on the shelves within the library.

Case study In-depth research study of an individual unit (e.g. a person, family, ward, practice setting or other identified social unit). Differs from case report, which is a descriptive report of a specific patient(s) case.

Catalogue A list of books and other graphic material in a library arranged in a specific order.

Citation database Citation databases contain structured and searchable lists of cited references for each documented publication, in addition to other bibliographic information. This makes it possible to evaluate how often a publication or an author has been cited and forms the basis for all bibliometric analysis.

Clinical academic A health professional who works concurrently in academic and clinical environments.

Clinical significance Determined through establishing how much benefit or harm results from a treatment or intervention; it is the practical impact of a treatment.

Colonisation The oftentimes violent process a dominant country uses to establish a colony by asserting control over and suppressing the Indigenous peoples in the area. It involves the appropriation of land, depopulation of people, economic and social marginalisation and loss of language and cultural practices.

Concurrent mixed methods Design in which the qualitative and quantitative data are collected at the same time, but independently of each other.

Concurrent validity Involves comparing a new test with an existing test (of the same nature) to see if they produce similar results.

Confidence interval Describes the range within which the supported value (i.e. size of the effect of an exposure) is expected to lie within a given degree of certainty (95% or 99%).

Confidentiality The privacy of written or spoken information, or observed behaviours through body language, acquired through privileged access.

Consent An agreement by a person to participate voluntarily in research after being fully informed about the study and the inherent risks and benefits of participation.

Control group A group that receives usual care or no intervention that provides a baseline to which a treatment or intervention group can be compared.

Co-production In research, this is when researchers and research teams collaborate with members of the public to design, develop, perform, analyse, evaluate and disseminate research. All persons involved are seen as equals in the research process. This helps to strengthen the research and make it more relevant and applicable to the community on which it is focused. Co-production adds credibility and trustworthiness to the research.

Correlation A relationship between variables or the process of establishing a relationship between variables.

Credibility Steps taken to make certain of accuracy, authenticity and validity of qualitative data.

Critical appraisal A structured process through which the strengths and limitations of research are evaluated and clinical relevance is established.

Critical thinking The process of questioning, interpreting, analysing, determining relevance and making judgments on information.

Culturally safe Culturally safe nursing practice recognises, respects and is inclusive of a patient's unique cultural identity. It is determined by the patient and their family feeling they have received respectful care that has included important cultural needs.

Culturally competent Refers to nurses' and midwives' having a comprehension of their own worldviews, sociocultural positioning and acting in respectful and responsive ways with people regardless of cultural background.

Data The plural term for information collected during a study.

Data collection The gathering of information necessary to address the research problem.

Data extraction Extracting and tabulating specific information.

Data immersion Repeated engagement with primary data to become familiar with its content, feeling and tone. This can mean listening and relistening to digitally recorded data and reading and rereading text (qualitative).

Data saturation A term used in qualitative research when further data reveals no new information than that which was already provided by the dataset.

Deductive reasoning Also called deduction; sets out with a general case from which specific instances are deduced.

Dependent variable A variable whose value depends on that of another.

Descriptive statistics Used to document the characteristics of a set of variables to classify or understand the scope of the topic of interest which provides the basis for further investigation.

Directional hypothesis A prediction made by a researcher regarding a positive or negative change, relationship or difference between two variables of a population.

Discrimination When people are treated unjustly and in unfair ways which are different or founded on unsubstantiated negative stereotypes based on age, sex and/or ethnic, social and cultural differences.

Distribution The distribution of a variable reflects the frequency of the occurrence of the range of values for variables in an observation.

Diversity The combination of our differences which are mainly age, race, religion, gender, disability, sexual orientation, socioeconomic status and social class. It is concerned with how these differences shape our view of the world and subsequently approach the society to which we belong. It is about valuing each other's differences and life experiences that make us who we are.

Electronic database A file of digitised information bibliographic records, abstracts, full-text documents, directory entries, images, statistics, etc. related to a specific subject or field, consisting of records of uniform format organised for ease and speed of search and retrieval and managed with the aid of database management system (DBMS) software.

Epistemology The study of knowledge; theorising about the nature and origin of knowledge.

Equity Recognises that each person has different situations, conditions and status and they are all afforded opportunities and resources in a fair and just manner to achieve an equal outcome.

Ethical principles Principles that describe what is expected in terms of right and correct and wrong or incorrect, in terms of behaviour and moral judgment.

Ethics The branch of knowledge that deals with doing what is right or morally acceptable.

Ethnography Qualitative research design that focuses on the worldview of an identified cultural group.

Evidence Proof or findings that can be used as the basis for decisions.

Evidence-based practice (EBP) An approach to care that combines the best available evidence with clinician judgment and personal/societal preferences for care.

Extraneous variables Any variable that is not being investigated but can potentially affect the outcomes of the research.

Face validity Whether an instrument appears to measure what it is supposed to measure.

Fidelity The extent to which an intervention is delivered as planned; the obligation to remain faithful to one's commitments to others, particularly promises given in confidence.

Focus groups A qualitative data collection technique, where groups of people who experience the phenomenon under investigation are interviewed together.

Focused mapping review and synthesis (FMRS) This review focuses on a field of knowledge to create a descriptive map of the findings rather than a synthesis.

Generalisation The ability to apply study results from the sample to the larger population.

Good Clinical Practice (GCP) Training for clinical trials based on principles derived from the World Medical Association's Declaration of Helsinki. The Declaration of Helsinki was used as a basis for the development of guidance for the conduct of clinical trials.

Grey literature Literature not formally published. It can appear in many forms, including government reports, statistics, patents, conference papers and even non-written resources such as posters and infographics.

Grounded theory Qualitative research that develops theoretical propositions about identified social/psychological processes from collected data.

Human rights The basic rights and freedoms that are inherent to everyone regardless of our background, where we live, sex, race, religion, language or any other status.

Hypothesis A predictive statement about the outcomes of a quantitative study.

Inclusion Occurs when individuals have the opportunity to contribute to society and fulfil their potential; when individuals have access to opportunities and resources; when they can contribute their own ideas and perspectives to improve a situation or meet an organisational aim; and when individuals have a sense of belonging to a group, organisation and society. It is a state of being made part of something and being socially and culturally accepted.

Inclusive research When researchers and practitioners work together with people such as those with intellectual disabilities, children, older people, survivors of mental health systems to plan and undertake research together rather than particular groups having research done 'on' them.

Independent variable A variable whose variation does not depend on that of another. In intervention studies it is this variable that is manipulated.

Index Historically used for a list of citations to periodicals and other publications such as newspapers and government or professional documents. Online indexes are now more commonly referred to as electronic databases.

Indigenous peoples The original inhabitants of a particular area. Also known as First Nations peoples.

Inductive reasoning Reasoning that moves from the particular to the general. It is a form of reasoning process in which a conclusion is drawn from particular cases (i.e. from the particular to the general) as opposed to deductive reasoning.

Inferential statistics To test theories or hypotheses about relationships or the effect of treatments, we need to make statistical inferences. Inferential statistics underpin decisions that allow researchers to estimate population characteristics from a sample of that population.

Information literacy The capacity to know when information is needed, and the ability to find, appraise, organise and use the information effectively.

Informed consent Communication in which permission is granted in full knowledge of the possible consequences, typically that which is given by a patient to a doctor or nurse for treatment with knowledge of the possible risks and benefits.

Instrument Device or technique used to collect data in research (e.g. biophysical instruments such as glucometers, psychological instruments such as questionnaires or interviews, behavioural instruments such as observation).

Integrative review A review method that summarises the literature to provide a comprehensive understanding of what is known about an issue or phenomenon.

Interlibrary loan/document delivery A service whereby a library sources items from other libraries for staff or student use.

Intersectionality The interrelated categorisation of people according to, for example, their race, class, gender, different abilities and socioeconomic status applied to individuals and groups of people. Intersectionality highlights those with privilege and can identify the compounding effects of disadvantage associated with each categorisation.

Intuition A 'gut feeling' or 'hunch' that comes from a place of personal experience and might not be explained or backed up easily by logic or facts; to have insight into the whole of a situation without possessing readily supportable or confirming data.

Journal A scholarly publication comprised of manuscripts written by researchers and other experts. May be peer reviewed or non-peer reviewed. *See also* peer reviewed.

Justice The concept that society has a responsibility to treat people fairly. This concept is considered in three categories: fair distribution of resources, respect for people's rights and respect for morally acceptable laws.

Knowledge translation (KT) The thought processes involved in reading, appraising and making a decision about using research findings in practice; a means of operating by understanding essential information about the world around us that allows us to function more effectively. *See also* research translation.

Lifeworld A term used by philosophers to describe the everyday world; that is, the real world as given to us by experience.

Literature review Critical summary of available literature on the selected topic.

Literature search Systematically retrieving the available literature on a selected topic.

Māori peoples The Indigenous peoples of Aotearoa New Zealand.

Method The specific means by which data are collected for a study (e.g. survey, interview).

Mentor A more-experienced researcher who acts as an adviser to a novice or less-experienced researcher.

Methodology Approach used by the researcher to guide the conduct of the study (e.g. phenomenology, grounded theory or randomised controlled trial).

Microform Consists of microfilm and microfiche that allows the reader to view different documents stored on film; for example, newspapers and historical records.

Mixed methods research Use of both qualitative and quantitative methods of data collection in a single study. For example, combining qualitative interviews and quantitative survey data collection.

Multimethod research Use of two or more data collection methods from the same research tradition. For example, participant observation and interviews (qualitative) or survey and population census data (quantitative).

Naturalistic paradigm Values subjectivity, is exploratory in nature, seeks to explore human experiences and associated meaning, and aims to describe and interpret these rather than quantify a research problem.

Normal distribution A continuous probability distribution that is symmetrical on both sides of the mean, so the right side of the centre is a mirror image of the left side.

Non-experimental research Quantitative research in which concepts are not manipulated, but are examined as they occur naturally.

Non-maleficence The concept of avoiding harm. This can vary according to context, and influences what we think and do to prevent harm to others.

Null hypothesis A hypothesis where there is no significant difference between specified populations with any observed difference being due to sampling or experimental error.

Nursing ethics Ethical and bioethical issues explored from the perspective of nursing theory and practice.

Peer reviewed A process whereby literature is subjected to a process of critical evaluation by one or more experts on the subject material prior to being published.

Phenomenology The study of lived experience. Its purpose is to understand and attribute meaning to the phenomenon of interest.

Phenomenon Some 'thing' that appears to us through our experiencing of it; an object of human experience.

PICO/PICO(T) A strategy for formulating questions and search strategies and for characterising clinical studies or meta-analyses. PICO stands for four different potential components of a clinical question. These four components are: Patient, Population or Problem; Intervention; Comparison; Outcome.

Sometimes T is added to make it PICO(T) to denote Timeframe or, less commonly, Type of study.

Power analysis To make inferences with statistical data, researchers need to reduce the risk of errors in the data and ensure the finding is probable or likely. This requires a power analysis. If we know the power of a statistical test is good, we know that our sample is large enough to reduce variability in responses, what our acceptable significance level is and how large we expect the effect of our intervention to be.

Predictive validity The extent to which it is valid to use a score on some scale or test to predict the value of some other variable in the future.

Primary research Research that collects original data directly from participants.

Privacy The expectation that information about participants will be kept confidential.

Probability The likelihood any given outcome will occur, given all of the possible outcomes.

Problem statement A concise and clear statement describing the problem or issues to be addressed in a study.

***p*-value** Denotes significance. A *p*-value of less than 0.05 is generally considered significant and tells us that there is less than a 5% chance that our hypothesis is incorrect.

Qualitative analysis A systematic search for meaning, which can include searching for patterns, categories and themes in qualitative data.

Qualitative descriptive research Focuses on exploring phenomena and contexts where there may be little known and describes the nature of that phenomenon.

Qualitative research Incorporates a range of methods of inquiry that, in the main, seek to explore the behaviour, perspectives and experiences of people through a systematic process of listening to and/or observing them.

Quantitative research Approaches that follow systematic logical processes to answer questions about measurable concepts.

Quasi-experimental research In a quasi-experimental design the sample is not randomly assigned. This makes it different from a true experiment where participants are randomly assigned to either the treatment or the control group.

Racism The prejudice, discrimination and expressions of dislike or hatred targeted towards a person or people who belong to racial or ethnic group(s), which are often minority or marginalised groups. Racism occurs in many forms and includes not only interpersonal racism but also in our systems and structures that perpetuate inequities in health outcomes.

Randomisation Refers to random assignment, which means there is an equal chance of being allocated into either the experimental or the control group, and that the allocation is done in a random way so that the researcher cannot influence or bias who is allocated into each group.

Realist review A theory-driven review of the literature that focuses on proving an explanation about why something does or doesn't work.

Reasoning Use of logical thought processes to solve problems. May be inductive or deductive in nature.

Reference collection Contains materials such as encyclopedias, dictionaries, statistical reports, directories, handbooks and other materials that are handy for quick reference.

Reflection A conscious process that involves exploration of thoughts, knowledge and practices to recognise inconsistencies, strengths and limitations and to identify where change and adjustments are required within ourselves, the healthcare environment and clinical practice.

Reflexivity In research, reflexivity is acknowledging your role as a researcher and how your assumptions, prior beliefs and experiences can affect your research. Through examination of your role, you can identify biases and improve credibility.

Reliability How consistently a method measures something. If the same result can be consistently achieved by using the same methods under the same circumstances, the measurement is considered reliable.

Research Systematic process using both inductive and deductive reasoning to confirm and refine existing knowledge and to build new knowledge.

Research capability The skills, ability, aptitude and knowledge of research.

Research capacity The ability to engage in and undertake quality research.

Research design The scheme or template used to provide a framework for the conduct of a study. Different designs have different attributes or components that have to be considered when deciding how to best conduct the study.

Research dissemination The process of circulating or releasing research reports, through means such as publication, conference presentation, social media or other means.

Research ethics The application of ethical principles to the design, conduct and reporting of research.

Research literacy The degree to which a person has the skills and capacity to become capable of making evidence-informed decisions to provide relevant care or to conduct a research project.

Research nurse/midwife Nurse or midwife who supports research through activities such as recruitment, informed consent, data collection and entry.

Research process The steps taken when conducting a study. The research process is a systematic approach used as a guide for the conduct of the study.

Research proposal A plan that sets out what the study seeks to do, how participants will be sampled and recruited, how the data will be collected, and methods of analysis and dissemination of findings.

Research question An interrogative statement that describes the issues to be explored by the research.

Research question (quantitative) Use of an interrogative format to identify the variables to be studied and possible relationships or differences between those variables.

Research translation The process of translating research findings into practice. *See also* knowledge translation.

Reserve collection Resources in high demand within a library that have limited borrowing conditions.

Risk The potential for participants' to be harmed.

Sample Subset of a population selected to participate in a study.

Scoping review A review that provides a preliminary assessment of the scope and volume of literature on a particular topic.

Search engine A software program used to find specific information online using keywords and phrases.

Search strategy An organised record of search activities undertaken including sources searched, keywords, subject headings, phrases and search techniques employed, to allow replication of the search.

Search terms Specific words and characters selected and entered into a search engine to explore a specific topic.

Seminal works Pivotal or landmark sources that are the first to describe a concept or idea that is of great importance to a field of study.

Sequential mixed methods Pivotal where the findings from one type of data collection method (e.g. interviews) provide a basis for the collection of a second set of data (e.g. survey).

Setting/field The physical location and conditions under which a study takes place.

Social media Media posted by the user. It takes many different forms; for example, forums, message boards, blogs, wikis and podcasts. Social media applications include Google, Facebook and YouTube.

Statistical significance Significance determined through testing a hypothesis and establishing probability.

Stereotypes A positive or negative image or set of characteristics believed to represent a particular type of person or thing. It can lead to assumptions and beliefs that persons will behave, act or present in a particular way.

Systematic review Data aggregation or integration to document available evidence, usually on the effectiveness of interventions, and tending to exclusively use empirical studies.

Systematic review with meta-analysis A systematic review uses a clearly defined, systematic method to gather all the literature about a specific research question. The meta-analysis is a statistical process of combining the data from several similar studies to draw an overall conclusion about the evidence.

Theoretical perspective/framework Informs the conduct of the study by providing a theoretical approach to underpin design, data collection and analysis.

Triangulation Use of two or more data sources, investigators, methods or theories in the study of a phenomenon. This may or may not involve the combination of qualitative and quantitative methods of data collection in a single study.

Trustworthiness The rigour of qualitative research, encapsulating the concepts of credibility, transferability, confirmability and dependability.

Type 1 error Occurs when the researcher rejects the null hypothesis when it's true. Also known as a 'false positive' or an α error.

Type 2 error Occurs when the researcher fails to reject the null hypothesis when it's false. Also known as a 'false negative' or β error.

Umbrella review A systematic review of the literature that only includes systematic reviews on a particular topic.

Validity How well the results among the study participants represent true findings among similar individuals outside the study.

Variable Identified concepts or traits that are measured, manipulated or controlled in a study.

Veracity When one's actions, speech and behaviour between individuals and groups of people are truthful and honest.

Vulnerability In research, this is when an individual's capacity to safeguard their own interest as a participant particularly through the informed consent process is compromised. It is not an inevitable consequence of possessing particular personal characteristics, but rather a failure to identify and address barriers to safe and ethical participation.

Worldview A system of knowledge that develops from birth and is shaped by the cultural, social and physical environment you grow up within.

INDEX